Social inclusion and mental health

Edited   ,

Helen

RCPsych Publications

© The Royal College of Psychiatrists 2010

RCPsych Publications is an imprint of the Royal College of Psychiatrists,
17 Belgrave Square, London SW1X 8PG
http://www.rcpsych.ac.uk

British Library Cataloguing-in-Publication Data.
A catalogue record for this book is available from the British Library.
ISBN 978 1 904671 87 9

Distributed in North America by Publishers Storage and Shipping Company.

The views presented in this book do not necessarily reflect those of the Royal College of
Psychiatrists, and the publishers are not responsible for any error of omission or fact.

The Royal College of Psychiatrists is a charity registered in England and Wales (228636)
and in Scotland (SC038369).

Printed by Bell & Bain Limited, Glasgow, UK.

Contents

Contributors

Jed Boardman Consultant and Senior Lecturer in Social Psychiatry at the South London and Maudsley NHS Foundation Trust and Institute of Psychiatry, King's College London, Senior Policy Advisor at Sainsbury Centre for Mental Health.

Susan Brook Reference Group Representative South West England (National Social Inclusion Programme), Expert Consultant (Inclusion Institute, University of Central Lancashire).

David Chang Carer and advocate for service improvement locally, regionally and nationally.

Tom K. J. Craig Professor of Social Psychiatry, Health Service and Population Research, Institute of Psychiatry, King's College London and Honorary Consultant Psychiatrist, South London and Maudsley NHS Foundation Trust.

Alan Currie Consultant in community psychiatry with the Northumberland, Tyne and Wear NHS Foundation Trust and an honorary lecturer at the University of Newcastle.

Helen Killaspy Senior Lecturer and Honorary Consultant in Rehabilitation Psychiatry, Royal Free and University College London Medical School and Camden and Islington NHS Foundation Trust.

Gillian Mezey Reader and Consultant in Forensic Psychiatry based at St George's, University of London.

Kwame McKenzie Professor in the Culture, Community and Mental Health Studies Program of the Department of Psychiatry, University of Toronto, Canada

Michael Osborne Service User Consultant (Voluntary), Nottinghamshire Healthcare NHS Trust, Nottingham, Fellow of the Institute of Mental Health, Chair of Mind Quality Review Panel.

Michael Parsonage Senior Policy Advisor, Sainsbury Centre for Mental Health.

Thomas Scharf Professor of Social Gerontology and Director, Irish Centre for Social Gerontology, National University of Ireland Galway; formerly Director, Centre for Social Gerontology, Keele University.

Geoff Shepherd Clinical Psychologist, Senior Policy Advisor, Sainsbury Centre for Mental Health, Visiting Professor, Health Services and Population Research Department, Institute of Psychiatry, and formerly Director of Partnerships and Service Development, Cambridgeshire and Peterborough Mental Health Foundation Trust.

Rosemary Wilson Mental Health Trainer from the user perspective, Solihull Mind, and Expert Advisor to the National Social Inclusion Programme and Shift.

Tables, boxes and figures

Foreword

Being part of society, contributing to it and, in return, being recognised and acknowledged, is a core need of human beings. The impact of social factors, whether they be isolation, unemployment, poor housing, financial hardship or debt, in the aetiology of mental and physical ill health and their role in its management cannot be underestimated. Whether an individual is egocentric or socio-centric, social inclusion is of great significance in ensuring that an individual feels part of the larger community. Mentally ill individuals often seek employment, housing and social contacts as their key priorities and it is essential that clinicians do not forget these goals. There is little doubt that social inclusion is often seen as a political or moral concept, but it is much more than that: it is a quintessential basic need that every individual has, to be accepted and to have the self-esteem and the self-confidence which will allow the individual to deal with stress. Social inclusion for individuals has many meanings, depending upon gender, age, sexual orientation, educational attainment or socio-economic status, among other things. The challenge for clinicians and policy makers is to make social inclusion work and not simply to rely on rhetoric. This book is doubly welcome for highlighting an important topic and for guiding practitioners and policy makers to encourage social inclusion. The book originates from a report which was developed by Jed Boardman, and for the book he has managed to attract a many eminent contributors. I hope that it will be of interest not only to clinicians but also to stakeholders, including politicians and policy makers.

Dinesh Bhugra
President, The Royal College of Psychiatrists

Preface

The origins of this book lie in the unpublished report written by the Social Inclusion Scoping Group of the Royal College of Psychiatrists. The Scoping Group was set up to examine the nature and extent of social exclusion in people with mental health problems and those with learning disabilities, the implications for the future organisation, structure and culture of mental health and learning disability services and for the practice and training of psychiatrists. The report was published in a shortened form as a position statement which summarised the findings and views of the Scoping Group (Royal College of Psychiatrists, 2009). The evidence amassed by the Group and their deliberations were considered too good to waste and have been adapted to produce this book, aimed primarily at psychiatrists but also of relevance to other mental health professionals and others working in mental health services. It should also be of value to those who have an interest in mental health policy and anyone who cares about the plight of those more vulnerable members of our society.

Included in the Scoping Group review was the full range of people with different diagnoses represented by the specialties within the Royal College of Psychiatrists, including learning disability, drug and alcohol problems, children and adolescents, older adults and mentally disordered offenders. In addition, people who have comorbid diagnoses such as psychotic or non-psychotic mental illness, alcohol and/or drug dependence, learning disability, personality disorder and adult neurodevelopmental disorders (Asperger's syndrome, autism, attention-deficit hyperactivity disorder) are included. The review also covered the full range of age groups and social identities – women, people from Black and minority ethnic groups, lesbian, gay and bisexual people, and faith groups. Most of these groups are represented by the various Faculties, Sections and Special Interest Groups of the College and they parallel many groups covered in the Equalities Review (2007). In addition, specific groups, including the homeless, refugees and asylum seekers with mental health problems, were highlighted by the Scoping Group as they are, by the nature of their circumstances, excluded by society.

The original Scoping Group report took a broad view of the socially inclusive perspective – anti-discrimination laws, equality and human rights, social justice and citizenship – in addition to a clinical perspective. The belief was that it is only from this standpoint that the importance of social inclusion for people with mental health problems and learning difficulties and the role that our social and political institutions have in creating exclusion can be truly appreciated. The report's title, *From Exclusion to Inclusion: The Transformation of Psychiatry in the 21st Century*, implied that change is needed if we are to move from 'exclusion' to 'inclusion'.

The aspiration for the Scoping Group was borrowed from the Equalities Review: that we wish 'to live in a society…which provides for each individual to realise his or her potential to the fullest' (p. 1). The Group confirmed what is already well established – that people with mental health problems and learning difficulties are excluded and discriminated against, and that this remains a blight on the status of a considerable number of citizens in our society. This book reports and expands on the findings of the Scoping Group, examining the ways in which this blight is manifest and how mental health professionals and services might respond to the challenges posed by the social exclusion of people with mental health problems and learning difficulties.

References

Equalities Review (2007) *Fairness and Freedom: The Final Report of the Equalities Review*. The Equalities Review (http://archive.cabinetoffice.gov.uk/equalitiesreview/publications.html).

Royal College of Psychiatrists' Social Inclusion Scoping Group (2009) *Mental Health and Social Inclusion: Making Psychiatry and Mental Health Services Fit for the 21st Century. Position Statement (PS01/2009)*. Royal College of Psychiatrists (http://www.rcpsych.ac.uk/publications/collegereports/positionstatements.aspx).

Jed Boardman, Alan Currie, Helen Killaspy and Gillian Mezey

Acknowledgements

Many people have generously shared their time and knowledge to help us write this book. The Scoping Group members have participated in the intense discussions that took place in the group's meetings, made comments on drafts of the original report and subsequent position statement, and helped write the report. In addition, the Faculties, Sections and Special Interest Groups of the Royal College of Psychiatrists all made contributions. Thanks are due to all of those and to Candace Gilles-Wright who provided administrative support.

In many ways the book is an output of collaborative efforts between many individuals from the College and several other organisations and most of the chapters contain some input from people other than the chapters' authors. Tania Burchardt and Tom Scharf both contributed to Chapter 2 through discussions on the concepts of exclusion; Tom also provided a summary paper. The section on philosophy was taken from George Ikkos's paper on philosophical concepts. For Chapter 3, Chris Phillipson provided a paper on the life course and Kwame McKenzie presented one on social capital. Tania Burchardt provided material on the capability approach and Glenn Roberts on recovery. Chapter 4 on policy covered all areas of psychiatry and material was shared by Liz Sayce, Tom Scharf, Susan Benbow, Robert Lindsay, Tom Carnwath, Roger Banks and Shaun Gravestock. The sections on the wider economic and social benefits of inclusion in Chapter 5 were based on material submitted by Michael Parsonage and Geoff Shepherd. Chapter 6 was based on material provided by members of the Royal College of Psychiatrists Faculties, including Child and Adolescent (Robert Lindsay), Liaison (George Ikkos), Psychotherapy (Ches Denman), Old Age (Susan Benbow), Addictions (Tom Carnwarth) and Learning Disability (Roger Banks and Shaun Gravestock). Paul Maklin provided information on physical health problems for Chapter 8. Bob Grove shared material from the evidence he gave to the *Foresight Review* and some material was provided by Robert Lindsay, Tom Carnwath, Susan Benbow and Tom Scharf. The material for Chapter 9 was provided by members of many of the College special interest groups and others with specialist expertise: women (Louise Howard), parents (Carol Henshaw), asylum seekers (Jo Stubley and Kam Bhui), sexual orientation (Michael King and Helen Killaspy), faith (Simon Dein), and homelessness (Phil Timms). Michael Parsonage and Max Rutherford from the Sainsbury Centre for Mental Health supplied material on the criminal justice system. Geoff Shepherd and Michael Parsonage shared information on the drivers of social exclusion for Chapter 10. The contributions from service users and carers in Chapters 11 and 12 were facilitated by Naomi Hankinson from the National Social Inclusion Programme. The unattributed quotes from service users in Chapter 11 were gathered by the chapter's authors from a range of people whom they had spoken to over several years. The quotes from service users used in Chapter 14 were all provided by Sophie Corlett from Mind, while Rene Cormac submitted the material on carers. Janey Antoniou gave us the information on service user involvement for Chapter 15. Glenn Roberts and Lisetta Lovett provided material on training for Chapter 16.

The Scoping Group on Social Inclusion, Royal College of Psychiatrists

Jed Boardman (Chair)
Sarah Davenport (Deputy Chair)
Maurice Arbuthnott (service user)
Kam Bhui (Queen Mary College, University of London)
Sophie Corlett (Mind)
Angela Greatley (Sainsbury Centre for Mental Health)
Bob Grove (Sainsbury Centre for Mental Health)
Naomi Hankinson (National Social Inclusion Programme)
Alison Mohammed (Rethink)
David Morris (National Social Inclusion Programme)
Nick Niven-Jenkins (later replaced by Rupert Lown) (Department for Work
    and Pensions)
Michael Parsonage (Sainsbury Centre for Mental Health)
Rachel Perkins (SW London and St George's Mental Health NHS Trust)
Chris Phillipson (Keele University)
Miles Rinaldi (SW London and St George's Mental Health NHS Trust)
Liz Sayce (RADAR)
Tom Scharf (Keele University)
Geoff Shepherd (Sainsbury Centre for Mental Health)

Royal College of Psychiatrists' Faculties' representatives:
Roger Banks (Learning Disabilities)
Susan Benbow (Psychiatry of Old Age)
Tom Carnwath (Addictions Psychiatry)
Alan Currie (General and Community)
Ches Denman (Psychotherapy)
Shaun Gravestock (Learning Disabilities)
George Ikkos (Liaison Psychiatry)
Helen Killaspy (Rehabilitation and Social Psychiatry)
Robert Lindsay (Child and Adolescent Psychiatry)
Gillian Mezey (Forensic Psychiatry)
Jo Stubley (Psychotherapy)

Part 1

What is social exclusion?

CHAPTER 1

Introduction

Jed Boardman, Alan Currie, Helen Killaspy and Gillian Mezey

Social exclusion is a term of relatively recent origin which has come into use in the area of social policy and has particular relevance for people with mental health problems and learning disability (Office of the Deputy Prime Minister, 2004). It encapsulates the position of many people with mental health problems and learning disability in contemporary society, as well as summarising their position in history. This book sets out to outline the meaning of social exclusion, the ways in which people with mental health problems and learning disability are excluded, and the implications of this for the training and practice of psychiatrists (and, by implication, other mental health professionals) and the services in which they work. The book seeks to inform by examining and evaluating the nature of social exclusion and the ways in which people with mental health problems and learning disability are excluded. In the subsequent chapters we build up a picture of social exclusion of those people in Britain in the 21st century. This picture illustrates that social exclusion is an objective reality in their lives; it is reflected in their own subjective experiences and is open to the independent scrutiny of health professionals.

In this book we set out a case for why social exclusion should be of concern to psychiatrists and others working in mental health services and why these services should be designed to be 'socially inclusive'. The nature of social exclusion and its relation to ill health makes it a legitimate concern to mental health professionals. However, this is only one of several possible standpoints from which the significance of social exclusion to mental health professionals can be assessed, which in turn raises the matter of professional values. A stream of possible actions follows from these concerns. How might the exclusion of people with mental health problems and learning disability be diminished? How might their participation in mainstream society be increased? What is the role of mental health services and mental health professionals in this? What are the implications for the training and practice of professionals, and the organisation, delivery and culture of mental health services? Finally, what should be the role of mental health professionals in influencing policy and public opinion?

This chapter introduces the concepts of social exclusion and inclusion, their importance for people with mental health problems and those with learning disability, and their relevance to professional practice and mental health services in the 21st century.

A note on terminology

Finding an acceptable summary term to describe the range of people with psychiatric diagnoses is fraught with difficulty. As this book was based on the Scoping Group on Social Inclusion review, the same range of diagnoses as was included in that review are represented here (see Preface).

In this book we emphasise the importance of regarding individuals who have a psychiatric diagnosis as being first and foremost people, regardless of the nature of their problems or disability. We have chosen to use the term 'mental health problem' to summarise most of the diagnoses listed above. However, learning disability is not in itself a mental health problem, although people with learning disabilities do have increased rates of mental illness, behaviour problems and pervasive developmental disorders. To help keep this in mind we sometimes refer to this group separately. We also recognise that the term mental health problem covers a heterogeneous collection of diagnoses and groups of people with very different experiences of exclusion, and where these groups need to be singled out then specific diagnostic categories and terms are used.

Context: society and contemporary mental health services

The context for this book lies in the changes in UK society, and in the delivery of mental health services, that have occurred since the 1940s. Although there have been undoubted improvements in the quality of life and in the standards of living, health, education and housing during the 20th century, the income gap between the richest and poorest in the population has widened (Wilkinson & Pickett, 2009). Inequalities have increased and the numbers in relative poverty reached a historic high in the 1990s. There has been some subsequent fall in those figures, but a high proportion of children still live in poor families and the reduction of child poverty remains a key government target.

For many people the experience of poverty, although unpleasant, is relatively brief. However, about 2–4% of the population live in persistent poverty and for others poverty may be a recurrent experience (see Chapter 7). People with multiple disadvantages are most at risk of poverty and social exclusion. Those who are jobless, older people, single parents, long-term sick and disabled are overrepresented among those who are multiply disadvantaged, as are those with mental health problems and people with learning disabilities. People from Black and minority ethnic groups are also more likely to experience social exclusion, especially if they are recent migrants or come from linguistically and/or culturally isolated groups.

There is little doubt that mental health services have changed, and in many ways improved, during the second half of the 20th century: the large institutions have closed and most services are now provided in a community setting. However, these arrangements are relatively new and it was only in the 1990s that the last large mental hospital closed in England and the first English national plan for mental services, the National Service Framework for Mental Health, was created (Department of Health, 1999). The evolution of mental health services during the 1990s was accompanied by an increasingly active and politicised disability movement, including people with mental health problems and those with learning disabilities, demanding not only improved services, but also equality, rights, participation and social and political action (Oliver, 1990; Sayce, 2000).

These three matters: the increasing demands of mental health service users and their families for just representation, their continuing exclusion from participating as full and active citizens, and the changing nature of mental health services are the main drivers behind the production of this book. There is no place for complacency and it is timely to examine the status and participation in society of people with mental health problems and those with learning disabilities and the ways in which the psychiatrists, other mental health professionals and services can respond to their social exclusion.

Social exclusion – old wine in new bottles?

Despite the relatively recent emergence of the term social exclusion, its origins are much older. Social exclusion is one way of conceptualising disadvantage, traditionally seen in terms of poverty, hardship, destitution, all of which focus on material deprivation and the consequent personal distress. These are matters familiar to people working in mental health services and will be encountered in their day-to-day practice. Efforts to improve the quality of life of service users have been seen as a legitimate role of mental health professionals and, historically, there have been notable attempts by professionals to counter the stigma, discrimination and injustice that are experienced by people with mental health problems and learning disabilities and to act as proponents for their human rights. This book therefore builds on much that we already know, but puts it in the context of current developments and the potential opportunities that face us.

Professional roles – healing and professionalism

The profession of medicine is changing. It is becoming more collaborative, with a greater emphasis on self-care and patient choice, and greater recognition of the contribution of patients as experts in their own conditions

(General Medical Council, 2006). This is reflected in the latest guidelines of *Good Psychiatric Practice* (Royal College of Psychiatrists, 2009a). Psychiatry has to face these challenges and each of the subspecialties will need to adapt its practice in different ways. In later chapters the idea of socially inclusive mental health services is discussed. The creation of these services, which will support individuals on their own unique journeys of recovery, represents a considerable challenge for psychiatrists, both as individual practitioners and as members of specialised teams. The implications of these changes are multiple. It is important that psychiatrists build on their existing skills, and adapt these to support socially inclusive practice and create new forms of relationships with service users and carers which are based on partnership.

As individual practitioners, psychiatrists are first and foremost doctors. Psychiatry is a medical specialty and psychiatrists are physicians but they also have a wider expertise in psychological and social dynamics in their broader forms. They are also people who experience health and personal difficulties as anyone else might, and who may be called upon to use their life experiences to inform their work. They therefore need to have a wide range of skills, significantly beyond the delivery of a traditional, biomedical model.

All the main mental health professional bodies have made explicit statements regarding social inclusion and mental health. The Royal College of Psychiatrists (2009b) has declared its position in regard to social exclusion and the importance of socially inclusive practice and has given clear support to the concepts of recovery (Royal College of Psychiatrists *et al*, 2007). Other mental health professional groups, including nurses, occupational therapists, clinical psychologists and social workers, have also indicated their support for socially inclusive and recovery-oriented practice (British Psychological Society Division of Clinical Psychology, 2000; College of Occupational Therapists, 2006; Department of Health, 2006; British Psychological Society Professional Practice Board Social Inclusion Group, 2008; Royal College of Nursing, 2009). The ideas of social exclusion and inclusion are fundamental to social work practice, which has traditionally occupied the space between the mainstream and the marginalised (Shepherd, 2006). Psychological therapists have often recognised the dilemma of working with individuals whose problems may be linked to wider social and economic factors, while leaving these wider factors unchallenged (Corey, 1991; Clark, 1993; Gordon, 1999). The way professionals work with excluded individuals, their social position, their empowerment and the effects of broader social, political and economic institutions are all legitimate concerns for mental health professionals.

What are the steps that psychiatrists and mental health workers can take to facilitate the social inclusion of people with mental health problems? Inevitably, many of the actions to be taken will go beyond those of individual practitioners and will involve changes at institutional, economic, political and social levels. Individually professionals may have a role in influencing these wider dimensions through the democratic process or through their own jobs. Their professional bodies may use their influence in campaigning and lobbying at the national level. An example of such a campaign is the College's 'Fair Deal for Mental Health' (Royal College of Psychiatrists, 2008), which is concerned with many of the elements of social inclusion (Box 1.1).

Individual practitioners do have a role to play in their professional life in facilitating action in relation to these collective dimensions as an integral part of inclusive practice. They may act by advocating for people with mental health problems who they see in the course of their daily practice, or by utilising their other roles as, for example, managers, teachers and researchers.

Inevitably, the way in which psychiatrists and other mental health professionals may have to alter their practice to face the challenges of exclusion raises questions about their roles as professionals and as healers. Both of these roles overlap (Fig. 1.1) and both can be maintained and enhanced by consideration of what may constitute 'socially inclusive practice'. The physician's roles of healer and professional are linked through ethics and values as well as through science, including social and political science (Cruess et al, 2002), all of which are considered in subsequent chapters.

Box 1.1 Royal College of Psychiatrists' Fair Deal campaign principles

- People with mental ill health and learning disability should live in a fair and just society where their human rights are respected and each individual is able to realise his or her own potential to the full.
- People with mental ill health and learning disability are entitled to an equitable distribution of the resources of the health and social care system. They should receive the same priority as patients with physical health problems wherever they present.
- There is no health without mental health. Mental health should be integrated into physical healthcare at all levels. This includes the mental health of patients with physical illness in the general hospital setting.
- Discrimination against people with mental health problems and learning disability can be tackled throughout the NHS. In particular, the quality of care must be the same irrespective of racial, religious or cultural background, gender, age, sexual orientation or diagnosis.
- The human rights of patients must be promoted and safeguarded. This applies particularly to those detained or deprived of liberty under mental health and mental capacity legislation.
- Healthcare to people with mental ill health and learning disability should promote social inclusion and be delivered jointly by health and social care services and an array of third-sector organisations.
- Service users and carers must play a central role in the design and delivery of services.

The Fair Deal campaign has several components that explicitly relate to social inclusion (http://www.rcpsych.ac.uk/campaigns/fairdeal.aspx).

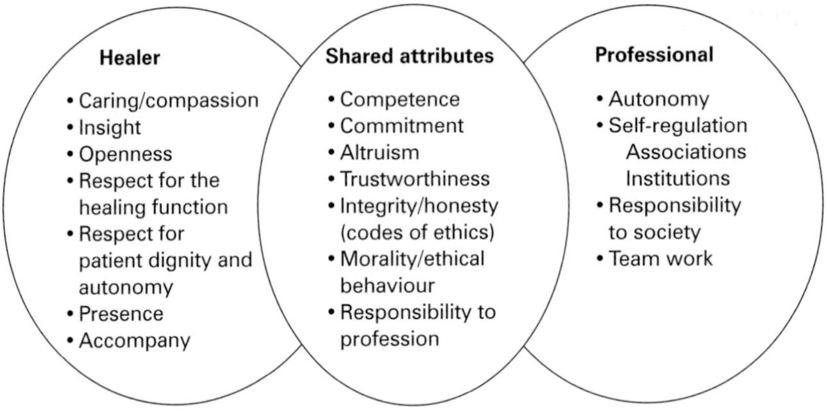

Fig. 1.1 Attributes of the healer and professional and their overlap. Adapted from Cruess & Cruess (2009), p. 13.

In addition to serving the best interests of the patient (by respecting patient autonomy and through viewing the doctor–patient relationship as a partnership), professionals have acquired an obligation to serve the wider society and be devoted to the public good, a form of 'civic professionalism' (Sullivan, 1995: p. 16; Cruess *et al*, 2002). At the individual level, the adoption of recovery-oriented practice (Shepherd *et al*, 2008) can enhance the healing role. The professional role may be strengthened through mental health workers and service users sharing a view of future mental healthcare at the same time as working to improve the rights and status of people with a mental disorder.

Summary

Social exclusion is one way of conceptualising disadvantage. It is not a new idea; it has its origins in the literature on poverty, hardship and destitution.

British society has changed during the 20th century, with improvements in the standards of living and quality of life. Nevertheless, a substantial number of people live in poverty and are socially excluded. The gap between rich and poor widened at the end of the century. Mental health services have also changed, becoming more community-based.

People with mental health problems and those with learning disabilities want to see improved health and social services and to have a greater voice in how these are run. They also seek greater opportunities for participation and emphasise the importance of equality and rights in promoting this.

Psychiatrists and other mental health workers can contribute to the social inclusion of people with mental health problems and learning disabilities and this is consistent with their professional roles and responsibilities.

References

British Psychological Society Division of Clinical Psychology (2000) *Recent Advances in Understanding Mental Illness and Psychotic Experiences*. British Psychological Society.

British Psychological Society Professional Practice Board Social Inclusion Group (2008) *Socially Inclusive Practice*. *Discussion Paper*. British Psychological Society.

Clark, C. R. (1993) Social responsibility ethics: doing right, doing good, doing well. *Ethics and Behaviour*, **3**, 303–327.

College of Occupational Therapists (2006) *Recovering Ordinary Lives: The Strategy for Occupational Therapy in Mental Health Services 2007–2017*. College of Occupational Therapists.

Corey, G. (1991) *Theory and Practice of Counselling and Psychotherapy (4th edn)*. Brooks Cole.

Cruess, R. L. & Cruess, S. R. (2009) The cognitive basis of professionalism. In *Teaching Medical Professionalism* (eds R. L. Cruess, S. R. Cruess & Y. Steinert). Cambridge University Press.

Cruess, S. R., Johnston, S. & Cruess, R. L. (2002) Professionalism for medicine: opportunities and obligations. *Medical Journal of Australia*, **177**, 208–211.

Department of Health (1999) *National Service Framework for Mental Health. Modern Standards and Service Models*. Department of Health.

Department of Health (2006) *From Values to Action: The Chief Nursing Officer's Review of Mental Health Nursing*. Department of Health.

General Medical Council (2006) *Good Medical Practice*. General Medical Council.

Gordon, P. (1999) *Face to Face: Therapy as Ethics*. Constable.

Office of the Deputy Prime Minister (2004) *Mental Health and Social Exclusion – Social Exclusion Report*. ODPM.

Oliver, M. (1990) *The Politics of Disablement: Critical Texts in Social Work and the Welfare State*. Palgrave Macmillan.

Royal College of Nursing (2009) *Socially Inclusive Practice for Nurses*. Royal College of Nursing.

Royal College of Psychiatrists (2008) *Fair Deal for Mental Health: Our Manifesto for a 3-Year Campaign Dedicated to Tackling Inequality in Mental Healthcare*. Royal College of Psychiatrists.

Royal College of Psychiatrists (2009a) *Good Psychiatric Practice (3rd edn)*. Royal College of Psychiatrists.

Royal College of Psychiatrists (2009b) *Mental Health and Social Inclusion: Making Psychiatry and Mental Health Services Fit for the 21st Century*. Royal College of Psychiatrists.

Royal College of Psychiatrists, Social Care Institute for Excellence & Care Services Improvement Partnership (2007) *A Common Purpose: Recovery in Future Mental Health Services*. Social Care Institute for Excellence.

Sayce, L. (2000) *From Psychiatric Patient to Citizen: Overcoming Discrimination and Social Exclusion*. Macmillan.

Shepherd, G., Boardman, J. & Slade, M. (2008) *Making Recovery a Reality*. Sainsbury Centre for Mental Health.

Shepherd, M. (2006) *Social Work and Social Exclusion: The Idea of Practice*. Ashgate.

Sullivan, W. (1995) *Work and Integrity: The Crisis and Promise of Professionalism in North America*. HarperCollins.

Wilkinson, R. & Pickett, K. (2009) *The Spirit Level: Why More Equal Societies Almost Always Do Better*. Penguin.

CHAPTER 2

Concepts of social exclusion

Jed Boardman

Before any consideration of what it means to be socially included can be made it is important to start with a consideration as to what is social exclusion? Social exclusion and its related concepts are mainly to be found in the social policy literature. This chapter does not intend to provide a complete review of the field but rather to give a brief outline of the concepts of social exclusion so that we may consider in subsequent chapters how this might be applied to people with mental health problems and those with learning disability. It also gives some brief consideration to three areas of political philosophy: citizenship, justice and human rights.

What is social exclusion?

Social exclusion has emerged as a concept relatively recently. It is thus not surprising that there is still a lack of clarity about its definition. Some believe that this lack of clarity has certain advantages: 'The expression is so evocative, ambiguous, multidimensional and elastic that it can be defined in many different ways [therefore] it can serve a variety of political purposes' (Silver, 1994: p. 536).

The modern use of the term social exclusion appears to have originated in France in the 1970s (Burchardt *et al*, 2002a; Morgan *et al*, 2007), referring to *les exclus*, people who have slipped through the net of the social insurance system and are thus administratively excluded by the state, such as those who are disabled, lone parents and the unemployed. Other versions of the concept have focused on it being an inherent characteristic of capitalism (Byrne, 1999), a lack of recognition of basic rights (Gore & Figueiredo, 1997) and the existence of an underclass (Murray, 1999). In distinction to the first two versions, the last version tends to place responsibility for being excluded on individuals themselves. In the political field some see the term social exclusion as providing an alternative means of speaking of poverty when this term has not been acceptable to politicians (Berghman, 1995). A widely held characterisation of social exclusion is that it refers to the extent to which individuals are unable to participate in key areas of the economic, social and cultural life of society.

Competing discourses of social exclusion

These competing conceptualisations of social exclusion reflect some of the complexities and contradictions inherent in the concept. They also suggest that the concept may be used in very different ways in both studying and measuring the problem of social exclusion and in considering its applications to social policy. In *The Inclusive Society?*, Levitas (1998) argues that there are at least three ways of thinking about social exclusion. These draw upon competing views about the ways in which exclusion can arise and are liable to generate different types of policy outcome.

- Redistributive discourse (RED): the origins of redistributive discourse can be traced to the critical social policy agenda of the last decades of the 20th century. Here emphasis is placed upon the way in which poverty limits social participation and the exercise of citizenship rights. Whereas poverty is perceived as a lack of material resources that restricts participation, exclusion refers to 'the dynamic process of being shut out, fully or partially, from any of the social, economic, political and cultural systems which determine the social integration of a person in society' (Walker & Walker, 1997: p. 8). In the literature relating to redistributive discourse, poverty is regarded as a major cause of exclusion, although this is compounded by other types of inequality.
- Moral underclass discourse (MUD): the emphasis is placed on the moral and cultural causes of poverty, with particular concern about the dependency of some on state benefits. This discourse bears similarities with notions of 'the underclass', expressed most forcefully in the work of those on the New Right (Murray, 1994).
- Social integrationist discourse (SID): the central feature is the social integration of people through paid employment. Involvement in the labour market is the key element of inclusion. Levitas suggests that this discourse covers up ways in which paid work can fail to prevent exclusion or can limit other forms of social participation. Social integrationist discourse tends to undervalue the contribution of unpaid work, such as informal caring.

Of course these three discourses are an oversimplification of a complex set of issues, but they do summarise what the excluded are seen as lacking: 'in RED they have no money, in SID they have no work, in MUD they have no morals' (Levitas, 1998: p. 27). Nevertheless, despite its oversimplification, this approach can be particularly helpful when reviewing social exclusion policy under the UK Labour government 1997–2010, in which elements of all three discourses can be seen in policy developments (Chapter 4). This can be applied to policies relating to people with mental health problems. On the one hand, there is the emphasis on promoting their labour market participation, for example welfare reform (HM Government 2005a,b, 2006); on the other, there are a variety of policies which focus on the behaviour of people with mental health problems, for example the reform of the Mental Health Act 1983 (Department of Health, 2004a).

11

Definitions of social exclusion

These different ways of thinking about social exclusion may help us to understand the breadth and complexities of the concept, but it is also useful to consider some definitions of exclusion that may assist in seeing how the ideas in this area may be applied to those with mental health problems and learning disability.

In government policy documents, such as *Opportunity for All* (Department of Social Security, 1999) and those from the Social Exclusion Unit (see Chapter 4), social exclusion was defined in descriptive terms and interrelation between different problems was emphasised:

> a shorthand term for what can happen when people or areas suffer from a combination of linked problems such as unemployment, poor skills, low incomes, poor housing, high crime, bad health and family breakdown (Social Exclusion Unit, 2001: p. 11).

This is a flexible definition that lists only some of the many problems associated with exclusion. The key point here is the perceived linkage between the cited problems: 'The most important characteristic of social exclusion is that these problems are linked and mutually reinforcing, and can combine to create a complex and fast moving vicious cycle' (Social Exclusion Unit, 2001: p. 11). The definition does not, however, identify a concept or element that brings these indicators or putative causal factors together.

The Centre for Analysis of Social Exclusion (CASE) at the London School of Economics adopted a working definition of social exclusion (Burchardt *et al*, 2002*b*: p. 30):

> An individual is socially excluded if he or she does not participate in key activities of the society in which he or she lives.

This working definition emphasises the central idea of participation and recognises that social exclusion is a concept relative to the time and place in question. In addition, there is an emphasis on lack of participation as being due to constraint, rather than choice. In their original definition, CASE included two further clauses: first, that the individual is not participating for reasons beyond his/her control, and second, that he or she would like to participate. In their simplified definition they omitted the matter of voluntary non-participation, arguing that this would be unlikely where the threshold for participation is set low; for example, few would choose to live on low incomes or with long-term sickness (Burchardt *et al*, 2002*b*).

This working definition, with its central theme of participation, may be particularly useful in helping us understand the position of people with mental health problems and learning disability in contemporary society, and forms the central definition of exclusion for the purposes of this book. But this concept demands further consideration.

Social exclusion may be seen as one recent attempt to conceptualise disadvantage, which has been traditionally set in terms of poverty, hardship, destitution, all of which focus on want and misery. A strong tradition in social policy research on disadvantage has been the examination of poverty and deprivation and it has influenced our thinking and policy in this area (Rowntree, 1901; Townsend, 1979). The social exclusion paradigm has been seen by some as adding to this tradition and social exclusion can be seen as a genuine extension of the traditional approach as it allows the phenomena of interest to extend beyond non-participation because of lack of material resources (Burchardt et al, 2002a). It extends the scope to the examination of multiple deprivations and broadens the range of indicators, while retaining the objective of identifying individuals who lack the resources to participate. Any indicators or measures of social exclusion should identify those whose non-participation arises in other ways, for example through discrimination, chronic illness or cultural identification (Gordon et al, 2000; Burchardt et al, 2002a; Levitas et al, 2007).

Social exclusion has also been seen as a more comprehensive and dynamic concept (Berghman, 1995), offering a change in emphasis rather than direction (Atkinson, 1998; Hills, 2002) and implying conceptual shifts: from consideration only of financial disadvantage to consideration of multiple dimensions of disadvantage; from a static to a dynamic analysis; from a concentration on the individual or the household to the local neighbourhood; and from a focus on distribution to a focus on social relations (Room, 1995, 1998, 2000). Importantly, it implies that we examine factors that separate people or groups from wider society.

There are three recurring features of social exclusion that emerge from reviews of its definitions (Atkinson, 1998):

1   Relativity – whether a person is socially excluded or included can only be judged in the context of their situation as a whole. Exclusion refers to a particular place and time. It can also be seen that exclusion is not absolute and can be considered as a matter of degree.

2   Agency – 'exclusion implies an act, with an agent or agents' (ibid, p. 14). Agency refers to the fact that someone or something is doing the exclusion and the different views about the causes of exclusion tend to reflect differing views about agency or who is 'doing' the excluding. Exclusion can be seen as the outcome of the system, with components of society, intentionally or unintentionally, acting as the excluding agents, including political, economic and social institutions. It is also concerned with power, with the excluded having a lack of autonomy or decision-making power and being at the mercy of the powerful (Burchardt et al, 2002a). However, all conceptions of social exclusion have had to contend with the possibility of voluntary or self-exclusion. Although it is possible for someone to exclude themselves, it may be difficult to determine when self-exclusion is truly voluntary in the presence of constraints to participation (Barry, 2002).

3   Dynamics – exclusion is seen as a dynamic process that operates across time, and potentially across generations. The causal models of exclusion are often not simple and represent the influences of the past (human, physical and financial capital) and those of the present

(constraints and choices), with the individual influenced at many levels, including family, community, national and global forces (Burchardt *et al*, 2002*a*). The levels interact, outcomes result and these become present influences which in turn feedback and affect constraints and opportunities. So, for example, a person may be excluded at one point in time because they lack work, but this exclusion could be exacerbated by the fact that they live in an area of high unemployment, that their family has been without work for many years and that there is a lack of future job prospects.

These matters of relativity, agency and dynamics are discussed further in the next chapter.

Empirical approaches to social exclusion have tended to adopt one of two methods: either to concentrate on specific problems or groups which are taken to be instances of exclusion (e.g. street homeless, single parents, long-term unemployed, or area abandonment), or to characterise social exclusion as lack of participation in key aspects of society. Approaches to providing a framework for understanding social exclusion are multidimensional and multifactorial.

Some philosophical matters underpinning social exclusion

Social exclusion and social inclusion are concepts with moral and political connotations, therefore it is worth briefly considering some aspects of political philosophy that have a bearing on this book. These may help to identify fair principles on which to promote social inclusion and the entitlements and obligations of those agreeing to these principles. Three areas will be briefly considered: citizenship, justice and human rights.

Citizenship

Consideration of the individual as a citizen is required if we view the individual as an active agent, rather than simply as passive recipient, in relation to society.

Historically there are two broad traditions of thinking about citizenship, the civic republican and the liberal. The former emphasises participation of citizens in the community for the mutual benefit of all, the latter emphasises protection of the liberty and property of the individual in relation to the actions of the state. Both traditions are relevant to psychiatry in general and social inclusion and psychiatry in particular.

Civic republican tradition

The civic republican tradition was first defined firmly by Aristotle and has evolved over the centuries through the work of thinkers such as Cicero, Machiavelli and Rousseau. More recently, it has influenced the current concerns in the UK about citizenship, multiculturalism and social integration.

Central to this tradition of thought is the definition of citizenship as the active involvement in public affairs for the mutual benefit of the citizen and the community. In addition, it emphasises the idea of obligation on the part of the citizen towards the community. The general picture is one of virtuous citizens developing concord and of well-functioning social institutions created through wisdom, dialogue and deliberation. Education of the young, participation of young people and adults in faith communities and the engagement of all in public festivals have been proposed as concrete examples of civic republican practice.

The civic republican tradition is of obvious relevance in thinking about the social inclusion of those with mental health problems and those with learning disability. It offers both opportunities and challenges. On the one hand, the definition of citizenship as participation in society places an obligation on the state and civic institutions to work actively towards ensuring that those with mental health problems are able to engage as citizens, for example in work and leisure. On the other hand, the sense of obligation in relation to citizenship may be an impossibly heavy burden for those with severe learning disability, long-term psychosis or dementia, unless relevant issues are thought through sensitively and constructively.

Liberal citizenship

The alternative tradition in thinking about citizenship is the liberal tradition. This tradition is more recent in origin (17th-century European Enlightenment) and has exercised greater influence in the Anglo-Saxon world.

John Locke, the 17th-century English philosopher, stands in relation to this tradition in the same way as Aristotle does in relation to the civic republican tradition. Other liberal thinkers include John Stuart Mill, Franz Hayek, Isaiah Berlin, Karl Popper and, more recently, liberal egalitarians such as John Rawls and libertarians such as Robert Nozick. The distinction between civic republicanism and liberalism is both artificial and an oversimplification. Furthermore, there is as much that divides thinkers within each of the traditions as unites them. For example, Rawls and Nozick both work within the liberal tradition but there is more that divides them than divides Rawls from Habermas, who works from within the civic republican tradition.

In contrast to the civic republican tradition, the liberal tradition considers citizenship as protection from unwarranted interference from the state. This is an important consideration when thinking about the social inclusion of those with psychiatric disabilities. The overzealous republican may well stray into what is not only inclusive but also intrusive or, even, coercive. Conversely, the overzealous liberal, in attempting to protect the disabled person from undue interference, may well stray into neglect of people in need.

15

The liberal political philosophical tradition is closely associated with ideas and practices of human rights. This flows from the centrality in this tradition of the protection of the liberty and property of the individual from undue interference from the state. It is important to be aware that social inclusion cannot be a coercive activity. Recent controversies in relation to proposed mental health legislation in England have focused significantly on human rights issues and the risks of stigmatisation of both patients and services that the proposed legislation would lead to.

John Rawls (1971) set out to work out the foundations of political institutions so as to allow a pluralism of 'conceptions of the good', or values (beliefs about ethics, religion, politics, etc.) that citizens may choose about their purposes or 'plans of life'. He saw a range of useful things, or 'primary goods' that are useful in furthering a wide range of life plans, such as health, intelligence, material resources, authority, opportunities, civil rights, and self-respect (Ikkos et al, 2006). This pluralism is helpful in that it provides fertile ground not only for personal choice, but also for flexibility when thinking about the citizenship of those with significant mental impairments. These 'conceptions of the good' and recognition of variety of 'plans of life' that people may want or be able to adopt can help us think flexibly, particularly about the obligations of people with disability and mental health problems. They are also useful in examining the importance of self-respect, mutuality, autonomy, and the exercise of people's realised capacities in relation to such things as mental health promotion and the value of meaningful activity in mental health (Ikkos et al, 2006).

Although the rights to property and civil rights are at the core of the liberal tradition, there is debate as to how far human rights extend beyond this. Marshall (1965), in particular, identified three categories of rights, civil (e.g. freedom of speech), political (e.g. freedom to participate as elector or elected citizen) and social (e.g. economic, education, cultural and security), which have arisen in England since the 18th century. To Marshall the fullest expression of citizenship requires a liberal welfare state to ensure participation and enjoyment of the common life of society (Kymlicka, 2002: p. 288). The extension of human rights to social rights brings the liberal tradition into close proximity to the civic republican tradition and confirms that the two traditions cannot be rigidly separated. Instead they are in constant dialogue and mutual cross-fertilisation.

Justice

Justice may relate to individuals, relations between individuals and relations taking place within the framework of social institutions, both at government level and beyond.

An individual may be just or unjust. For Aristotle, justice consists of all the elements of disposition, character and behaviour that constitute the good and virtuous citizen. He argued these include courage, moderation, liberality (but not excess), pride (but not vanity) and good temper, honesty, faithfulness, integrity and trustworthiness. Relations between individuals may also be just or unjust. Here justice is closely related to the notion of fairness. In relations between individuals, fairness may pertain to distributive justice (fair shares) or corrective justice (fair punishment and recompense).

Distributive justice

Distributive justice is at the core of social exclusion and social inclusion of people with mental health problems. Psychiatrists and other mental health professionals often make assumptions and, at times, deliberate on issues that relate to access to resources. It is the assumptions that professionals may make that may be prejudicial or discriminating that are of concern here and may lead to unfair relations between professional and patient and adverse outcomes for the patient. The Ten Essential Shared Capabilities (Department of Health, 2004b; also Chapter 14) may be an important starting point in addressing relevant issues, from the point of training and clinical practice.

Whether fair deliberations by professionals lead to fair outcomes for mental health service users depends on fair social opportunities and welfare arrangements being in place. Of specific relevance here is the issue of disability rights, with emphasis on the need to make social arrangements such as to allow disabled people to overcome the obstacles that exclude them from an equitable share of activities and resources in society (Oliver, 1990; Sayce, 2000; Sayce & Boardman, 2003). The social arrangements necessary for outcomes may need to be sophisticated. For example, many employers confirm that they are in favour of employing disabled people with mental health conditions, but success for such ventures may require additional, appropriate, evidence-based support from the state and other civic institutions.

One strand of thinking about social exclusion concerns exclusion from work and employment. Although some mental health service users also think along the same lines, others worry about unfair coercion to work or loss of benefits. Indeed, some have argued that emphasis on return to work may result in other important areas of social inclusion being neglected. It is not just return to work, but also the more general issue of welfare benefits, insurance and pension entitlements because of inability to work that is of interest here. For example, in relation to state or private insurance and pension schemes, the suspicion remains that there may be selective instruction of mental health experts so that the result is prejudicial rejection of applications for retirement or other benefits. Such prejudicial rejections are discriminatory. In addition, there is the issue of fairness of many private health insurance schemes, which specifically exclude or limit psychiatric treatment in terms of benefits. The question here is how informed are the choices prospective policy-holders make and how such practices may contribute to social exclusion and discrimination against those with psychiatric problems. In their implementation of policy, the NSIP have attempted to balance employment with other domains of inclusion (National Social Inclusion Programme, 2009).

Corrective justice

Complementary to distributive justice is corrective justice. People with learning disability and/or mental health problems may be the perpetrators and/or the victims of offending behaviour, although they are in fact more likely to be victims than perpetrators of criminal offences (Hiday *et al*, 1999; Walsh *et al*, 2003; Teplin *et al*, 2005). Protection of vulnerable adults and their access to both administrative and judicial systems are relevant. However, like work, the issue of corrective justice is also multifaceted. For example, some people with a diagnosis of mental illness, though more likely to be victims than perpetrators, may also be perpetrators of serious violent offences. For violent offenders with mental health problems, the question arises not so much as to whether they would wish to be included in society, but whether society is ready and willing to accept them. It could be argued that, through their offending behaviour, they have effectively opted for 'self-exclusion'. Another view may be that they are excluded because of their illness ('illness-excluded'), and it is this point that we should be concerned with here.

Relevant issues to consider for those with mental health problems who also commit offences include the quality of psychiatric care in prisons, the quality of psychiatric care of people with mental health problems who have committed criminal offences, and criminality in society and its impact on psychiatric practice. Consideration of issues of justice highlights the need to balance the rights of individuals and the public.

Human rights

Human rights may be conceived as emanating from God, Nature, the 'Law within', the inherent dignity of the human person or, simply, from empathy with the suffering of others. Whatever their origins, human rights are enshrined in formal declarations and law.

The United Nations' Universal Declaration of Human Rights (1948) confirms that everyone is born free and equal in dignity and rights and no one shall be subjected to inhuman or degrading treatment or to arbitrary interference with privacy, family or home. It further declares that everyone has the right to work, rest, leisure and education and freely to participate in the cultural life of the community, to enjoy the arts and to share in scientific advancement and its benefits.

The declaration also states: 'everyone has duties to the community in which alone the free and full development of his personality is possible'. This is an indication how, since the end of the Second World War, there has been an evolution of ideas of human rights from a focus on protections of the liberty and property of the individual to a substantive web of reciprocal obligations between individuals, a civic republican approach.

An example of the widening conception of human rights since the War is the United Nations' International Covenant on Economic, Social and Cultural Rights (1966). This affirms that everyone has a right to just and favourable conditions at work, social security, an adequate standard of living, the highest attainable standard of physical and mental health, and a right to education, cultural and scientific life. This must include those with disability arising out of psychiatric conditions. The European Social Charter (1961) also affirms that everyone has the right to just conditions at work, the right to appropriate facilities for vocational guidance and training and the right to 'benefit from all measures enabling him to enjoy the highest possible standard of health attainable'.

Conclusion

Here we have set out the main features of the concept of social exclusion and central to these is the definition of exclusion which we will adopt in this book. This definition emphasises a lack of participation in society, which is seen as the central feature of social exclusion. Notwithstanding the matter of people excluding themselves from society, which we will return to in subsequent chapters, this definition highlights constraint rather than choice as being the main driver of reduced participation. In the next chapter we will begin to examine the concepts and influences of exclusion that are of most relevance to people with mental health problems and learning disability.

Summary

Social exclusion is a relatively recently developed concept which refers to the extent to which individuals are unable to participate in key areas of economic, social and cultural life. There is an emphasis on non-participation arising from constraint rather than choice.

Social exclusion is one way of conceptualising disadvantage, which has been traditionally set in terms of 'poverty', 'hardship', 'destitution', all of which focus on want and misery. Social exclusion extends this traditional approach beyond non-participation due to lack of material resources. This allows expansion of a range of indicators, while retaining the objective of identifying individuals who lack the resources to participate, identifying those whose non-participation arises in other ways, for example through discrimination, chronic illness or cultural identification.

Social exclusion and inclusion are concepts with moral and political connotations, particularly those relating to citizenship, justice and human rights.

References

Atkinson, A. B. (1998) Social exclusion, poverty and unemployment. In *Exclusion, Employment and Opportunity, CASE Paper 4* (eds A. B. Atkinson & J. Hills), pp. 1–20. Centre for Analysis of Social Exclusion, London School of Economics.

Barry, B. (2002) Social exclusion, social isolation, and the distribution of income. In *Understanding Social Exclusion* (eds J. Hills, J. Le Grand & D. Piachaud). Oxford University Press.

Berghman, J. (1995) Social exclusion in Europe: policy context and analytic framework. In *Beyond the Threshold* (ed. G. Room). Polity Press.

Burchardt, T., Le Grand, J. & Piachaud, D. (2002a) Introduction. In *Understanding Social Exclusion* (eds J. Hills, J. Le Grand & D. Piachaud). Oxford University Press.

Burchardt, T., Le Grand, J. & Piachaud, D. (2002b) Degrees of exclusion: developing a dynamic, multidimensional measure. In *Understanding Social Exclusion* (eds J. Hills, J. Le Grand & D. Piachaud). Oxford University Press.

Byrne, D. (1999) *Social Exclusion*. Oxford University Press.

Department of Health (2004a) *Improving Mental Health Law: Towards a New Mental Health Act*. Department of Health.

Department of Health (2004b) *The Ten Essential Shared Capabilities: A Framework for the Whole of the Mental Health Workforce*. Department of Health.

Department of Social Security (1999) *Opportunity for All: Tackling Poverty and Social Exclusion*. First Annual Report. TSO (The Stationery Office).

Gordon, D., Levitas, R., Pantazis, C., *et al* (2000) *Poverty and Social Exclusion in Britain*. Joseph Rowntree Foundation.

Gore, C. & Figueiredo, J. (eds) (1997) *Social Exclusion and Anti-Poverty Policy: A Debate (RS 110)*. International Labour Organization.

Hiday, V. A., Swartz, M. S., Swanson, J. W., *et al* (1999) Criminal victimization of persons with severe mental illness. *Psychiatric Services*, **50**, 62–68.

Hills, J. (2002) Does a focus on 'social inclusion' change the policy response? In *Understanding Social Exclusion* (eds J. Hills, J. Le Grand & D. Piachaud). Oxford University Press.

HM Government (2005a) *Health, Work and Well-Being: Caring for Our Future. A Strategy for the Health and Well-Being of Working Age People*. TSO (The Stationery Office).

HM Government (2005b) *Department for Work and Pensions' Five Year Strategy: Opportunity and Security throughout Life (CM 6447)*. TSO (The Stationery Office).

HM Government (2006) *A New Deal for Welfare: Empowering People to Work* (Green Paper, CM6730). TSO (The Stationery Office).

Ikkos, G., Boardman, J. & Zigmond, T. (2006) Talking liberties: John Rawls's theory of justice and psychiatric practice. *Advances in Psychiatric Treatment*, **12**, 202–210.

Kymlicka, W. (2002) *Contemporary Political Philosophy: An Introduction (2nd edn)*. Oxford University Press.

Levitas, R. (1998) *The Inclusive Society? Social Exclusion and New Labour*. Macmillan.

Levitas, R., Pantazis, C., Fahmy, E., *et al* (2007) *The Multidimensional Analysis of Social Exclusion: A Research Report for the Social Exclusion Task Force*. The Cabinet Office.

Marshall, T. H. (1965) *Class, Citizenship and Social Development*. Anchor.

Morgan, C., Burns, T., Fitzpatrick, R., *et al* (2007) Social exclusion and mental health: conceptual and methodological review. *British Journal of Psychiatry*, **191**, 477–483.

Murray, C. (1994) *Underclass: The Crisis Deepens*. Institute of Economic Affairs.

Murray, C. (1999) *The Underclass Revisited*. Institute of Economic Affairs.

National Social inclusion Programme (2009) *Vision and Progress: Social Inclusion and Mental Health*. National Social inclusion Programme.

Oliver, M. (1990) *The Politics of Disablement*. Macmillan.

Rawls, J. (1971) *A Theory of Justice*. Oxford University Press.

Room, G. (1995) *Beyond the Threshold*. Polity Press.

Room, G. (1998) Social exclusion, solidarity and the challenge of globalisation. *International Journal of Social Welfare*, **8**, 166–174.

Room, G. (2000) Trajectories of social exclusion. In *Breadline Europe* (eds D. Gordon & P. Townsend). Polity Press.

Rowntree, B. S. (1901) *Poverty: A Study of Town Life*. Macmillan (reprinted 2000, Policy Press).

Sayce, L. (2000) *From Psychiatric Patient to Citizen: Overcoming Discrimination and Social Exclusion*. Macmillan.

Sayce, L. & Boardman, J. (2003) The Disability Discrimination Act 1995: implications for psychiatrists. *Advances in Psychiatric Treatment*, **9**, 397–404.

Silver, H. (1994) Social exclusion and social solidarity: three paradigms. *International Labour Review*, **133**, 531–578.

Social Exclusion Unit (2001) *Preventing Social Exclusion*. TSO (The Stationery Office).

Teplin, L., McClelland, G., Abram, K., *et al* (2005) Crime victimisation in adults with severe mental illness: comparison with the National Crime Victimization Survey. *Archives of General Psychiatry*, **62**, 911–921.

Townsend, P. (1979) *Poverty in the United Kingdom*. Penguin.

Walker, A. & Walker, C. (eds) (1997) *Britain Divided: The Growth of Social Exclusion in the 1980s and 1990s*. Child Poverty Action Group.

Walsh, E., Moran, P., Scott, C., *et al* (2003) Prevalence of violent victimisation in severe mental illness. *British Journal of Psychiatry*, **183**, 233–238.

CHAPTER 3

Social exclusion of people with mental health problems and learning disabilities: key aspects

Jed Boardman

Throughout this book the central characteristic of social exclusion is seen as the non-participation of people in the key activities of society. This allows us to examine what factors affect social exclusion, its scope, and the evidence for its extent. Many people working in mental health and learning disability services will recognise that disadvantage and exclusion from participation are common experiences for users of services and that reducing these aspects of social exclusion can bring about significant improvements to their lives. In this chapter we expand upon these and outline how these might help us to understand their application to people with mental health problems and learning disabilities.

Social exclusion and mental health problems

What we are concerned with here are the concepts associated with social exclusion that are useful in providing a means of understanding the importance of the links between exclusion and mental health problems or learning disability. These are summarised in Box 3.1.

Concepts and applications

The concept of social exclusion has been applied to a range of specific groups, including people who are unemployed, single parents, the homeless, refugees and asylum seekers, and people living in deprived areas. It has also been extended to people with disabilities (Blaxter, 1980; Martin & White, 1988) and thus includes people with mental health problems and learning disabilities. People from specific social identity groups (e.g. women, people from Black and minority ethnic groups, gay and lesbian people) who also have mental health problems are likely to experience social exclusion (Chapter 9).

Box 3.1   Central concepts of social exclusion relevant to people with mental health problems and learning disabilities

Elements of social exclusion:

- a relative concept
- has been applied to a range of specific groups – including those with disabilities
- based on concepts of poverty and deprivation
- emphasises agency and processes
- has a dynamic dimension
- central role of participation
- multifactorial causal framework
- life course and longitudinal perspective
- links to choice and access
- stigma and discrimination
- equality and human rights
- citizenship
- social capital
- recovery.

As a relative concept, an analysis of social exclusion can be applied to the UK in the 21st century and to those with mental health problems and learning disabilities who live in the UK. Further to this, the analysis of exclusion and its associated concepts can help to develop a vision for society and mental health services in the future. It can also help us view the historical changes that have occurred in mental health services and the position of people with mental health problems and learning disabilities in society.

The ideas of social exclusion are based on concepts of poverty and deprivation, but represent an extended concept which can be readily applied to disability and its multifactorial causal components that relate to social exclusion. Many people with mental ill health or learning disability are materially deprived, but many recognise that they are excluded in other important ways which relate to such matters as stigma and discrimination, and these multiple factors can readily be seen to interact.

The central role of participation

We have adopted a working definition of social exclusion where the central component is participation in society. But, in practice, what does this mean and how might it help in assessing the extent of exclusion?

Several authors have identified the dimensions of participation that define the ways in which people may be excluded from society and also assist in developing measures of exclusion (Box 3.2). The examples shown in Box 3.2 are similar to each other and have several dimensions in common. The dimensions relate to income poverty and exclusion from material resources, exclusion from productive activity, exclusion from social relations and neighbourhoods, and exclusion from civic participation or political decision-making.

Each of these dimensions helps us to define social exclusion and point to objective ways of measuring exclusion. It is important to consider that the dimensions interact, and lack of participation in any one dimension is sufficient for a person or group to be considered as socially excluded. Each of the dimensions represents a general outcome that is important in its own right and thus, in this sense, social inclusion is reflected by the absence of exclusion on all of the dimensions. In addition, exclusion on any of the dimensions is not likely to be absolute, but rather is a matter of degree – the less the participation, the greater the degree of exclusion. For measurement purposes, the dimensions (or exclusion) represent an outcome and what are often regarded as indicators of exclusion (e.g. having a mental illness or disability, being a member of an ethnic minority, living in a deprived area) are the causes of, or risk factors for, exclusion.

Box 3.2   Dimensions of social exclusion

From Burchardt *et al* (2002*b*):

- consumption – capacity to purchase goods and services (income poverty)
- production – participation in economically or socially valuable activities (employment, education, etc.)
- social interaction – interaction with family, friends, community (isolated networks)
- political engagement – involvement in local or national decision-making (having a voice, choice and control).

From Gordon *et al* (2000):

- impoverishment – exclusion from adequate income or material resources;
- labour market exclusion – lack of attachment to the labour market
- service exclusion – lack of access to basic services, in the home (e.g., power or water supplies) or outside it (e.g. transport, shops, financial services)
- exclusion from social relations – non-participation in common social activities, isolation, lack of support, disengagement and confinement.

From Scharf *et al* (2005):

- exclusion from material resources – income and material security
- exclusion from social relations – ability to engage in meaningful relationships with others
- exclusion from (socially valued) productive activity – labour market participation, informal caring and potentially retirement
- exclusion from civic participation – engaging civil society and decision-making processes
- service exclusion – access to services in and beyond the home
- neighbourhood exclusion – the immediate residential setting.

The details of these broad dimensions may vary according to different demographic groups. For example, Scharf *et al*'s (2005) list (Box 3.2) relates to the exclusion of older people and encompasses equivalent roles beyond the labour market, including informal caring and retirement. Gordon *et al* (2000) include in their list (Box 3.2) service exclusion or lack of access to basic services, which may be subsumed by others under material resources, but nevertheless serves to remind us that many people with mental health problems (particularly long-term psychoses) and learning disabilities find health services difficult to access (Mencap, 2004; Disability Rights Commission, 2006; Mencap, 2007), and for these groups this additional dimension should be considered.

This problem of access to basic services, especially mainstream services, may be particularly pertinent for people with learning disabilities. O'Brien (1989) has highlighted the difficulties experienced in achieving and sustaining social inclusion, suggesting that prejudice towards people with severe disabilities is perpetuated by their exclusion from 'ordinary classrooms, workplaces and homes'. In what have come to be known as 'O'Brien's five accomplishments', he defines the quality of supported lives of people with learning disabilities in relation to valued inclusive experiences of growing in relationships, contributing, making choice, having the dignity of valued social roles, and sharing ordinary places and environments. These accomplishments are phrased in terms of exclusion, rather than inclusion, and each accomplishment is seen as 'challeng(ing) and strengthen(ing) the relationship between people with disabilities and other community members' (O'Brien, 1989).

For people with mental health problems and learning disabilities, the dimensions of participation may be summarised as:

- consumption (exclusion from material resources) – capacity to purchase goods and services (income poverty)
- production (exclusion from (socially valued) productive activity) – participation in economically or socially valuable activities (employment, education, etc.)
- social interaction (exclusion from social relations and neighbourhoods) – interaction with family, friends, community (isolated networks)
- political engagement (exclusion from civic participation) – involvement in local or national decision-making (having a voice, choice and control)
- health and health service engagement (exclusion from health and health services) – having good health and accessing appropriate services.

Examples of how people with mental health problems and learning disabilities are excluded in these dimensions are given in Chapter 8.

Agency and process

The emphasis on agency and processes, outlined in Chapter 2, allows us to identify those institutions and social processes which play a part in exclusion. This corresponds to the 'social model of disability', which stresses the role of social and environmental barriers in producing disability (Oliver, 1983,1990,1996; Barnes, 2000). This model is important to consider in relation to the application of the concepts of social exclusion to people with mental health problems and learning disabilities.

The social model of disability places the problems of disability within society, rather than the individual:

> disability, according to the social model, is all the things that impose restrictions on disabled people; ranging from individual prejudice to institutional discrimination, from inaccessible public buildings to unusable transport systems, from segregated education to excluding work arrangements, and so on (Oliver, 1996: p. 33).

This view is distinguished from individual models of disability, which locate disability within people themselves. It does acknowledge the reality of peoples' impairments and the pain associated with them, but it separates the experience of impairments from those of disability and sees no necessary causal relationship between the two. In this way it points our attention away from the individual to focus on matters of discrimination, exclusion and oppression (Mulvany, 2000). This separation has been disputed by some (Williams, 1991; French, 1993), but the advocates of the social model remain adamant that,

> Disability is seen as wholly and exclusively social ... it is a consequence of social oppression (Oliver, 1996: p. 35).

The essential arguments for this model have been conceptual (identifying the causes of disability within the social world and separating this from the causes of impairment) and pragmatic (it is an attempt to identify matters that may be addressed through collective action). But, in addition and importantly, the model is viewed by people who are disabled as a clear representation of their own experiences and the diversity of this experience.

This model provides the same helpful framework for describing the experiences of people with mental health problems and learning disabilities and the social barriers that they face. The model provides a base for much of what is discussed in this book as we try and identify the social barriers and other factors which are implicated in the pathways to the undesirable outcome of social exclusion. However, as a model and not a social theory it cannot explain everything, but it does provide a descriptive framework.

An example of how this approach may be of advantage to people with mental health problems can be seen in the area of employment. In this setting, it offers a more helpful conceptual basis for understanding and promoting employment opportunities for people who use mental health services and offers more hope for the recovery of social roles; it better captures the experience of discrimination and exclusion central to the lives of many mental health service users and addresses the barriers to employment; it is consistent with government policy (e.g. the Disability

Discrimination Act 1995); it is consistent with the views of users and people with disabilities; and it assists in achieving dialogue with employers (Boardman, 2003).

For people with mental health problems, framing the wider social problems associated with having a mental health problem as disabilities, not only highlights many of their own experiences, but also has the advantage that the individuals with these problems have rights to particular benefits rather than being considered as the 'worthy poor' to receive discriminatory charity (Thornicroft, 2006). This approach offers 'disabled people a feeling of self-worth, as well as offering them a collective identity and a stronger political organisation' (Butler & Bowlby, 1997: p. 412).

Dynamic dimension

As indicated in Chapter 2, the causal models of exclusion are complex, involving factors at several levels and feedback loops. A further dynamic dimension is seen when exclusion is not viewed as a fixed state, but rather as one that people move into and out of as the conditions that lead to exclusion change (Smith & Middleton, 2007); this may be seen with conditions of poverty (see Chapter 7). Similarly, many people with mental health problems have 'fluctuating conditions' which are both difficult for the individual to cope with and are also not always readily tolerated by others, and may lead to loss of employment or other social roles. These dynamics and the associated social responses are commonly experienced by people with mental health problems.

A further dynamic component of exclusion may be seen within families, through early life experiences which may provide the basis for an individual's later exclusion and also by the transmission of exclusion across generations. This may be a familiar experience for people who develop mental health problems at an early stage of their life or who grow up in a family whose members have mental health problems or other forms of disability. This is taken up later in Part 2 and can be illustrated in terms of cycles of disadvantage or deprivation (Chapter 10). Importantly, viewing the dynamic of exclusion in this way means that possible causal factors can be identified, which makes these states potentially amenable to intervention.

Causality, a life course and longitudinal perspective

The causal framework for understanding social exclusion reveals complex and multifactorial influences acting on individuals (Chapter 10). To understand these influences it is helpful to take a life course and longitudinal perspective to examine the effects of early variables in determining exclusion and of important intergenerational and intragenerational aspects of transmission of social exclusion (Centre for Longitudinal Studies, 2008). Put simply, all present influences are products of the past and the past is 'the starting point for the present' (Burchardt et al, 2002a: p. 8). The 'present influences' are generally seen as external (current constraints facing the individual or community) or internal (choices that individuals or communities make).

Data from cohort studies are required if we are to provide the evidence for a longitudinal perspective on social exclusion. In Britain several major population-based cohort studies provide data that are of relevance here, providing repeated measures of samples of people born in certain years: the British 1946 Birth Cohort, the 1958 National Child Development Study, the British 1970 Birth Cohort and the Millennium Cohort study (Douglas, 1964; Chamberlain, et al, 1975, 1978; Osborn et al, 1984; Wadsworth, 1991; Bynner et al, 1997; Dex & Joshi, 2005). These studies were not designed specifically to examine the development and effect of mental health problems, but they do provide information on such things as health, education and skills, family life, gender and the workplace, inequality and life chances. In particular, they give us insights into the effect of early life chances on adult outcomes and the factors that reinforce positive and negative developments in people's lives (Sainsbury Centre for Mental Health, 2009). In other words, they provide important data to support the life course perspective. Other influences on the cohort are related to the periods of history in which the cohort is raised and enters adulthood; thus the 1946 cohort will be subjected to different external influences than those born in 1970 or 2000. Not only do people change over time, but so does the environment around them. This perspective may also be illuminated by data from repeated cross-sectional studies such as the General Household Survey (set up in 1971), the British Social Attitudes Survey (set up in 1983), and the British Crime Survey (set up in 1982), or panel studies such as the British Household Panel (set up in 1991) or the English Longitudinal study of Ageing (done since 2002).

A life course approach outlines the links between childhood circumstance and the outcomes in adult life. The approach highlights critical points of transition in a person's life and these transitions through the life course may lead to experiences of social inclusion or exclusion. The idea of 'transition' refers to changes or 'turning points' at key points of the individual's life, such as going to or leaving school, starting work, redundancy, retirement and bereavement. Transitions may themselves be simple or complex, depending on the range of social and cultural institutions involved. They may be clearly marked with formal rites of passage or, as is the case with most adult transitions, left open for individual negotiation. In some cases they may be relatively insulated from social and economic change, whereas in others they may be driven and largely constructed by external forces.

The life course perspective makes an important distinction between *trajectories* on the one side and transitions on the other:

> A long view of the life course takes the perspective of trajectories with sequences of family and work roles, among others. A shorter view focuses on life transitions that represent a change in state(s), such as when children leave home. Some transitions involve multiple changes in a multi-phasic process.

Disillusionment in marriage may lead to separation and then divorce... or birth control may be used to prevent unwanted pregnancies. At each stage of the process, the selection of certain options over others results in a different course. Transitions are embedded within larger trajectories (Elder & Johnson, 2003: p. 54–55).

It is obvious to mental health professionals that key events can severely disrupt these transitions and produce a negative impact on an individual's development and life outcomes. For example, traumatic experiences in early life (such as sexual abuse) are associated with later onset of mental health problems, and the onset of mental health problems during the key life phase of adolescence may have long-term consequences for later life chances.

When considering the life course approach, ageing individuals and cohorts are viewed across their entire lifetime, taking into account the influences of historical, social, economic and environmental factors that occur at earlier ages (Elder, 1974; Settersten, 2003). Ageing is considered to occur from birth to death, involving social, psychological and biological processes, and the experiences of ageing to be shaped by factors related to the period in which a person is born and raised (cohort effects) (Passuth & Bengston, 1988).

These cohort effects may be seen in relation to mid-age and older people. Transitions occurring in later life will be different from those in earlier periods of development; for example, the larger trajectory may involve a changing orientation to employment and a growing awareness about impending retirement. People taking on new responsibilities in relation to care work for parents and/or grandchildren may accompany these personal changes of orientation. Transitions after the age of 50 years appear increasingly complex in respect of the range of statuses and institutions involved. They may overlap in a variety of ways and include several activities, including paid work, care work and leisure. There may also be opposing trends in operation, for example, family transitions associated with divorce in midlife may foster a desire to maintain a presence within the labour force, an expansion of care tasks may lead to an individual withdrawing from work, or new leisure interests may lead to a reassessment of the priority accorded to paid work. Mid and later life seems to be becoming more 'crowded' in relation to demographic and occupational change, such as divorce, earlier retirement or new caring responsibilities. But at the same time, society has become less interventionist in terms of the range of supports that appear to be on offer (Phillipson, 2002). This may reflect what has been called the 'post-traditional life course', in which self-development is a more individualised, but deinstitutionalised, process (Giddens, 1991). What has changed over time is that employment has become a less stable experience, with the rise of what has been described as 'contingent work' and the decline of the traditional working career; family experiences are also changing, with an increasing proportion of 50-year-olds living alone (around 13% of men), and a rise in divorce rates. The implications of such developments are that new types of social integration will emerge for men and women moving through their fifties: work may become less important, whereas personal networks, leisure experiences and voluntary activities may matter rather more and there will be new forms of social exclusion as well as inclusion.

Social exclusion of people in middle and later life may arise through increasingly pronounced inequalities in cumulative advantage and disadvantage. Research also suggests that social divisions related to class, gender, cohort and ethnic divides also become more pronounced in later life (Walker, 1996; Casey & Yamada, 2002; Scharf *et al*, 2002; Price & Ginn, 2003). There is growing understanding of the extent of diversity and inequality within cohorts, with evidence for wide variations in income and consumption prospects in retirement, these reflecting educational, occupational, gender, class and other social factors.

Social inclusion or exclusion may also be fostered by patterns of 'age integration' or 'age segregation' over the life course. Some commentators suggest evidence for a greater mix of age groups in social networks (age integration), giving a 'blurring' in age divisions and the tendency for adulthood to be interspersed with periods of education and leisure rather than wholly devoted to the sphere of work (Neugarten & Neugarten, 1986; Riley & Riley, 1994). This relaxation of age divisions may be affected by changing patterns of consumption in middle and later life, and the development of lifestyles which cross traditional generational boundaries (Gilleard & Higgs, 2002). On the other hand, there is some evidence for continuing age segregation and age homogeneity in social networks, with younger network members being drawn overwhelmingly from kin. Uhlenberg & de Jong (2004) noted 'a deficit of young adults in the networks of older people' (p. 22), and social networks being made up of people of similar ages. The trends for the future remain uncertain, but there are some trends which might promote exclusion through later life transitions, including: continuing alarmism about the implications of demographic change; threats to the funding of state pensions and other types of support; and the possible lack of recognition of emotional needs associated with the changes running through the life course.

Choice and access

Choice and access are implicit in social exclusion. Choice refers to the power to make decisions and as such is a key part of the political engagement dimension of participation outlined earlier. Choice may also be seen in a more limited, consumerist way, as a way of making services more responsive to the needs and demands of the people who use them and making these services more accessible – in this sense it is a means to an end. In a wider sense, choice is a manifestation of the rights and responsibilities of adult citizens which goes beyond the use of health services, to people's life choices and engagement in wider politics, and being treated with dignity and respect – in this sense it is an end in itself (Rankin, 2005). Both these senses of choice must be taken into account when considering the social inclusion of people with mental health problems and learning disability.

Choice has been central to government policies in health and social care, and set out under the banner of creating a patient-led NHS (e.g. Department of Health, 2003, 2004). Much of this has, however, been concerned with financial systems such as payment by results or practice-based commissioning, or referral systems such as 'choose and book'. For mental health services the vision for patient choice has been set out in *Our Choices in Mental Health* (Care Services Improvement Partnership, 2005) and for learning disability in *Valuing People* (Department of Health, 2001a). These policies are aspirational but are also associated with market mechanisms. For example, giving people more choice over the services they receive is expected to empower them and reduce inequalities by providing choices to all service users, but also to increase the range of available services and providers, and improve standards through competition (Sainsbury Centre for Mental Health, 2006). Choice here may be linked to diverse markets, when otherwise more universal coverage may be more welcome. In addition, increasing choice may have the paradoxical effect of reducing a sense of control and the associated increase in expectations may be debilitating (Schwartz, 2004).

The disability rights movement has often welcomed the place of choice in the policy agenda as it has been seen to make it more difficult for the government to dismiss their views (Oliver, 1996; Barnes *et al*, 1999; Rankin, 2005). This applies to people with mental health problems and may have beneficial effects in areas of treatment choice, access and engagement, involvement in service planning, community services, collective choices, and life choices (Rankin, 2005; Sainsbury Centre for Mental Health, 2006; Samele *et al*, 2007). Several of these matters relate to the ideas of recovery, which will be taken up later in this chapter. They may also be of particular significance to people with longer-term and severe mental health problems whose experiences of the coercive aspects of services have overshadowed their views of contact with mental health services (Perkins & Repper, 1998).

Rankin (2005) has helpfully highlighted two aspects of choice that face clinicians and people with mental health problems. The first relates to risk and the making of choices by service users that mental health workers and others may find unpalatable. Professionals often have to accept that service users make choices that they may not like, something that they do not deny to other people, nor to themselves. In addition, there is also a political nettle that has yet to be grasped: a policy based around the voice of the consumer, with its associated rising expectations, may lead to demands that cannot be met when resources are restricted. Unpalatable choices may thus face the government.

The second aspect of choice leads us back to the notion of self-exclusion. People with mental health problems may choose to disengage or shun attempts at a more structured life or increasing participation. This may be a way of coping with the harsh realities of life for those on the margins, but it may also be informed by limited experiences and narrow perspectives and by a limited knowledge of possible options. Rankin points out that these are false choices and may be considered as no choice at all. She quotes Le Grand's example of a false choice as an illustration of this (Rankin, 2005):

> If an individual only has two unpalatable choices (your money or your life) then if he or she chooses only one of them (such as giving up money), it would be odd to judge the outcome as promoting individual welfare or even a just one, simply because it was the product of a choice (Le Grand, 2003: p. 5).

For people with mental health problems or those with learning disabilities, choice is a key component of social inclusion, but without increasing participation many choices may be devoid of meaning or may even be counterproductive.

Stigma (ignorance, prejudice and discrimination)

One of the most widely recognised barriers to participation for people with mental health problems and learning disabilities is the stigma associated with their conditions. There is a large literature on the subject of stigma, too voluminous to cover here – the reader is referred to Thornicroft (2006), who provides an up-to-date summary of the subject as well as reviewing some of the shortcomings of models of stigma. In summary, Thornicroft (2006) argues that although the concept of stigma may be important in helping to develop an understanding of the experiences of social exclusion, it tends to locate the problem within the individual rather than in the social world; as such, the concept of stigma requires revision if it is to allow us to examine the importance of stigma as a barrier to participation and inclusion. He suggests that three related issues need to be considered: ignorance, prejudice and discrimination.

This emphasis on ignorance, prejudice and discrimination has several advantages: it shifts attention from intentions to behaviours; interventions to change behaviour towards individuals with mental health problems can be developed and tested; it implies parity for people with mental ill health with others who have physical disabilities and so they may benefit from anti-discriminatory laws and provisions; and it requires a change from seeing things from the viewpoint of those in the 'in group' to those in the 'out group'.

In the past, the solution for some has been seen as one of reducing stigma, but for others it has been about retaining the basic rights of citizenship (Chamberlin, 2006). This shift in the focus of the solution may be a more helpful aid in considering how to alter the focus from exclusion to inclusion for people with mental health problems and those with learning disabilities. One consequence of this limited solution to stigma has been anti-stigma campaigns that focus on encouraging people to engage in treatment. This may be valuable when discriminating attitudes limit access to areas that others without a diagnosis of mental ill health have greater entry to, but treatment may be a part of the problem and there are many other areas, including employment, education, civil participation, to which access is limited. This is aptly summarised by Chamberlin (2006: p. xii):

> The attitudes that most people hold towards those labelled with mental illness are…major barriers to their being able to lead the lives they want – to hold down jobs they are qualified for, to live in ordinary housing, to engage in social relations and to enjoy their basic rights as citizens.

Equality and human rights

The notion of discrimination points to a need for a focus on human rights and injustice experienced by people with mental health problems and learning disabilities. Associated with social exclusion are the concepts of equality and human rights. Equality of some kind is important in its own right and this places a value on people getting the same, or being treated the same, in some respect (Burchardt, 2006). The human rights approach, although not necessarily eschewing equality, is unconditional as entitlement is on the basis of one's humanity. Both equality and human rights are matters that fit in the scope of social exclusion.

Until recently, the Commission for Racial Equality, the Disability Rights Commission and the Equal Opportunities Commission have focused attention on preventing discrimination along the lines of the social identity characteristics of ethnicity, disability and gender. The new Equality and Human Rights Commission (EHRC), which brought together the three rights commissions, has added further social identity groups: sexual orientation, religion and faith, transgender and age. People with disabilities caused by mental ill health, intellectual impairment, and the other social groups listed above all have representation in the Royal College of Psychiatrists through the faculties and special interest groups. Chapter 9 highlights the same groups covered by the EHRC and is consistent with recent developments. This offers a means of highlighting not only the broad constituency of people with mental health problems and learning disabilities, but also of those with specific social identity characteristics who also have these problems (people with 'multiple diversities').

Capability approach

Central to the idea of equality is the question of 'Equality of what?' We do not have sufficient space in this book to do justice to this question, but it is helpful to consider the approach used by the Equalities Review (2007) – the capability approach (Sen, 1992; Burchardt, 2006; Burchardt & Vizard, 2007; Vizard & Burchardt, 2007).

The capability approach proposes that a key aspect of human freedom relates to the substantive opportunity that a person has to have a life they value and choose, and have reasons to value and choose – and that social and economic arrangements ought to be evaluated and judged from this

33

perspective. The approach focuses on substantive freedom (also referred to as substantive capabilities), that is what people are able to do, or be, in their lives. In this context, if the question 'Equality of what?' is posed, the answer is the 'Equality of substantive freedoms'. Substantive freedom may be limited by a lack of personal resources in which the individual is operating (i.e. economic, social, political, cultural, environmental conditions) which determine what she or he can achieve given her or his endowments and entitlements. This is consistent with the social model of disability discussed earlier. Central and valuable capabilities are the important things people can do, or be, in life, which make their lives go well (e.g. being healthy, keeping safe, etc.).

The capability approach to equality has advantages over other approaches (Burchardt, 2006; Burchardt & Vizard, 2007). First, it focuses on the central and important things in life that people can actually do, and thus it is concerned with what matters to people, for example being healthy, participating and enjoying self-respect. This makes it intuitively attractive as it is something we can all understand and that is raised time and time again in clinicians' interactions with the people who use health and social services. Second, it is concerned with people being treated in the same manner (e.g. equality of respect) and thus it can incorporate many aspects of an equality of process, as well as outcome. This has often been raised in the narrative accounts of people who use mental health services and in the surveys of opinions of service users about mental health services – they place great emphasis on being treated with dignity and respect. Third, it accommodates variations in need, recognising that individuals who have greater needs will need more flexible institutional arrangements and greater material resources in order to have access to the same capability set than the person without those needs. This variation in needs has always been recognised by clinicians and others and it is recognised that resources need to be directed accordingly. A fourth advantage of the capability approach is that it adds to the recognition of the variation in needs as it focuses on the substantive freedoms that individuals have to achieve valuable objectives rather than on the outcomes themselves; thus, it supports a diversity of goals, values and preferences. This recognises that being able to shape one's own life is valuable in itself, so an objective of equality is the exercise of choice and control (people have real freedom to formulate and pursue their own objectives), something that is important in the concepts of recovery that are discussed later in this chapter.

In addition, the capability approach acknowledges the accumulation of advantages and disadvantages over a lifetime and thus recognises the life course and longitudinal perspective and the multiple causes of social exclusion. It also places an emphasis on barriers, constraints, structures and processes and is thus consistent with the definition of social exclusion outlined in Chapter 2 and the emphasis on external constraints. Although the capability approach is an individualistic model, it nevertheless emphasises the importance of a person's situation, such as the constraints they operate under and the institutions, structures and processes. These kinds of constraints are seen to limit what a person can do or be – that is, their real freedoms. It also has the potential to point to ways in which action can be taken to increase real freedoms. However, the capability approach is not without its problems and distinguishing between differences in outcome that originate from differences in underlying values and preferences from those of opportunity remains a difficulty for the capability approach.

Regardless of this limitation, the capability approach does appear to be consistent with the elements of social exclusion discussed in this chapter and it also has additional advantages. It allows us to capture and suggest ways of measuring the substantive freedoms or real opportunities that people with mental health problems have to live the kind of life they value and would choose. The ten domains of central and valuable capabilities, identified for the Equalities Review for the purposes of conceptualisation and measuring inequality, provide a useful means of listing the areas in which people with mental health problems experience discrimination and exclusion: life; physical security; health; education; standard of living; productive and valued activities; individual, family and social life; participation, influence and voice; identity expression and self-respect; legal security. These domains are consistent with the dimensions of participation discussed earlier and offer a way by which inequality can be measured and by which policy initiatives can be targeted. In addition, these may be separately examined by social identity characteristics or broad diagnostic groups (and/or context and resources).

Citizenship

People with disabilities should have the same rights to active citizenship as everyone else in society. This is related to, and implied by, the rights approach and the social disability model. Some of the philosophical aspects of citizenship have been discussed in Chapter 1. In the context of social exclusion, the idea of citizenship offers several advantages (Thornicroft, 2006). For example, it allows service users to challenge the narrow disease-based definitions of disability and to highlight the social barriers that create disability, and acts as a point of reference in calls for social change. It also supports the assumption that the human rights of people with mental health problems and learning disabilities should be respected, and offers a benchmark to assess the success of measures of self-determination. Finally, it fixes responsibility with governments to respond to legitimate demands for parity of treatment and to respond by committing resources.

Social capital and associated concepts

Social capital is a complex theory with a number of definitions. Essentially, it is a way of describing the linkages in society that allow it to work for the common good. These linkages can be psychological as well as structural and occur at a number of levels. The most commonly used definition of social capital in the health sciences originates from the political scientist Robert Putnam (1993). His description consists of five principal characteristics:

1   networks (community, voluntary, state, personal) and density
2   civic engagement, participation and use of civic networks
3   local civic identity – sense of belonging, solidarity and equality with local community members
4   reciprocity and norms of cooperation, a sense of obligation to help others and confidence in return of assistance
5   trust in the community.

Others have included community efficacy – the ability of communities to come together to fight for a common cause (for instance, to stop a hospital closing) – as an important facet of social capital (see Bandura, 1997, 2000). As well as measuring social cohesion and organisation, community efficacy measures the sociopolitical organisation of a country which enables groups to access power.

Associated with social capital is the concept of social quality (Berman & Phillips, 2000; Huxley & Thornicroft, 2003), which refers to 'the extent to which citizens are able to participate in the social and economic life of their communities under conditions which enhance their well-being and individual potential' (Beck et al, 1997, quoted in Huxley & Thornicroft, 2003: p. 290). It overlaps with concepts of social exclusion and socioeconomic security, social cohesion and empowerment (Putnam, 2000; Social Exclusion Unit, 2000) and concepts of community (McMillan & Chavis, 1986; Crow & Allan, 1994).

Both social inclusion and social capital focus, to varying degrees, on participation in social networks, which may facilitate or frustrate access to different kinds of resources (Phillipson et al, 2004; Morgan et al, 2007). Social capital may refer to the benefits that arise from membership of social networks and other kinds of social structures. In this way social capital may promote social inclusion by tying people to others in the wider community. In general, social networks are viewed as positive; people with smaller social networks may experience disadvantage and have worse health and general well-being. Lower social involvement in the community may produce adverse health effects (Wilkinson, 2005) and adverse effects on people whose poverty acts as a barrier to social involvement. Social networks give access to a range of material and psychological resources and to social capital and in this way help you stay healthy. On the other hand, high-density social networks may be 'exclusive' and may demand conformity, leading to the marginalisation of certain groups, including those with mental illness (Crow, 2004).

Social networks, social integration and social fragmentation all overlap with social capital and exclusion. Also linked is the goal of social cohesion which has emerged as a major policy objective in the UK and Europe (Levitas, 2005).

Recovery

Although recovery is not a concept that is traditionally part of the general literature on social exclusion, it does have particular currency among people with mental health problems and learning disabilities, and may operate as a means of promoting their inclusion. At the individual level, recovery is concerned with what matters to people with mental ill health, which parallels the discussion about the advantages of the capability approach to equality.

What is meant by recovery? There is a considerable literature on recovery and this is summarised in several publications (Repper & Perkins, 2003; Roberts & Wolfson 2004; Roberts *et al*, 2006; Shepherd *et al*, 2008; Slade, 2009). What we will present in this chapter is a brief summary of the concepts of recovery and consideration of its importance for mental health practice, particularly its relation to social inclusion.

The ideas of recovery have been largely formulated by, and for, service users to describe their own life experiences. One widely agreed definition states that recovery is

> a deeply personal, unique process of changing one's attitudes, values, feelings, goals, skills and/or roles. It is a way of living a satisfying, hopeful and contributing life, even with the limitations caused by illness. Recovery involves the development of new meaning and purpose in one's life as one grows beyond the catastrophic effects of mental illness (Anthony, 1993: p. 14).

Recovery in the sense used here does not necessarily mean 'clinical recovery' (usually defined in terms of symptoms and resolution), but rather it concerns 'social recovery', the idea of building a life beyond illness, of recovering one's life without necessarily achieving a clinical recovery. In this way recovery from mental health problems has a theme in common with other chronic illnesses such as diabetes, asthma and arthritis. People can and do recover, even from the most serious and long-term mental health problems (Harrison *et al*, 2001; Trieman & Leff, 2002).

Recovery can be seen as a process, the main components of which have been summarised in Box 3.3. It is often seen as a unique and individual experience. Some people, particularly those who experience more long-term problems, say that recovery is about more than the absence of symptoms. For some it is about regaining control and possibly having a different relationship to their symptoms. For others it means recovery from the impact of an illness. It is not necessarily an end point, but is often termed a 'journey', and thus people are not seen as 'recovered', but as 'recovering' or 'in recovery' (Repper & Perkins, 2003). Such an understanding of what recovery means is fundamentally different from the traditional clinical sense of recovery. The journey of recovery may have ups and downs but a period of illness does not necessarily mean that recovery stops – it may in fact be part of the longer-term process of growth and development.

Box 3.3   Components of the process of recovery

- Finding and maintaining hope – believing in oneself; having a sense of personal agency; being optimistic about the future
- Re-establishment of a positive identity – finding a new identity which incorporates illness, but retains a core, positive sense of self
- Building a meaningful life – making sense of illness; finding a meaning in life, despite illness; being engaged in life
- Taking responsibility and control – feeling in control of illness and in control of life

Source: Andresen *et al* (2003).

Three concepts make up the central aspects of recovery ideas: hope (sustaining motivation and supporting expectations of an individually fulfilled life), agency (recovering a sense of personal control) and opportunity (using circumstances to gain favourable ends). Further recovery principles are shown in Box 3.4. Recovery also involves self-management and self-determination.

1   Hope is a central aspect of recovery and some would say that recovery is impossible without hope. Essentially this seems to mean that if you cannot see the possibility of a decent future for yourself, then what is the point in trying? Relationships are important to hope, as it is difficult to believe in yourself if everyone around you thinks you will never amount to very much, and when you find it hard to believe in yourself, you need others to believe in you.

2   Agency, in the sense used here, is concerned with who is in control and refers to service users taking control over their own problems, their life and their future. It means taking control over such matters as the way they understand what has happened to them, their problems and the help they receive, what they do in their lives and their dreams and ambitions.

3   Opportunity, the third concept, links us with the concept of social inclusion or participation in a wider society. Social inclusion is important for recovery as people with mental health problems and learning disabilities wish to be part of our communities, to be their valued members, to have access to the opportunities that exist within them, and to have the opportunity to contribute.

Recovery is not a new term, rather it is an idea whose time has come (Shepherd *et al*, 2008). Some of the ideas of recovery date back to the 18th century and 'moral treatment'. There are parallels with the therapeutic communities of the 1950s and 1960s. A more recent impetus came from the consumer and survivor movements of the 1980s and 1990s, which themselves grew from the civil rights movements of the 1960s and 1970s and were based on self-help, empowerment and advocacy. Despite their

Box 3.4   Principles of recovery

- Recovery is about building a meaningful and satisfying life, as defined by the person themselves, whether or not there are ongoing or recurring symptoms or problems.
- Recovery represents a movement away from pathology, illness and symptoms to health, strengths and wellness.
- Hope is central to recovery and can be enhanced by each person seeing how they can have more active control over their lives ('agency') and by seeing how others have found a way forward.
- Self-management is encouraged and facilitated. The processes of self-management are similar, but what works may be very different for each individual. No 'one size fits all'.
- The helping relationship between clinicians and patients moves away from being expert/patient to being 'coaches' or 'partners' on a journey of discovery. Clinicians are there to be 'on tap, not on top'.
- People do not recover in isolation. Recovery is closely associated with social inclusion and being able to take on meaningful and satisfying social roles within local communities, rather than in segregated services.
- Recovery is about discovering – or re-discovering – a sense of personal identity, separate from illness or disability.
- The language used and the stories and meanings that are constructed have great significance as mediators of the recovery process. These shared meanings either support a sense of hope and possibility, or invite pessimism and chronicity.
- The development of recovery-based services emphasises the personal qualities of staff as much as their formal qualifications. It seeks to cultivate their capacity for hope, creativity, care, compassion, realism and resilience.
- Family and other supporters are often crucial to recovery and they should be included as partners wherever possible. For many people peer support is central in their recovery.

Source: Shepherd *et al* (2008). Adapted from *Recovery: Concepts and Application*, by Laurie Davidson, the Devon Recovery Group.

long history, the ideas of recovery are especially pertinent at the turn of the 21st century when in England the asylums are closed, most mental health services are provided in a community setting and there is an ever-strengthening service user movement which has developed a more confident voice.

Although these concepts have been largely formulated by, and for, service users to describe their own life experiences, for recovery to have the impact that it deserves, professionals need to understand what it means and, together with service users and others, actively support its implementation across services. This will require changing the way in which professionals work, adapting the structure of mental health services and the culture of these services to be recovery-oriented.

In mental health services, recovery ideas have received most attention in relation to working-age adults, but can be applied to anyone who experiences a significant mental health problem at any age. They can be applied in specialist areas such as forensic mental health services, brain disorders and drug and alcohol services (indeed some of them are embedded in the approach of Alcoholics Anonymous). There are also strong connections to rehabilitation services – recovery offers a new conceptual framework for rehabilitation practice (Roberts *et al*, 2006). In physical health services, recovery ideas can be applied to any long-term health problem and the management of these conditions now relies on the provision of information and self-management in addition to treatment and symptom control.

Recovery provides a new rationale for mental health services and has radical implications for the design and operation of mental health services. The concepts of recovery have already been taken up by policy initiatives in several countries: New Zealand (Mental Health Commission, 1998), Australia (Australian Government, 2003), the USA (Department of Health and Human Services, 2003), Ireland (Mental Health Commission, 2005), Scotland (Scotland Government, 2006). In England these ideas are supported by Department of Health policies that promote self-management and choice (Department of Health, 2001*b*,2006*a*,2007). In the UK, the representative bodies of all the main mental health professionals have given support to the ideas of recovery: the Royal College of Psychiatrists, in the position paper *A Common Purpose* (Royal College of Psychiatrists *et al*, 2007); nurses, in a review *From Values to Action* (Department of Health, 2006*b*); occupational therapists, in *Recovering Ordinary Lives* (College of Occupational Therapists, 2006); and clinical psychologists, in *Recent Advances in Understanding Mental Illness and Psychotic Experiences* (British Psychological Society Division of Clinical Psychology, 2000).

From a practice and service perspective, a recovery-oriented approach provides an important way for mental health professionals and mental health services to contribute to combating the social exclusion experienced by people with mental illness. Recovery ideas and recovery-oriented practice have the potential to radically transform mental health services and to alter traditional power relationships. In later chapters we consider how the recovery approach can be put into practice and what services need to do to make it happen. Although most of the ideas of recovery have been developed in the context of general adult and rehabilitation services, there is no reason why they could not be integrated into the subspecialty services, and it is important that these ideas are adapted to these services using the often already established principles of these subspecialties.

Recovery has implications for the organisation of mental health services and the approaches adopted by those who work in them (Shepherd *et al*, 2008). Recovery is about a person's own personal coming to terms with their illness, their reaction and adaptation to it. Recovery-oriented services have an important role to play in instilling and holding hope for that person who is trying to come to terms with the potentially devastating consequences of a diagnosis of a severe and enduring mental health problem. The content of recovery is therefore different for different people, but recovery-oriented practice should have common, shared concepts and an overarching ethos which can support an individual (and their family) through the often slow or even lifelong process of recovery.

Recovery and social inclusion

Opportunity and optimism are key ingredients for both social inclusion and recovery. There is a creative synthesis between these two approaches: recovery both requires and allows social inclusion and social inclusion helps to promote recovery. Both are key concepts for modern consultant and other clinician roles and for modern psychiatric practice.

Recovery-oriented practice should promote social inclusion and challenge marginalisation and stigmatising views/behaviours within our own services and in wider society. Many of the 'markers of recovery' are, in reality, markers of social inclusion: working, studying and participating in leisure activities in mainstream settings; good family relationships; living independently; having control of one's self-care, medication and money; having a social life; taking part in the local community; and satisfaction with life (Liberman & Kopelowicz, 2002). In promoting social inclusion, clinicians will also be promoting opportunities for their patients to achieve their full potential as they recover, and, in so doing, the service will be embracing some of the core components of recovery-oriented practice.

The development of recovery ideas provides a means of changing professional practice, as it requires a different relationship between service user and professional. But this also necessitates a modification of the way mental health services are organised, emphasising more the objectives of housing, employment, education and participation in mainstream community and leisure activities, and the role the services themselves play in identifying and driving developments in these key domains.

Conclusion

Several concepts related to social exclusion relevant to people with mental health problems and those with learning disability have been outlined in this chapter. These highlight the political and civil nature of exclusion (citizenship, equality and human rights, choice); the importance of material (poverty and deprivation), social (social capital, stigma and discrimination) and individual factors (participation, choice and agency); and a means of identifying and describing causal factors for social exclusion (agency and process, dynamic dimensions, multifactorial causes, life course and longitudinal perspectives). The additional concept, or more accurately set of concepts, of recovery do not fit into the conventional social exclusion literature, but do provide the bridge between the literature on social exclusion and that on mental health problems. Importantly, the concepts of recovery spring from a literature dominated by accounts of the service users' and help to emphasise the importance of examining both objective and subjective aspects of exclusion. The concepts highlighted here also reflect a set of values that are important to consider in relation to psychiatry and mental health services.

Summary

Several central and associated concepts of social exclusion are of key importance to people with mental health problems and learning disabilities, including participation, citizenship, equality and human rights, stigma and discrimination.

The recovery approach, although not traditionally part of the social exclusion literature, plays an important part in promoting inclusion and participation for people with mental health problems and learning disabilities.

References

Andresen, R., Oades, L. & Caputi, P. (2003) The experience of recovery from schizophrenia: towards an empirically validated stage model. *Australian and New Zealand Journal of Psychiatry*, **37**, 586–594.

Anthony, W. A. (1993) Recovery from mental illness: the guiding vision of the mental health service system in the 1990s. *Psychosocial Rehabilitation Journal*, **16**, 11–23.

Australian Government (2003) *Australian Health Minister's National Mental Health Plan 2003–2008*. Australian Government.

Bandura, A. (1997) *Self-Efficacy in Changing Societies*. Cambridge University Press.

Bandura, A. (2000) Exercise of human agency through cognitive efficacy. *Current Directions in Psychological Science*, **9**, 75–78.

Barnes, C. (2000) A working social model? Disability, work and disability politics in the 21st century. *Critical Social Policy*, **20**, 441–457.

Barnes, M., Harrison, S., Mort, M., *et al* (1999) *Unequal Partners: User Groups and Community Care*. Polity Press.

Berman, Y. & Phillips, D. (2000) Indicators of social quality and social exclusion at national and community level. *Social Indicators Research*, **50**, 329–350.

Blaxter, M. (1980) *The Meaning of Disability*. Heinemann.

Boardman, J. (2003) Work, employment and psychiatric disability. *Advances in Psychiatric Treatment*, **9**, 327–334.

British Psychological Society Division of Clinical Psychology (2000) *Recent Advances in Understanding Mental Illness and Psychotic Experiences*. British Psychological Society.

Burchardt, T. (2006) *Foundations for Measuring Equality (A Discussion Paper for the Equalities Review)*. ESRC Research Centre for Analysis of Social Exclusion, London School of Economics.

Burchardt, T. & Vizard, P. (2007) *Definition of Equality and Framework for Measurement. Final Recommendations of the Equalities Review Steering Group on Measurement. Paper 1*. The Equalities Review.

Burchardt, T., Le Grand, J. & Piachaud, D. (2002a) Introduction. In *Understanding Social Exclusion* (eds J. Hills, J. Le Grand & D. Piachaud). Oxford University Press.

Burchardt, T., Le Grand, J. & Piachaud, D. (2002b) Degrees of exclusion: developing a dynamic, multidimensional measure. In *Understanding Social Exclusion* (eds J. Hills, J. Le Grand & D. Piachaud). Oxford University Press.

Butler, R. & Bowlby, S. (1997) Bodies and spaces: an exploration of disabled people's experiences of public space. *Environment and Planning D: Society and Space*, **15**, 379–504.

Bynner, J., Ferri, E. & Shepherd, P. (1997) *Twenty-Something in the 90s: Getting on, Getting by, Getting Nowhere*. Dartmouth Press.

Care Services Improvement Partnership (2005) *Our Choices in Mental Health*. CSIP.

Casey, B. & Yamada, A. (2002) The Public–Private Mix of Retirement Income in Nine OECD Countries: Some Evidence from Micro Data and an Exploration of its Implications. In *Rethinking the Welfare State: The Political Economy of Pension Reform* (eds M. Rein & W. Schmähl), pp. 395–411. Edward Elgar.

Centre for Longitudinal Studies (2008) *Now We are 50: Key Findings from the National Child Development Study*. Centre for Longitudinal Studies.

Chamberlain, G., Philipp, E., Howlett, B. C., et al (1978) British Births 1970. *Vol. 2: Obstetric Care*. Heinemann Medical Books.

Chamberlain, R., Chamberlain, G., Howlett, B. C., et al (1975) *British Births 1970. Vol. 1: The First Week of Life*. Heinemann Medical Books.

Chamberlin, J. (2006) Foreword. In *Shunned: Discrimination Against People with Mental Illness* (G. Thornicroft). Oxford University Press.

College of Occupational Therapists (2006) *Recovering Ordinary Lives: The Strategy for Occupational Therapy in Mental Health Services 2007–2017*. College of Occupational Therapists.

Crow, G. (2004) Social networks and social exclusion: an overview of the debate. In *Social Networks and Social Exclusion* (eds C. Phillipson, G. Allan & D. Morgan). Ashgate.

Crow, G. & Allan, G. (1994) *Community Life*. Harvester Wheatsheaf.

Department of Health (2001a) *Valuing People: A New Strategy for Learning Disability for the 21st Century – Long Report* (White Paper). HMSO.

Department of Health (2001b) *The Expert Patient*. Department of Health.

Department of Health (2003) *Developing Choice, Responsiveness and Equity in Health and Social Care: A National Consultation Exercise*. Department of Health.

Department of Health (2004) *Better Information, Better Choices, Better Health: Putting Information at the Centre of Health*. Department of Health.

Department of Health (2006a) *Our Health, Our Care, Our Say*. Department of Health.

Department of Health (2006b) *From Values to Action: The Chief Nursing Officer's Review of Mental Health Nursing*. Department of Health.

Department of Health (2007) *Commissioning Framework for Health and Well-Being*. Department of Health.

Department of Health and Human Services (2003) *Achieving the Promise: Transforming Mental Health Care in America*. President's New Freedom Commission on Mental Health, pub no. SMA–03–3832. Department of Health and Human Services.

Dex, S. & Joshi, H. (2005) *Children of the 21st Century: From Birth to Nine Months*. Polity Press.

Disability Rights Commission (2006) *Equal Treatment: Closing the Gap. A Formal Investigation into Physical Health Inequalities Experienced by People with Learning Disabilities and/or Mental Health Problems*. Disability Rights Commission.

Douglas, J. W. B. (1964) *The Home and the School*. MacGibbon and Kee.

Elder, G. H. (1974) *Children of the Great Depression: Social Change in Life Experience*. University of Chicago Press.

Elder, G. H. & Johnson, M. (2003) The life course and aging: challenges, lessons and new directions. In *Invitation to the Life Course: Toward New Understandings of Later Life* (ed. R. A. Settersten Jr), pp. 49–81. Baywood Publishing.

Equalities Review (2007) *Fairness and Freedom: The Final Report of the Equalities Review*. The Equalities Review (http://archive.cabinetoffice.gov.uk/equalitiesreview/publications. html).

French, S. (1993) Disability, impairment or something in between? In *Disabling Barriers – Enabling Environments* (eds J. Swain, V. Finkelstein & M. Oliver). Sage.

Giddens, A. (1991) *Modernity and Self-Identity*. Polity Press.

Gilleard, C. & Higgs, P. (2002) *Cultures of Ageing: Self, Citizen and the Body*. Prentice-Hall.

Gordon, D., Levitas, R., Pantazis, C., *et al* (2000) *Poverty and Social Exclusion in Britain.* Joseph Rowntree Foundation.

Harrison, G., Hopper, K., Craig, T., *et al* (2001) Recovery from psychotic illness: a 15- and 25-year international follow-up study. *British Journal of Psychiatry*, **178**, 506–517.

Huxley, P. & Thornicroft, G. (2003) Social inclusion, social quality and mental illness. *British Journal of Psychiatry*, **182**, 289–290.

Le Grand, J. (2003) *Choice and Social Exclusion (Case Paper 75).* ESRC Research Centre for Analysis of Social Exclusion, London School of Economics.

Levitas, R. (2005) *The Inclusive Society and New Labour (2nd edn).* Palgrave Macmillan.

Liberman, R. P. & Kopelowicz, A. (2002) Recovery from schizophrenia: a challenge for the 21st century. *International Review of Psychiatry*, **14**, 245–255.

Martin, J. & White, A. (1988) *OPCS Surveys of Disability in Great Britain, Report 2: The Financial Circumstances of Disabled Adults Living in Private Households.* HMSO.

McMillan, D. & Charvis, D. (1986) Sense of community: a definition and theory. *Journal of Community Psychology*, **14**, 6–23.

Mencap (2004) *Treat Me Right! Better Healthcare for People with Learning Disability.* Mencap.

Mencap (2007) *Death by Indifference: Following up the Treat Me Right! Report.* Mencap.

Mental Health Commission (1998) *Blueprint for Mental Health Services in New Zealand.* Mental Health Commission.

Mental Health Commission (2005) *A Vision for a Recovery Model in Irish Mental Health Services.* Mental Health Commission.

Morgan, C., Burns, T., Fitzpatrick, R., *et al* (2007) Social exclusion and mental health: conceptual and methodological review. *British Journal of Psychiatry*, **191**, 477–483.

Mulvany J. (2000) Disability, impairment or illness? The relevance of the social model of disability to the study of mental disorder. *Sociology of Health and Illness*, **22**, 582–601.

Neugarten, B. & Neugarten, D. (1986) Changing meanings of age in the aging society. In *Our Ageing Society: Paradox and Promise* (eds A. Pifer & L. Bronte), pp. 33–52. Norton.

O'Brien, J. (1989) *What's worth working for? Leadership for better quality human services.* Responsive Systems Associates.

Oliver, M. (1983) *Social Work and Disabled People.* Macmillan.

Oliver, M. (1990) *The Politics of Disablement.* Macmillan.

Oliver, M. (1996) *Understanding Disability: From Theory to Practice.* Palgrave Macmillan.

Osborn, A. F., Butler, N. R. & Power, C. (1984) *The Social Life of Britain's Five-Year-Olds: A Report of the Child Health and Education Study.* Routledge and Kegan Paul.

Passuth, P. & Bengtson, V. L. (1988) Sociological theories of aging: current perspectives and future directions. In *Emergent Theories of Aging* (eds J. E. Birren & V. L. Bengtson), pp. 333–355. Springer.

Perkins, R. & Repper, J. (1998) *Dilemmas in Community Mental Health Practice: Choice or Control?* Radcliffe.

Phillipson, C. (2002) *Transitions from Work to Retirement: Developing a New Social Contract.* Policy Press.

Phillipson, C., Allan, G. & Morgan, D. (2004) *Social Networks and Social Exclusion.* Ashgate

Price, D. & Ginn, J. (2003) Sharing the crust: gender, partnership, status and inequalities in pension accumulation. In *Gender and Ageing* (eds S. Arber, K. Davidson & J. Ginn), pp. 127–146. Open University Press.

Putnam, R. D. (1993) The prosperous community: social capital and public life. *The American Prospect*, **13**, 35–42.

Putnam, R. F. (2000) *Bowling Alone: The Collapse and Revival of American Community.* Simon & Schuster.

Rankin, J. (2005) *Mental Health in the Mainstream: A Good Choice for Mental Health (Working Paper 3).* Institute for Public Policy Research.

Repper, J. & Perkins, R. (2003) *Social Inclusion and Recovery: A Model for Mental Health Practice.* Ballière Tindall.

Riley, M. W. & Riley, J. W. Jr. (1994) Structural lag. In *Age and Structural Lag* (eds M. W. Riley, R. L. Kahn & A. and Foner), pp. 15–36. Wiley.

Roberts, G. & Wolfson, P. (2004) The rediscovery of recovery: open to all. *Advances in Psychiatric Treatment*, **10**, 37–49.

Roberts, G., Davenport, S., Holloway, F., *et al* (2006) *Enabling Recovery: The Principles and Practice of Rehabilitation Psychiatry*. Gaskell.

Royal College of Psychiatrists, Social Care Institute for Excellence & Care Services Improvement Partnership (2007) *A Common Purpose: Recovery in Future Mental Health Services*. Social Care Institute for Excellence.

Samele, C., Lawton-Smith, S., Warner, L., *et al* (2007) Patient choice in psychiatry. *British Journal of Psychiatry*, **191**, 1–2.

Sainsbury Centre for Mental Health (2006) *Choice in Mental Health Care (Briefing Paper 31)*. Sainsbury Centre for Mental Health.

Sainsbury Centre for Mental Health (2009) *Childhood Mental Health and Life Chances in Post-War Britain: Insights from Three National Birth Cohort Studies (Executive Summary)*. Sainsbury Centre for Mental Health.

Scharf, T., Phillipson, C., Smith, A. E., *et al* (2002) *Growing Older in Socially Deprived Areas: Social Exclusion in Later Life*. Help the Aged.

Scharf, T., Phillipson, C. & Smith, A. E. (2005) Social exclusion of older people in deprived urban communities of England. *European Journal of Ageing*, **2**, 76–87.

Schwartz, B. (2004) *The Paradox of Choice: Why More is Less*. HarperCollins.

Scotland Government (2006) *Rights, Relationships and Recovery: the Report of the National Review of Mental Health Nursing in Scotland*. Scotland Government (http://www.scotland.gov.uk/Publications/2006/04/18164814/0).

Sen, A. K. (1992) *Inequality Re-Examined*. Clarendon Press.

Settersten, R. A. Jr (ed) (2003) *Invitation to the Life Course: Toward New Understandings of Later Life*. Baywood Press.

Shepherd, G., Boardman, J. & Slade, M. (2008) *Making Recovery a Reality*. Sainsbury Centre for Mental Health.

Slade, M. (2009) *Personal Recovery and Mental Illness*. Cambridge University Press.

Smith, N. & Middleton, S. (2007) *A Review of Poverty Dynamics Research in the UK*. Joseph Rowntree Foundation.

Social Exclusion Unit (2000) *Minority Ethnic Issues in Social Exclusion and Neighbourhood Renewal*. Cabinet Office.

Thornicroft, G. (2006) *Shunned: Discrimination Against People with Mental Illness*. Oxford University Press.

Trieman, N. & Leff, J. (2002) Long-term outcome of long-stay psychiatric in-patients considered unsuitable to live in the community: TAPS Project 44. *British Journal of Psychiatry*, **181**, 428–432.

Uhlenberg, P. & De Jong, G. J. (2004) Age segregation in later life: an examination of personal networks. *Ageing and Society*, **24**, 5–28.

Vizard, P. & Burchardt, T. (2007) *Developing a Capability List: Final Recommendations of the Equalities Review Steering Group on Measurement, Paper 2*. The Equalities Review.

Wadsworth, M. (1991) *The Imprint of Time*. Clarendon Press.

Walker, A. (ed) (1996) *The New Generational Contract*. UCL Press.

Wilkinson, R. (2005) *The Impact of Inequality: How to Make Sick Societies Healthier*. The New Press.

Williams, G. H. (1991) Disablement and the ideological crisis in health care. *Social Science and Medicine*, **33**, 517–524.

CHAPTER 4

Policy and social exclusion

Jed Boardman

Over the past 20 years there has been a considerable increase in UK government policy initiatives in the area of mental health, as witnessed by the number of official documents produced on mental health policy (Boardman, 2005). It is not the intention in this chapter to review mental health policy, but to give an overview of aspects of health policy that relate to social inclusion and recovery. However, as shown in the previous chapter, the components of social exclusion go beyond those traditionally dealt with by health services and cover several different government departments, such as those that deal with justice, employment, housing and education. It is therefore inevitable that we should examine cross-cutting aspects of policy and some of the policy initiatives since 1997, when the Labour government was elected, that have focused on social exclusion and poverty reduction. The focus of the chapter is on policy in the UK, but some European policy is relevant and therefore included.

Equality and rights

Human rights

Before 1997 there was no codified human rights in UK domestic law, although the UK had ratified the European Convention on Human Rights (ECHR) in 1951, which meant it was bound by international law to observe the ECHR and was accountable for violations. The European Court of Human Rights in Strasbourg had been set up to consider cases brought by people who claim that their rights under the Convention have been broken or breached and consequently may rule that the British government has breached the Convention.

Equality and human rights were part of the Labour election manifesto in 1997. The Human Rights Act 1998, which came into force in October 2000, gave UK citizens certain basic human rights which government and public authorities are legally obliged to respect (Box 4.1). It gives legal effect in the UK to 15 of the fundamental civil and political rights and freedoms contained in the ECHR (sometimes referred to as the Convention),

Box 4.1   Fundamental rights and freedoms from the European Convention on Human Rights which are protected by the Human Rights Act 1998

Article 2: Right to life

Article 3: Prohibition on torture

Article 4: Prohibition on slavery and forced labour

Article 5: Right to liberty and security

Article 6: Right to a fair trial

Article 7: No punishment without law

Article 8: Right to respect for private and family life

Article 9: Freedom of thought, conscience and religion

Article 10: Right to freedom of expression

Article 11: Freedom of assembly and association

Article 12: Right to marry and found a family

Article 14: Prohibition on discrimination

Article 1 of the First Protocol: Protection of property

Article 2 of the First Protocol: Right to education

Article 3 of the First Protocol: Right to free elections

originally written in 1950. The rights granted by the Human Rights Act are often referred to as 'Convention rights'. This means that the Convention rights can be enforced in UK courts, which can make judicial declarations of incompatibility.

Importantly, the Human Rights Act 1998 says that public authorities must respect people's Convention rights and that it is unlawful for them to act in a way that is 'incompatible with a convention right'. Public authorities include government departments, the police, local councils, the prison service, education, health and Social Services. It is possible for some organisations to be considered public authorities at some times but not at others. For example, a security company is a public authority when it is working for the prison service but not when it is doing private security work.

The rights in the ECHR are set out as separate articles, but since the Convention was written new protocols have been added, introducing new rights to the ECHR or dealing with procedure (Council of Europe, 2003). The articles or protocols of the Human Rights Act are like a series of principles. Not all of the rights set out in the ECHR and its protocols are incorporated into British law by the Human Rights Act 1998 (Box

4.1), which includes the rights in Articles 2 to 12 and Article 14 of the ECHR, plus those in the First Protocol. Article 1 of the Convention is the 'Obligation to respect human rights'. Article 13 is the 'Right to an effective remedy', which provides that people whose rights under the Convention have been breached should have the right to effective redress. This was not included in the Human Rights Act 1998 as it was thought that the Act itself would meet the requirements of the article by giving people the right to take proceedings in the British courts if they considered that their Convention rights had been breached.

There are three different categories of Convention rights: absolute rights, qualified rights, and limited rights. Absolute rights cannot be infringed under any circumstances, for example Article 3, 'Prohibition of torture' (Curtice, 2008). Qualified rights are rights that the state can lawfully interfere with in certain circumstances. Generally in such articles, the right is set out at the start and then qualified by certain criteria, such as: whether the interference is in accordance with the law; whether it is in pursuit of a legitimate aim; and whether it is necessary in a democratic society. Examples of this are Article 8, 'The right to respect for your private life' (Curtice, 2009), and Article 10, 'The right to freedom of expression'. Limited rights are those where the circumstances of the right can be limited and the limitations are set out in the text of the article itself. Article 5, 'Right to liberty and security', is a limited right.

The Human Rights Act 1998 covers civil and political rights and one socioeconomic right under Protocol 1, but does not include broader rights, such as children's rights, and key economic and social rights, such as a right to health (Vizard, 2009). For example, the United Nations Convention on Rights of the Child is not incorporated into domestic law. However, the UK Ministry of Justice has consulted on a British Statement of Values and Bill of Rights which may include codification of these broader rights in the future (Ministry of Justice, 2007; Vizard, 2009).

For people with disabilities, the Convention on the Rights of Persons with Disabilities and its Optional Protocol were adopted by the United Nations General Assembly in December 2006 (www.un.org/disabilities/convention/conventionfull.shtml). Article 1 states that the purpose of the convention is to 'promote, protect and ensure the full and equal enjoyment of all human rights and fundamental freedoms by all persons with disabilities, and to promote respect for their inherent dignity.'

The Convention regards people with disabilities to include 'those who have long-term physical, mental, intellectual or sensory impairments which in interaction with various barriers may hinder their full and effective participation in society on an equal basis with others'.

Equality and Human Rights Commission

In October 2007, the Equality and Human Rights Commission (EHRC), established by the Equality Act 2006, came into existence (see Chapter 3). It covers England, Scotland and Wales, with statutory committees responsible for the work of the EHRC in Scotland and Wales.

The EHRC has taken on all of the powers of the previous commissions as well as new powers to enforce legislation more effectively and promote equality for all. The government is committed to single equality legislation, designed to bring coherence to equalities legislation. This is likely to mean the EHRC will in time be tasked with promoting positive equalities duties covering all six strands (gender, race, disability, sexual orientation, age and religion/belief). The EHRC is also tasked with promoting human rights, which could encompass issues such as rights to dignity, privacy and family life, for example in health and social care facilities. It will also promote awareness and understanding of human rights and encourage good practice by public authorities in meeting their Human Rights Act obligations. Finally, the EHRC aims to promote good relations between groups and communities. Although this has been largely discussed in relation to ethnic and faith communities, it might be applied, for example, to countering NIMBY (not in my back yard) campaigns.

In 2008 the government announced its plans for the Equality Bill (HM Government, 2008) and published the Bill the following year (Government Equalities Office, 2009). The Bill completed its passage through Parliament in April 2010, becoming the Equality Act 2010. The Bill brings together in one piece of legislation the different strands of equality law, such as the Equal Pay Act 1970, the Sex Discrimination Act 1975 and the Disability Discrimination Act 1995. It introduces a new single Equality Duty requiring public bodies to consider the needs of diverse groups including those related to gender, race, disability, sexual orientation, belief and age.

Disability rights

Anti-discrimination law has underpinned citizenship for disabled people in Britain, including people with psychiatric conditions, since 1995, when the Disability Discrimination Act was introduced. Before the Act there was no law to prevent discrimination, but the Disabled Persons (Employment) Act did allow for some positive discrimination for disabled workers in the form of a quota system. The Disability Discrimination Act was amended in 2001 and 2005. It is an important piece of legislation that has demonstrated its potential to protect the rights of disabled people in employment, education and access to goods and services (Sayce & Boardman, 2008). It covers direct forms of discrimination, where there is less favourable treatment because of a person's disability. More recently coverage has been extended to transport and public functions (for example, decisions on planning permission).

The Act provides for people with a physical or mental impairment that has a substantial and long-term adverse effect on a person's ability to carry out normal day-to-day activities. The Act has been important in providing individual redress in cases of discrimination and in setting a framework for good practice on the part of employers, educationalists and service providers.

It can also stimulate more systemic change: through formal investigations of organisations or whole sectors; and through the Disability Equality Duty, in force since December 2006, which requires public sector organisations to proactively promote equality rather than responding to discrimination after the event. The Disability Discrimination Act has implications for people working in mental health and learning disability services when they are considering employment and educational opportunities for service users and how to redress systemic disadvantage, including inequalities in physical health (Sayce, 2000; Sayce & Boardman, 2003, 2008). The Act assumes a predominantly individual model of disability (Barnes, 2000) and does not necessarily tolerate differences between groups or individuals (Fredman, 2005). Wheat (2007: p. 201) argues for an approach 'that treats disabled people as non-disabled people should be treated: as unique individuals'.

The Disability Discrimination Act is now incorporated into the Equality Act 2010. The Act has new rules to discourage employers from asking job applicants disability-related questions.

Social exclusion

When the Labour government came to power in 1997, levels of poverty and inequality were higher than at any time since 1945. They had no intention of going back to the previous Labour commitments of tax and spend, and, from 1997, the Labour government set out a social policy programme to tackle poverty and social exclusion that covered a range of areas from child poverty, older people, ethnic minorities, employment, education, health, and neighbourhoods (Hills & Stewart, 2005; Joseph Rowntree Foundation, 2005; Hills et al, 2009). However, the government did not formally define social exclusion; their concern seemed to be with multiple deprivation (Stewart et al, 2009).

Before the 1997 election it was not clear what New Labour's intention was in relation to poverty and disadvantage, but an early speech by the Prime Minister at a Peckham housing estate in June 1997 indicated that these matters were part of the government's policy programme (Toynbee & Walker, 2001; Stewart et al, 2009). Soon after this the Social Exclusion Unit was established (see below). In 1999, Opportunity for All (Department of Social Security, 1999) was published, setting out the range of problems that were associated with poverty and social exclusion (Box 4.2), all of which are of relevance to people with mental health problems and learning disability. The report set out four policy priorities as a response to these problems. They were to tackle childhood deprivation, promote employment, alleviate the plight of pensioners and pursue area-based solutions to exclusion (Department of Social Security, 1999). The report detailed a range of indicators against which they would monitor the progress of the policies. Since 1999 the government has produced an annual Opportunity for All report detailing progress against these indicators. The last set of indicators

> Box 4.2   Key features of the complex multidimensional problems of poverty and social exclusion from *Opportunity for All* (Department of Social Security, 1999)
>
> - lack of opportunities to work
> - lack of opportunities to acquire education and skills
> - childhood deprivation
> - disrupted families
> - barriers to older people living active, fulfilling and healthy lives
> - inequalities in housing
> - poor housing
> - poor neighbourhoods
> - fear of crime
> - disadvantage or discrimination on grounds of age, ethnicity, gender or disability

was published in 2007 (Department for Work and Pensions, 2007*a*). The biannual *National Action Plan on Social Inclusion* (Department for Work and Pensions, 2006*a*), produced to align with agreements reached at the European Union (EU) summits in Lisbon and Nice, summarises the UK government's approach to tackling poverty and social exclusion. Hills *et al* (2009) have produced a comprehensive account of the changes in poverty and inequality since 1997 which summarises the *Opportunity for All* indicators and is discussed further in Chapter 7.

The 1997–2010 Labour government's main strategies to reduce material poverty and improve redistribution were controlled through the Treasury (Sefton *et al*, 2009; Stewart, 2009; Stewart *et al*, 2009). The use of tax credits (e.g. working families' tax credit, children's tax credit) has played a strategic role, as well as the establishing of the national minimum wage. There has been a reliance on employment as a means of escaping poverty (see below) through 'welfare to work' programmes such as the New Deal for Young People and the New Deal for Lone Parents. In addition, the importance of the damaging effects of poverty and disadvantage in childhood on later life opportunities has been reflected in policy initiatives, particularly the setting of targets to reduce child poverty by a quarter by 2004/2005 and by half by 2010 (eradicating it by 2020). Behind these targets seems to lie a vision of the values of a just society of 'equal worth, opportunity for all, responsibility and community' (Blair, 1998, quoted in Stewart *et al*, 2009: p. 10).

Social Exclusion Unit

The Social Exclusion Unit was set up in the Cabinet Office in 1997. In May 2002 the Unit moved to the Office of the Deputy Prime Minister as part of government restructuring. The Unit produced the first ever report on mental health and social exclusion (ODPM, 2004*a*), followed by an action plan on mental health and social exclusion (ODPM, 2004b), which then evolved into the National Social Inclusion Programme run within the National Institute for Mental Health in England (NIMHE). The Social Exclusion Unit produced reports on communities (ODPM, 2005a; ODPM & Department of Health, 2005), young people (ODPM, 2005b), older people (OPDM, 2006) and mental health (OPDM, 2004a,b).

The Unit was closed in 2006 and its work transferred to a smaller Social Exclusion Task Force in the Cabinet Office, which aimed to focus on the most severely excluded, particularly on hard to reach children and families (HM Government, 2006a). They have also run a pilot programme on adults facing chronic exclusion to tackle long-term exclusion among the most marginalised members of society. An interim evaluation in 2009 showed only limited progress of the individuals in the 12 pilots (Cattell *et al*, 2009). More recently the Social Exclusion Task Force and the Department of Health have focused on the primary healthcare needs of people with learning disability as well as homeless people, sex workers and gypsies and travellers (Cabinet Office & Department of Health, 2010; Department of Health, 2010).

Public Service Agreements

In the 1998 Comprehensive Spending Review the government introduced Public Service Agreements, which are the government's top delivery priorities and commitments to improve outcomes. Each Public Service Agreement is a broad-based statement of desired outcomes (for example, no. 25: Reducing the harm caused by alcohol and drugs) and is supported by measurable performance indicators and targets to assess progress, which are subject to regular public reporting and scrutiny. The responsibility for the Agreements cuts across government departments. The form has evolved over time, reducing in number and being increasingly focused on outcomes. In October 2007, 30 new Agreements were introduced in the Comprehensive Spending Review, covering the period 2008–2011 (Box 4.3).

Several of the Agreements shown in Box 4.3 are relevant to social exclusion and to people with mental health problems across all age ranges, but two are particularly pertinent. Agreement no. 16 aims to increase the proportion of socially excluded adults in settled accommodation and employment, education or training, with particular reference to adults in contact with mental health services, adults with moderate to severe learning disabilities, care leavers and offenders. Agreement no. 15 aims to address the disadvantage that individuals experience because of their gender, race, disability, age, sexual orientation, religion or belief in all aspects of their lives, including healthcare provision and employment.

The Agreements have implications for local services as local authorities have to choose the top 35 delivery targets from the Agreements on which to be measured and in each local authority there will be a senior manager

Box 4.3   Public Service Agreements for 2008–2011

Sustainable growth and prosperity

1   Raise the productivity of the UK economy
2   Improve the skills of the population, on the way to ensuring a world-class skills base by 2020
3   Ensure controlled, fair migration that protects the public and contributes to economic growth
4   Promote world-class science and innovation in the UK
5   Deliver reliable and efficient transport networks that support economic growth
6   Deliver the conditions for business success in the UK
7   Improve the economic performance of all English regions and reduce the gap in economic growth rates between regions

Fairness and opportunity for all

8   Maximise employment opportunity for all
9   Halve the number of children in poverty by 2010–11, on the way to eradicating child poverty by 2020
10   Raise the educational achievement of all children and young people
11   Narrow the gap in educational achievement between children from low-income and disadvantaged backgrounds and their peers
12   Improve the health and well-being of children and young people
13   Improve children and young people´s safety
14   Increase the number of children and young people on the path to success
15   Address the disadvantage that individuals experience because of their gender, race, disability, age, sexual orientation, religion or belief
16   Increase the proportion of socially excluded adults in settled accommodation and employment, education or training
17   Tackle poverty and promote greater independence and well-being in later life

Stronger communities and a better quality of life

18   Promote better health and well-being for all
19   Ensure better care for all
20   Increase long-term housing supply and affordability
21   Build more cohesive, empowered and active communities
22   Deliver a successful Olympic Games and Paralympic Games with a sustainable legacy and get more children and young people taking part in high-quality physical education and sport
23   Make communities safer
24   Deliver a more effective, transparent and responsive criminal justice system for victims and the public
25   Reduce the harm caused by alcohol and drugs
26   Reduce the risk to the UK and its interests overseas from international terrorism

A more secure, fair and environmentally sustainable world

27   Lead the global effort to avoid dangerous climate change
28   Secure a healthy natural environment for today and the future
29   Reduce poverty in poorer countries through quicker progress towards the United Nations' Millennium Development Goals
30   Reduce the impact of conflict through enhanced UK and international efforts.

responsible for the health communities and older people section of the Local Area Agreement, the priorities for which are agreed with primary care trust commissioners and NHS providers. There are resources attached to the Public Service Agreement adopted by the local authority and performance is measured against the targets.

Employment and welfare benefits

The view that employment is an effective means of getting out of poverty has figured highly in government policy. Plans to increase employment opportunities and changes to welfare benefits have had particular relevance for people with disabilities. During their time in office, the Labour government had been concerned about the increasing numbers of people receiving incapacity benefit, of which the highest single proportion were people with mental health problems. With the increasing levels of employment seen in the late 1990s, the government aimed to increase the overall employment rate by reducing the number of jobless people (mainly those on incapacity benefit and lone parents) (HM Government, 2005a,b). Several initiatives were undertaken, including restructuring of Jobcentres, a Pathways to Work scheme targeted on those newly placed on incapacity benefit, and reform of the welfare system which includes the replacement of incapacity benefit with a new benefit, Employment Support Allowance and the introduction of work-focused interviews and benefit sanctions (Department for Work and Pensions, 2006a,b, 2007b). The Welfare Reform Act 2007 introduced Employment Support Allowance in 2008 (to replace incapacity benefit and income support based on incapacity or disability) and the work capability assessment (to replace the old personal capability assessment) to assess an individual's entitlement for benefits.

In 2008, a Green Paper (Department for Work and Pensions, 2008a) sought views on the next steps for the government's welfare reform and later that year the government produced its White Paper *Raising Expectations and Increasing Support: Reforming Welfare for the Future* (Department for Work and Pensions, 2008b), which built on two independent reviews: the Freud report (Freud, 2007) and the Gregg review (Gregg, 2008). Although the focus of supporting the jobless back into work may be of benefit to people with mental health problems, there are some possible disadvantages, not least the fact that because of its populist emphasis on the 'work-shy' the new system captures within its remit many people with mental health problems. Importantly, it accepts the introduction of conditions and sanctions (what is often described as 'conditionality') applied to the receiving of Employment Support Allowance, and these will mean that claimants must attend job-focused interviews in order to receive benefits. In addition, the schemes to support people back to work will be offered to a greater range of independent providers. Both these aspects of the Welfare Reform Bill 2009 have implications for people with mental health problems in view of the fluctuating nature of their conditions and the possibility of 'cherry picking' the groups who are easier to work with in a contracted out system of support (Rangarajan *et al*, 2008).

In addition, the Department for Work and Pensions has been concerned with health and well-being at work (HM Government, 2005*b*) and the Department of Health with stigma and discrimination at work (Department of Health, 2006*a*). In 2008 the former published a review of the health of the working age population (Black, 2008), which included a review of mental health and work (Lelliott *et al*, 2008). The following year, the Boorman Report on the health of NHS staff was published (Boorman, 2009).

Among the recommendations of the Black review was the introduction of a new 'fit for work' service which aimed to get people with health conditions back to work (introduced and ongoing until 2011) and a 'fit note' (introduced in April 2010) to replace the old medical 'sick' certificate (Harvey *et al*, 2009).

Following the Black review, in December 2009 the government published its first-ever national mental health and employment strategy, *Working Our Way to Better Mental Health* (Secretaries of State of the Department for Work and Pensions & Department of Health, 2009). The publication of this strategy coincided with two related documents on employment support for people in contact with secondary mental health services: the Perkins review (Perkins *et al*, 2009) and *Work, Recovery and Inclusion* (HM Government, 2009*a*) which set out the government's response to Perkins. The recommendations of the Perkins review included the widespread use of employment specialists and individual placement and support (IPS) schemes (see Chapter 13) in health services, the monitoring of work outcomes as standard in mental health services, and the creation of more effective links between employment, health and social service organisations. The publication of these three employment documents coincided with the launch of New Horizons (Department of Health, 2009*a*) in an attempt to emphasise the need for a cross-government approach to tackling the problems of ill health and work.

The economic downturn has increased the likelihood of rising unemployment in the UK population and the possibility of returning to the high levels of unemployment, particularly long-term unemployment, seen in the 1980s (Barnes *et al*, 2009; Cabinet Office, 2009; HM Government, 2009*b*). These threats may particularly affect younger people. The measures set out in the 2009 White Paper, *Building Britain's Recovery* (HM Government, 2009*c*), aim to help bring down unemployment more quickly than in previous recessions, with measures aimed at supporting young people back to work.

Health and social care

In the second part of the 20th century, overall health and social policies have had to contend with the rising costs of providing health and social services, increasing demands and expectations, and the rising numbers of older people in the population. In recent years, and of relevance to social inclusion, there has been an emphasis on patient choice and participation, self-care and a focus on health inequalities.

In 2003, following public consultation, the government produced a strategy paper *Choice, Responsiveness and Equity*, which was mainly concerned with health records, information services and booking appointments (Secretary of State for Health, 2003). *The NHS Improvement Plan* (Department of Health, 2004a) emphasised the idea of personalised care and set out the priorities for the NHS 2004–2008, supporting the reforms laid out in *The NHS Plan* (Secretary of State for Health, 2000).

The problems of health inequalities were highlighted by the Black report in 1980 (Townsend & Davidson, 1982) and were an early concern for the Labour government. Donald Acheson headed up an independent inquiry into health inequalities (Department of Health, 1998) which confirmed most of what was written in the Black report. The White Paper, *Saving Lives: Our Healthier Nation* (Department of Health, 1999a) and the associated action report (Department of Health, 1999b) set out the policy and strategy. *The NHS Plan* announced national targets for reducing health inequalities which were issued in 2001. In 2003, the government assessed their progress since the Acheson inquiry and set out their programme for tackling health inequalities (Department of Health, 2003a) and achieving national targets for 2010 to reduce the gap in infant mortality across social groups, and raise life expectancy in the most disadvantaged areas. Little seems to have changed and in November 2008 the government announced a strategic review of health inequalities led by Michael Marmot (the Marmot review) to assist in developing the strategic approach after 2010. The completed review, *Fair Society, Healthy Lives* (Marmot, 2010) highlighted the social gradient in health (the lower a person's social position, the worse their health) and the relationship between health and social inequalities. Its recomendations for action focused on early childhood intervention and prevention, employment, the social environment and healthy communities and interventions across the social gradient.

The public health White Paper (Department of Health, 2004b) emphasised the promotion of well-being and the central role of promoting participation, inclusion and employment in achieving this. *The Expert Patient* (Department of Health, 2001a) set out the role of self-care in chronic disease management and is supported by the *National Service Framework for Long-Term Conditions* and other self-care initiatives (Department of Health, 2003b, 2005a,b). Many of these documents support the concepts underlying recovery, as does the Chief Nursing Officer's review of mental health nursing (Department of Health, 2006b).

The social care Green Paper set out plans to give service users more independence, choice and control (Department of Health, 2005c). The White Paper *Our Health, Our Care, Our Say* (Secretary of State for Health, 2006) outlined the key elements of reform in the adult social care system in

England, emphasising partnership between local authorities, the NHS and third sector and private sector agencies. It gave an emphasis to providing local social care and NHS services in the communities where they live and to a person-centred approach to supporting independence with self-directed support and personal budgets. The concordat *Putting People First* was signed by several government departments and local authority and social care organisations in December 2007 (HM Government, 2007).

In 2008, the government published its 5-year *Independent Living Strategy* (Office for Disability Issues, 2008), which emphasised having choice and control over support. The report contained the government's commitment,

> [to] delivering on full and equal citizenship for disabled people and sees independent living as being part of the way we advance this. Independent living enables disabled people to fulfil the roles and responsibilities of citizenship (Executive Summary: p. 1).

The 2010 White Paper, *Building the National Care Service* (HM Government, 2010), set out the government's plans for the reform of the care and support system in England over the 5 years after 2010. This covers care for older people and working-age adults. The emphasis is again on independence and personalised care and support (through a personal budget).

European policy

Policies focusing on social exclusion have been a feature in several European countries (Burchardt *et al*, 2002) and in 1991 the EU set up an observatory on national policies to combat social exclusion, which requests national governments to submit annual reports on how they are tackling exclusion.

The Mental Health Declaration and Mental Health Action Plan for Europe (WHO Europe, 2005) placed emphasis on human rights, provisions to tackle stigma, discrimination and inequity, and the promotion of inclusion of people with mental illness, and recognised that mental health is fundamental to the quality of life and the productivity of individuals, families, communities and nations. The EU was asked for support to take this forward. The publication of the EU Green Paper (European Commission, 2005) was the first step in the EU's response, followed by an analysis of national reports from EU states on the promotion of social inclusion (Mental Health Europe, 2008).

The House of Lords European Union Committee (2007) urged a wider public recognition of the 'considerable body of evidence which indicates the substantial social and economic impact of mental health problems' and the role of the EU in facilitating exchange of information and best practice.

The EU disability strategy recognises that there are 44.6 million people in the EU aged between 16 and 64 who report a long-standing health problem or disability. There are four pillars to the strategy: EU anti-discrimination legislation, the mainstreaming of disability issues, accessibility and dialogue with relevant stakeholders ('nothing about people with disabilities without people with disabilities').

Mental health policy

The publication of the *National Service Framework for Mental Health* (Department of Health, 1999c) set out for the first time a set of officially sanctioned minimum standards which mental health services were expected to attain. Standard 1 outlines those relating to mental health promotion, discrimination and exclusion. Some of the subsequent policy implementation guides were focused on services for women, ethnic minorities and support, time and recovery workers (Department of Health, 2002a, 2003c,d, 2004c). The National Institute for Mental Health in England was established to implement the framework; it was later subsumed into the Care Services Improvement Partnership (CSIP), but was wound up in April 2009 as the lifespan of the framework was coming to a close.

The social exclusion of people with mental health problems has featured in policy documents of several government departments, including the Office of the Deputy Prime Minister Social Exclusion Unit's report on mental health and social exclusion (OPDM, 2004a). The recommendations of the Social Exclusion Unit have been taken up by the National Social Inclusion Programme (part of NIMHE) for implementation. In addition, the Department of Health has published guidelines on day services and vocational services (Department of Health, 2006c,d; Department of Health & Department for Work and Pensions, 2006). Specific groups have been given particular attention, including Black and ethnic minorities (Department of Health, 2003e, 2005d), prisoners (Department of Health & HM Prison Services, 2001), people with personality disorders (NIMHE, 2003), women (Department of Health, 2002a, 2003d, 2006d) and carers (Department of Health, 2002b). There have also been programmes on improving access to psychological therapies (Department of Health, 2008), patient and public involvement (CSIP, 2006), direct payments (Department of Health, 2006e; National Mental Health Development Unit, 2010), mental health promotion (Department of Health, 2001b, 2006f), and stigma (NIMHE, 2004; www.seemescotland.org.uk).

The Mental Health Act has been a controversial area for reform, with the government's original plans for a new Mental Health Act (Department of Health, 2004d) being abandoned in favour of amending the 1983 Act (Department of Health, 2006g).

The *National Framework for Mental Health* (Department of Health, 1999c) ran its course by 2010 and at the end of 2009 the government published its future intentions in New Horizons (HM Government, 2009a). This vision for mental health policy for working-age adults aimed to be cross-cutting and for the first time set out plans for a public mental health policy aimed at improving the mental health and well-being of the population. Its twin aim was to improve the quality and accessibility of mental health services. The document set out guiding principles, which included equality and justice, and emphasised the importance of prevention, early intervention and tackling stigma. It highlighted Recovery as central to improving mental health services.

Policy and older people

Opportunity Age (Department for Work and Pensions, 2005) is the government's overarching strategy for an ageing society. The annual *Opportunity for All* reports (e.g. Department for Work and Pensions, 2007a) chart progress in meeting targets aimed at reducing poverty and exclusion. The *Opportunity for All* indicators relating to older people highlight what government regards as priority areas in relation to later life, which include tackling low income, healthy life expectancy, being helped to live independently, improving housing and reducing fear of crime.

Opportunity Age aims to end the perception of older people as dependent, ensure that a longer life is healthy and fulfilling, and that older people can participate fully in society. The priority areas for action are: first, to achieve higher employment rates overall and greater flexibility for over 50-year-olds in continuing careers, to manage any health conditions and to combine work with family and other commitments; second, to enable older people to play a full and active role in society, with an adequate income and decent housing; and third, to allow people to keep their independence and control over their lives as they grow older, even if constrained by associated health problems. Progress in meeting these aims, all of which can be regarded as preventative and having a bearing on mental health, has been monitored by a range of indicators. However, progress in tackling the problems of some of the most disadvantaged older people, including those with mental health conditions, appears slow (OPDM, 2004c).

Opportunity Age refers specifically to the need 'to continue to strengthen services for old age conditions, including giving priority to tackling mental health problems in older people' (p. 56). Two specific examples of progress in this area are identified: a substantial increase in the numbers of consultants in old age psychiatry and medicine (since 1991), and progress in the early detection of treatable illnesses through the single assessment process. However, *Opportunity Age* acknowledges that more needs to be done in relation to improving coordination between health and local authorities; anticipating and preventing ill health; building capacity to deliver more responsive, timely services; improving mental health services; and better managing complex and long-term conditions (p. 56).

The need to improve mental health services was also identified in a wide-ranging review of the impact of government policies aimed at reducing social exclusion among older people (Phillipson & Scharf 2004: p. 64).

Reporting on Social Service Inspectorate inspections over 2002–2003, Bainbridge & Ricketts (2003) identified several common problems in relation to mental health services for older people. They noted that the mental health needs of Black and minority ethnic elders were often unmet, particularly for intensive services. There was also a lack of strategic grasp, practical planning and shortfalls in the availability of services, sometimes resulting in placements or provision that did not meet the needs of older people. Indeed, institutional options were often seen as the mainstay of provision, older people's mental health services were usually unable to access intermediate care, some areas with community mental health teams lacked provider services and there was little focus on the needs of older people with functional mental health needs.

The Social Exclusion Unit's *Sure Start to Later Life* report (OPDM, 2006) takes *Opportunity Age* a stage further in its focus on preventing negative outcomes for some of Britain's most disadvantaged older people. Taking a broad view of disadvantage through the life course, it highlights the problems faced by older people with mental health problems and their informal carers in relation to formal service provision (p. 40). *Sure Start to Later Life* has resulted in eight LinkAge Plus pilot projects designed to improve the coordination of services for older people. The LinkAge Plus pilots share a number of similarities with the Department of Health's (2006i) *Partnership for Older People Projects*, especially in relation to the emphasis on low-level services and prevention. The *Partnership for Older People Projects* aimed at promoting health, well-being and independence for older people and preventing or delaying the need for higher-intensity or institutional care. An evaluation conducted in 29 local authority pilot sites found that a diverse range of projects resulted in improved quality of life for the project participants, cost savings and better local working partnerships across agencies (Windle *et al*, 2009).

One of the eight standards of the *National Service Framework for Older People* (Department of Health, 2001c) specifically addresses mental health. As with other standards, it suggests service models, provides guidance for implementation and suggests national performance milestones. This framework was followed in 2006 by *A New Ambition for Old Age: Next Steps in Implementing the National Service Framework for Older People* (Philp, 2006), which outlined new work to coordinate planning, commissioning and delivery under the themes of dignity in care, system reform and active ageing. *A Recipe for Care: Not a Single Ingredient* (Department of Health, 2007) reinforced the need for specialist services for older people, as outlined in the national service framework. In addition, *Everybody's Business* (CSIP, 2005) is a service development guide which extends the model of older people's mental health in the national service framework and its philosophy is in accord with the principles of social inclusion. *Everybody's Business* stresses the importance of respect and dignity, having a purpose and meaning in life, a person-centred approach, improving quality of life, the importance of social networks, combating social isolation, ensuring financial security, providing access to adequate housing, and providing people with the integrated support and assistance.

The National Dementia Strategy, published in 2009 (Department of Health, 2009b) included in its 17 objectives the development of structured peer support and learning networks, improved community personal support services, a carers' strategy and consideration of the potential for housing support, housing-related services and telecare to support people with dementia and their carers.

Policies for children and young people

Over the past decade there has been an increasing awareness of the effects on society of poor mental health in children and young people, reflected in policy development in the UK. The posts of Children's Commissioners for England and Wales and Scotland's Commissioner for Children and Young People have been created to advise government in this process. Particular attention has been paid to the rights of children to influence their own lives, especially if being raised in care or experiencing the various forms of social and personal disadvantage. There has been a series of initiatives in England since the start of the century, including the establishment of the Children's Fund in 2000, which gives direct funding to local authorities, with the aim of tackling disadvantage through enhanced cooperation between agencies and increased user involvement.

The Every Child Matters: Change for Children programme (www.everychildmatters.gov.uk) highlights mental health as being of core importance in child welfare and raises specific concerns about the vulnerability of young people in local authority care. That this group carries a particularly high psychiatric morbidity is reflected in one of the first reports by Scotland's Commissioner for Children and Young People which described the problems facing young people who are leaving care. The rights of young people with mental health problems are better protected under the revision of mental health legislation in England and Wales but are extended to the children of parents with psychiatric disorder under the Mental Health (Care and Treatment) Scotland Act 2003.

The National Service Framework for children (Department of Health, 2004e) sets a series of standards for children's healthcare services (including mental health) as provided by the NHS and Social Services in England. There has been release of core funding to help health authorities reach these standards in recognition of the fact that child and adolescent mental health services (CAMHS) are underprovided for in most areas of the country. Similarly in Scotland, the shortfall in CAMHS was described in a report by The Scottish Executive (2005). The report's recommendations have been accepted by the government in Scotland but are yet to be implemented. These included the doubling of the CAMHS workforce over a period of 10 years, which, if achieved, would almost bring parity with England and Wales and would approach recommended levels.

The creation of the UK Department for Children, Schools and Families in 2007 is encouraging in the attention that this brings to children and young people. The Department has an ambitious programme of social improvement under the Children's Plan, which aims to cut child poverty in half by 2010 and eradicate it altogether by 2020 (see Chapter 7). This will be achieved through a range of measures including the offer of parenting support and by maintaining young people in education.

The Social Exclusion Task Force has focused on families at risk of exclusion. They have seen these families to have multiple and complex problems, such as joblessness, poor mental health or substance misuse. The review aimed to identify means of reducing the impact of parental problems on children's life chances. The interim analysis report, *Reaching Out: Think Family* (Cabinet Office, 2007), provided an initial analysis of who the families at risk are, and the final report, *Think Family: Improving the Life Chances of Families at Risk* (Cabinet Office, 2008), set out possible means of breaking the cycle of disadvantage. The work on families at risk was taken up by the Department for Children, Schools and Families under the Family Pathfinder programme (www.dcsf.gov.uk/everychildmatters/strategy/parents/pathfinders/familypathfinders/).

Alcohol and drug policies

The government's 10-year drug strategy includes a number of components aimed at encouraging the social reintegration of drug users and their families (Home Office, 2008). These include focusing on families where parents misuse drugs, intervening early to prevent harm to children, prioritising parents' access to treatment where children are at risk, providing intensive parenting guidance, and supporting family members, such as grandparents, who take on caring responsibilities. The strategy also draws plans to develop packages of support to help people in drug treatment to complete treatment to re-establish their lives, for instance ensuring local arrangements are in place to refer people from Jobcentres to sources of housing advice, advocacy and appropriate treatment. There are also opportunities presented by the benefits system to support people in re-integrating into society and gaining employment. These are associated with commitments to examine how claimants can be incentivised to engage with treatment and other services, and to pilot new approaches which allow a more flexible and effective use of resources, including individual budgets, to meet treatment and wider support needs.

The strategy builds on a number of previously established initiatives. Since April 2003, those who misuse substances have been able to receive assistance for their housing needs through the Supporting People programme (Sullivan, 2004). Another initiative, Positive Futures, is a national social inclusion programme using sport and leisure activities to engage with disadvantaged and socially marginalised young people. The Integrated Drug

Treatment Strategy was introduced into many prisons in 2007 with the aim of preventing recidivism by providing continuity between treatment inside and outside prison. The Drug Intervention Project provides crucial support in the first few weeks immediately after release. Specific community sentences, such as Drug and Alcohol Rehabilitation Requirements, provide alternatives to prison and associated social exclusion. *Hidden Harm* (Advisory Council on the Misuse of Drugs, 2003, 2007) is an influential report on the harm suffered by children of those misusing alcohol and drugs. Its recommendations have been accepted by the government and should in future lead to substantial resources being deployed to support families and alternative care systems, in a bid to prevent the cycle of deprivation. In contrast, funding for drug treatment in the 1990s largely stemmed from the drive to prevent the spread of HIV and hepatitis, and in the early 2000s from a desire to reduce crime. This progression indicates a move towards social integration as a key component of drug treatment policy.

The *Alcohol Harm Reduction Strategy for England* (Cabinet Office, 2004) acknowledged that damage to health, crime and disorder, and the loss of work productivity resulting from alcohol misuse cost around £20 billion per year in England and Wales, and that associated unemployment, imprisonment, poor health and inadequate parental care were a potent cause of social exclusion. However, up to now the government's response has focused mostly on supply-side measures and education about safe drinking (Home Office, 2007). In 2004, the Alcohol Needs Assessment Research Project discovered that in some parts of the country less than 1% of dependent drinkers were receiving treatment (Department of Health, 2004*f*). The situation has not improved greatly since that time. For many heavy drinkers adequate treatment is an essential first step in physical and social rehabilitation, but is currently not available.

Learning disabilities

The development of services for people with learning disabilities over the past 30 years, and in particular the move from institutional to community care, has been underpinned by overt and strong philosophies of social inclusion, including normalisation (Wolfensberger, 1972), social role valorisation (Wolfensberger, 1983), ordinary living (King's Fund, 1980), service accomplishments (O'Brien, 1989), needs assessments and essential lifestyle planning/person-centred planning principles and approaches.

The Department of Health's *Valuing People* White Paper for England (2001*d*, 2005*e*) set out aspirational values for the future lives and service delivery for all people with learning disabilities: rights as citizens, inclusion in local communities, choices in daily life and real chances for independence. According to the strategy, the appropriateness of mainstream primary care, secondary care, mental health, social care and other services for people with learning disabilities should be determined through multiprofessional/

interagency individual needs-led, person-centred planning principles and approaches. Despite these aspirations, clinically many people with learning disabilities and mental health needs will still require access to specialist, community-based, out-patient, in-patient and secure mental health or learning disabilities services. Such people with learning disabilities include those with moderate to profound learning disabilities and limited verbal communication skills and those with continuing complex mental health (and other) needs including severe enduring mental illness, personality disorders, challenging or offending behaviours, autism, dementia, and complex genetic and neuropsychiatric disorders including epilepsy. In 2006, the Department of Health issued a paper clarifying the nature and extent of existing government policy in relation to adults with an autistic spectrum disorder (Department of Health, 2006*h*).

Conclusion

There has been an array of policies that have addressed social exclusion and the exclusion of people with mental health problems and learning disability. A sceptical reader may question the degree to which these policies are effective in achieving change. There is no doubt that many aspects of mental health services have improved, for example the funding of services has increased (Boardman & Parsonage, 2007). But there is less evidence as to how the exclusion of people with mental health problems has changed. There is also some evidence that policies aimed at improving equalities have achieved some success. In their review of government policy and the progress made since 1997 towards a 'more equal' society, Hills *et al* show that there have been 'clear, if sometimes slow, movements towards greater equality in some important aspects, but not in others' (2009: p. 349): the gaps have narrowed between neighbourhoods (in education, crime, employment and local perceptions), but there have been no reductions in health inequalities and reductions in poverty have showed mixed changes. If the government's official assessment of changes detailed in their annual poverty reports (*Opportunity for All*) is used to assess progress, then for 55 of the indicators in 2007, 40 have improved since 1997 or 1998, 8 were steady and 7 deteriorated. Using an independent analysis, almost half the indicators improved, a quarter worsened and the remainder did not change (Hills *et al*, 2009). Thus, some progress has been made and this mainly reflects policy initiatives: 'Where significant policy initiatives were taken, the outcomes generally moved in the right direction, if not always as rapidly as policy makers and others might have hoped' (Hills *et al*, 2009: p. 358).

References

Advisory Council on the Misuse of Drugs (2003) *Hidden Harm: Responding to the Needs of Children of Problem Drug Users*. ACMD.
Advisory Council on the Misuse of Drugs (2007) *Hidden Harm Three Years On*. ACMD.

Summary

UK policy which has an impact on social exclusion and people with mental health problems and learning disabilities ranges from human rights and disability rights, to specific policies relating to exclusion, welfare reform, and health and social care.

For adults of working age the *National Service Framework for Mental Health* set out for the first time a set of officially sanctioned minimum standards which mental health services were expected to attain. This and the associated policies were supportive of recovery and social inclusion. Similar policies exist for children, older adults, people with learning disabilities and people with addictions.

Since 1997, the UK government has had an array of policies directed at reducing exclusion. These policies have been largely successful, but with some notable exceptions.

Bainbridge, I. & Ricketts, A. (2003) *Improving Older People's Services: An Overview of Performance*. Social Services Inspectorate.

Barnes, C. (2000) A working social model? Disability, work and disability politics in the 21st century. *Critical Social Policy*, **20**, 441–457.

Barnes, M., Mansour, A., Tomaszewski, W., *et al* (2009) *Social Impacts of Recession: The Impact of Job Loss and Job Insecurity on Social Disadvantage*. National Centre for Social Research.

Black, C. (2008) *Working for a Healthier Tomorrow*. TSO (The Stationery Office).

Boardman, J. (2005) New services for old: an overview of mental health policy. In *Beyond the Water Towers. The Unfinished Revolution in Mental Health Services1985–2005* (eds A. Bell & P. Lindley). Sainsbury Centre for Mental Health.

Boardman, J. & Parsonage, M. (2007) *Delivering the Government's Mental Health Policies: Service Staffing and Costs*. Sainsbury Centre for Mental Health.

Boorman, S. (2009) *NHS Health and Wellbeing, Final Report*. Department of Health.

Burchardt, T., Le Grand, J. & Piachaud, D. (2002) Introduction. In *Understanding Social Exclusion* (eds J. Hills, J. Le Grand & D. Piachaud). Oxford University Press.

Cabinet Office (2004) *Alcohol Harm Reduction Strategy for England*. Cabinet Office.

Cabinet Office (2007) *Reaching Out: Think Family*. Cabinet Office.

Cabinet Office (2008) *Think Family: Improving the Life Chances of Families at Risk*. Cabinet Office.

Cabinet Office (2009) *Learning from the Past: Working Together to Tackle the Social Consequences of the Recession. Evidence Pack*. Social Exclusion Task Force.

Cabinet Office & Department of Health (2010) *Inclusion Health: Evidence Pack*. Social Exclusion Task Force.

Care Services Improvement Partnership (2005) *Everybody's Business: Integrated Mental Health Service for Older Adults: A Service Development Guide*. Department of Health.

Care Services Improvement Partnership (2006) *Our Choices in Mental Health: A Framework for Improving Choice for People Who Use Mental Health Services and Their Carers*. Department of Health.

Cattell, J., Hutchins, T. & Mackie, A. (2009) *Care Services Improvement Partnership (CSIP) ACE evaluation interim report*. Matrix Insight.

Council of Europe (2003) *Convention for the Protection of Human Rights and Fundamental Freedoms as Amended by Protocol No. 11 with Protocol Nos. 1, 4, 6, 7, 12, and 13*. European Court of Human Rights.

Curtice, M. (2008) Article 3 of the Human Rights Act 1998: implications for clinical practice. *Advances in Psychiatric Treatment*, **14**, 389–397.

Curtice, M. (2009) Article 8 of the Human Rights Act 1998: implications for clinical practice. *Advances in Psychiatric Treatment*, **15**, 23–31.

Department of Health (1998) *Independent Inquiry into Inequalities in Health Report*. Department of Health.

Department of Health (1999*a*) *Saving Lives: Our Healthier Nation*. Department of Health.

Department of Health (1999*b*) *Reducing Health Inequalities: An Action Report*. Department of Health.

Department of Health (1999*c*) *National Service Framework for Mental Health: Modern Standards and Service Models*. Department of Health.

Department of Health (2001*a*) *The Expert Patient: A New Approach to Chronic Disease Management for the 21st Century*. Department of Health.

Department of Health (2001*b*) *Making it Happen: A Guide to Delivering Mental Health Promotion*. Department of Health.

Department of Health (2001*c*) *National Service Framework for Older People*. Department of Health.

Department of Health (2001*d*) *Valuing People: A New Strategy for Learning Disability for the 21st Century – Long Report* (White Paper). HMSO.

Department of Health (2002*a*) *Women's Mental Health: Into the Mainstream (Draft Strategy)*. Department of Health.

Department of Health (2002*b*) *Developing Services for Carers and Families of People with Mental Illness*. Department of Health.

Department of Health (2003*a*) *Tackling Health Inequalities: A Programme for Action*. Department of Health.

Department of Health (2003*b*) *Improving Chronic Disease Management*. Department of Health.

Department of Health (2003*c*) *Mental Health Policy Implementation Guide: Support, Time and Recovery (STR) Workers*. Department of Health.

Department of Health (2003*d*) *Mainstreaming Gender and Women's Mental Health: Implementation Guidance*. Department of Health.

Department of Health (2003*e*) *Delivering Race Equality: A Framework for Action. Mental Health Services Consultation Document*. Department of Health.

Department of Health (2004*a*) *The NHS Improvement Plan: Putting People at the Heart of Public Services*. TSO (The Stationery Office).

Department of Health (2004*b*) *Choosing Health: Making Healthier Choices Easier (Public Health White Paper)*. Department of Health.

Department of Health (2004*c*) *Policy Implementation Guide: Community Development Workers for Black and Minority Ethnic Communities (Interim Guidance)*. Department of Health.

Department of Health (2004*d*) *Improving Mental Health Law: Towards a New Mental Health Act*. Department of Health.

Department of Health (2004*e*) *National Service Framework for Children, Young People and Maternity Services*. Department of Health.

Department of Health (2004*f*) *Alcohol Needs Assessment Research Project (ANARP): The 2004 National Alcohol Needs Assessment for England*. Department of Health.

Department of Health (2005*a*) *Self Care – a Real Choice, Self Care Support – a Practical Option*. Department of Health.

Department of Health (2005*b*) *The National Service Framework for Long Term Conditions*. Department of Health.

Department of Health (2005*c*) *Independence, Well Being and Choice: Our Vision for the Future of Social Care for Adults in England* (CM6499, Social Care Green Paper). TSO (The Stationery Office).

Department of Health (2005*d*) *Delivering Race Equality in Mental Health Care: An Action Plan for Reform Inside and Outside Services and the Government's Response to the Independent Inquiry into the Death of David Bennett*. Department of Health.

Department of Health (2005*e*) *Valuing People: The Story So Far ... A New Strategy for Learning Disability for the 21st Century (Long Report)*. Department of Health.

Department of Health (2006a) *Action on Stigma: Promoting Mental Health, Ending Discrimination at Work*. Department of Health.

Department of Health (2006b) *From Values to Action: The Chief Nursing Officer's Review of Mental Health Nursing*. Department of Health.

Department of Health (2006c) *From Segregation to Inclusion: Commissioning Guidance on Day Services for People with Mental Health Problems*. Department of Health.

Department of Health (2006d) *Supporting Women into the Mainstream: Commissioning Women-Only Community Day Services*. Department of Health.

Department of Health (2006e) *Direct Payments for People with Mental Health Problems: A Guide to Action*. Department of Health.

Department of Health (2006f) *Choosing Health: Supporting the Physical Health Needs of People with Severe Mental Illness (Commissioning Framework)*. Department of Health.

Department of Health (2006g) *The Mental Health Bill: Plans to Amend the Mental Health Act 1983. Briefing Sheet: Implementing Government Policies on Mental Health Law*. Department of Health.

Department of Health (2006h) *Better Services for People with Autistic Spectrum Disorders*. Department of Health.

Department of Health (2006i) *Partnership for Older People Projects: Making the Shift to Prevention*. Department of Health.

Department of Health (2007) *A Recipe for Care: Not a Single Ingredient*. Department of Health.

Department of Health (2008) *Improving Access to Psychological Therapies, Implementation Plan: National Guidelines for Regional Delivery*. Department of Health.

Department of Health (2009a) *New Horizons: Towards a Shared Vision for Mental Health*. Department of Health.

Department of Health (2009b) *Living Well with Dementia: A National Dementia Strategy*. Department of Health.

Department of Health (2010) *Inclusion Health: Improving Primary Care for Socially Excluded People*. Department of Health.

Department of Health & Department for Work and Pensions (2006) *Vocational Services for People with Severe Mental Health Problems: Commissioning Guidance*. Department of Health.

Department of Health & HM Prison Service (2001) *Changing the Outlook: A Strategy for Developing and Modernising Mental Health Services in Prisons*. Department of Health.

Department of Social Security (1999) *Opportunity for All: Tackling Poverty and Social Exclusion – First Annual Report*. (TSO) The Stationery Office.

Department for Work and Pensions (2005) *Opportunity Age: Meeting the Challenges of Ageing in the 21st Century* (CM 6466i). TSO (The Stationery Office).

Department for Work and Pensions (2006a) *UK National Report on Strategies for Social Protection and Social Inclusion 2006–2008*. Department for Work and Pensions.

Department for Work and Pensions (2006b) *Transformation of the Personal Capability Assessment*. Department for Work and Pensions.

Department for Work and Pensions (2007a) *Opportunity for All: Indicators Update 2007*. Department for Work and Pensions.

Department for Work and Pensions (2007b) *In Work, Better Off: Next Steps to Full Employment* (Green Paper). Department for Work and Pensions.

Department for Work and Pensions (2008a) *No One Written off: Reforming Welfare to Reward Responsibility*. Department for Work and Pensions.

Department for Work and Pensions (2008b) *Raising Expectations and Increasing Support: Reforming Welfare for the Future*. Department for Work and Pensions.

European Commission (2005) *Improving the Mental Health of the Population: Towards a Strategy on Mental Health for the European Union* (Green Paper COM(2005)484). European Communities.

European Union Committee (2007) *Improving the Mental Health of the Population: Can the European Union help? Volume 1: Report*. TSO (The Stationery Office).

Fredman, S. (2005) Disability equality and the existing paradigm. In *Disability Rights in Europe* (eds A. Lawson & C. Gooding): pp. 203–208. Hart.

Freud, D. (2007) *Reducing Dependency, Increasing Opportunity: Options for the Future of Welfare to Work. An Independent Report to the Department for Work and Pensions*. Department for Work and Pensions.

Government Equalities Office (2009) *A Fairer Future: The Equality Bill and Other Action to Make Equality a Reality*. Government Equalities Office.

Gregg, P. (2008) *Realising Potential: A Vision for Personalised Conditionality and Support. An Independent Report to the Department for Work and Pensions*. Department for Work and Pensions.

Harvey, S. B., Henderson, M., Lelliott, P., et al (2009) Mental health and employment: much work still to be done. *British Journal of Psychiatry*, **194**, 201–203.

Hills, J. & Stewart, K. (2005) *A More Equal Society? New Labour, Inequality and Exclusion*. Policy Press.

Hills, J., Sefton, T. & Stewart, K. (2009) *Towards a More Equal Society? Poverty, Inequality and Policy since 1997*. Policy Press.

HM Government (2005a) *Department for Work and Pensions Five Year Strategy: Opportunity and Security throughout Life* (CM 6447). TSO (The Stationery Office).

HM Government (2005b) *Health, Work and Well-Being: Caring for Our Future, a Strategy for the Health and Well-Being of Working Age People*. TSO (The Stationery Office).

HM Government (2006a) *Reaching Out: An Action Plan on Social Exclusion*. Cabinet Office.

HM Government (2006b) *A New Deal for Welfare: Empowering People to Work* (Green Paper CM6730). TSO (The Stationery Office).

HM Government (2007) *Putting People First: A Shared Vision and Commitment to the Transformation of Adult Social Care*. TSO (The Stationery Office).

HM Government (2008) *Framework for a Fairer Future: the Equality Bill*. TSO (The Stationery Office).

HM Government (2009a) *Work, Recovery and Inclusion: Employment Support for People in Contact with Secondary Mental Health Services*. National Mental Health Development Unit.

HM Government (2009b) *Learning from the Past: Tackling Worklessness and the Social Impacts of Recession*. Cabinet Office.

HM Government (2009c) *Building Britain's Recovery: Achieving Full Employment*. Department for Work and Pensions.

HM Government (2010) *Building the National Care Service* (White Paper). TSO (The Stationery Office).

Home Office (2007) *Safe, Sensible, Social: The Next Steps in the National Alcohol Strategy*. Home Office.

Home Office (2008) *Drugs: Protecting Families and Communities, 2008–2018 Strategy*. Home Office.

Joseph Rowntree Foundation (2005) *Policies towards Poverty, Inequality and Exclusion since 1997*. Joseph Rowntree Foundation.

King's Fund (1980) *An Ordinary Life: Comprehensive Locally-Based Residential Services for Mentally Handicapped People*. King's Fund Centre.

Lelliott, P., Boardman, J., Harvey, S., et al (2008) *Mental Health and Work: A Report for the National Director for Work and Health*. TSO (The Stationery Office).

Marmot, M. (2010) *Fair Society, Healthy Lives: The Marmot Review. Strategic Review of Health Inequalities in England post-2010*. University College London.

Mental Health Europe (2008) *From Exclusion to Inclusion: The Way Forward to Promoting Social Inclusion of People with Mental Health Problems in Europe*. Mental Health Europe.

Ministry of Justice (2007) *The Governance of Britain: Constitutional Renewal*. Ministry of Justice.

National Mental Health Development Unit (2010) *Paths to Personalisation in Mental Health*. NMHDU.

NIMHE (2003) *Personality Disorder No Longer a Diagnosis of Exclusion: Policy Implementation Guidance for the Development of Services for People with Personality Disorder*. Department of Health.

NIMHE (2004) *From Here to Equality: A Strategic Plan to Tackle Stigma and Discrimination on Mental Health Grounds, 2004–2009*. NIMHE.

O'Brien, J. (1989) *What's Worth Working for? Leadership for Better Quality Human Services*. Responsive Systems Associates.

Office of the Deputy Prime Minister (2004*a*) *Mental Health and Social Exclusion*. ODPM.

Office of the Deputy Prime Minister (2004*b*) *Action on Mental Health: A Guide to Promoting Social Inclusion*. ODPM.

Office of the Deputy Prime Minister (2004*c*) *Breaking the Cycle: Taking Stock of Progress*. TSO (The Stationery Office).

Office of the Deputy Prime Minister (2005*a*) *Multiple Exclusion and Quality of Life amongst Excluded Older People in Disadvantaged Neighbourhoods*. ODPM.

Office of the Deputy Prime Minister (2005*b*) *Transitions, Young Adults with Complex Needs: A Social Exclusion Unit Final Report*. ODPM.

Office of the Deputy Prime Minister (2006) *Sure Start to Later Life: Ending Inequalities for Older People*. ODPM.

Office of the Deputy Prime Minister & Department of Health (2005) *Creating Healthier Communities: A Resource Pack for Local Partnerships*. ODPM.

Office for Disability Issues (2008) *Independent Living: A Cross-Government Strategy about Independent Living for Disabled People*. Office for Disability Issues.

Perkins, R., Farmer, P. & Litchfield, P. (2009) *Realising Ambitions: Better Employment Support for People with a Mental Health Condition*. Department for Work and Pensions.

Phillipson, C. & Scharf, T. (2004) *The Impact of Government Policy on Social Exclusion of Older People: A Review of the Literature*. ODPM.

Philp, I. (2006) *A New Ambition for Old Age: Next Steps in Implementing the National Service Framework for Older People*. Department of Health.

Rangarajan, A., Wittenburg, D., Honeycutt, T., *et al* (2008) *Programmes to Promote Employment for Disabled People: Lessons from the United States (Research Report no. 548)*. Department for Work and Pensions.

Sayce, L. (2000) *From Psychiatric Patient to Citizen: Overcoming Discrimination and Social Exclusion*. Macmillan.

Sayce, L. & Boardman, J. (2003) The Disability Discrimination Act 1995: implications for psychiatrists. *Advances in Psychiatric Treatment*, **9**, 397–404.

Sayce, L. & Boardman, J. (2008) Disability rights and mental health in the UK: recent developments of the Disability Discrimination Act. *Advances in Psychiatric Treatment*, **14**, 265–275.

The Scottish Executive (2005) *The Mental Health of Children and Young People: A Framework for Promotion, Prevention and Care*. The Scottish Executive.

Secretaries of State of the Department for Work and Pensions & the Department of Health (2009) *Working Our Way to Better Mental Health: A Framework for Action*. TSO (The Stationery Office).

Secretary of State for Health (2000) *The NHS Plan: A Plan for Investment, a Plan for Reform* (Cm 4818-I). TSO (The Stationery Office).

Secretary of State for Health (2003) *Building on the Best: Choice, Responsiveness and Equity in the NHS*. TSO (The Stationery Office).

Secretary of State for Health (2006) *Our Health, Our Care, Our Say: A New Direction for Community Services* (White Paper CM6737). TSO (The Stationery Office).

Sefton, T., Hills, J. & Sutherland, H. (2009) Poverty, inequality and redistribution. In *Towards a More Equal Society? Poverty, Inequality and Policy since 1997* (eds J. Hills, T. Sefton, & K. Stewart). Policy Press.

Stewart, K. (2009) Poverty, inequaliy and child well-being in international context: still bottom of the pack? In *Towards a More Equal Society? Poverty, Inequality and Policy since 1997* (eds J. Hills, T. Sefton, & K. Stewart). Policy Press.

Stewart, K., Sefton, T., Hills, J. (2009) Introduction. In *Towards a More Equal Society? Poverty, Inequality and Policy since 1997* (eds J. Hills, T. Sefton, & K. Stewart). Policy Press.

Sullivan, E. (2004) *Review of the Supporting People Programme*. ODPM.

Townsend, P & Davidson, N. (eds) *(1982) Inequalities in Health: The Black Report.* Penguin.

Toynbee, P. & Walker, D. (2001) *Did Things Get Better? An Audit of Labour's Successes and Failures.* Penguin.

Vizard, P. (2009) The Equality and Human Rights Commission: a new point of departure in the battle against discrimination and disadvantage. In *Towards a More Equal Society? Poverty, Inequality and Policy since 1997* (eds J. Hills, T. Sefton, & K. Stewart). Policy Press.

Wheat, K. (2007) Mental health in the workplace. 2: Mental health and discrimination in employment. *Journal of Mental Health Law*, **November**, 194–208.

WHO Europe (2005) *Mental Health Declaration for Europe: Facing the Challenge, Building Solutions.* WHO Europe.

Windle, K., Wagland, R., Forder, J., *et al* (2009) *National Evaluation of Partnerships for Older People Projects: Final Report.* Personal Social Services Research Unit (http://www.pssru. ac.uk/pdf/dp2700.pdf).

Wolfensberger, W. (1972) *The Principle of Normalization in Human Services.* National Institute on Mental Retardation.

Wolfensberger, W. (1983) Social role valorisation: a proposed new term for the principle of normalization. *Mental Retardation*, **21**, 234–239.

CHAPTER 5

How is social exlusion relevant to psychiatry?

Jed Boardman and Helen Killaspy

In previous chapters we have outlined the concepts of inclusion and the components of exclusion that are relevant to people with mental health problems and learning disability. It is clear that exclusion refers to the position of these groups in relation to society and their status as citizens with access to the same rights and freedoms as others. It is also clear that many of these components of exclusion have been part of social and mental health policy over the past 10 years or more.

In Part 2 of this book we will turn to examine the scope of the problems: the extent of disadvantage, poverty and exclusion in the population of the UK, of people with mental health problems and with learning disability, and in specific social identity groups with mental health problems. To some degree this chapter anticipates Part 2, by setting out the arguments as to why psychiatry should be concerned with social exclusion. However, it is possible to answer this question simply and directly – it is because people with mental health problems (especially those with severe problems) and with learning disability are among the most socially excluded and stigmatised groups in our society. Social exclusion is not only a result of having mental health problems or learning disability, but it is also a cause of mental and physical ill health. It may be worth reflecting at this stage that the key features of the complex multidimensional problems of poverty and social exclusion listed in Box 4.2 (p. 51) all apply to people with mental health problems or learning disability.

For the purposes of this chapter the term psychiatry refers to the individual practice of psychiatrists and to the collective body of psychiatrists as, for example, represented by professional bodies such as the Royal College of Psychiatrists. It encompasses the range of specialties of psychiatric practice including adult, child and adolescent and old age psychiatry, rehabilitation, forensic, addictions and liaison psychiatry, psychotherapy and the psychiatry of learning disability. We outline the general reasons why psychiatry should be concerned with social exclusion. Central to this is what are increasingly being referred to as the recovery-oriented approach and/or socially inclusive practice, and the benefits of these approaches to clinicians, service users and the wider collective.

Why should psychiatry be concerned with social exclusion?

One of the general thrusts of this book is to argue for a level platform for people with mental health problems and learning disability in relation to others in society. Contained in this argument is a view that social inclusion is something that applies to all members of society and that social justice should occupy a central place in social policy with values such as freedom, equality, dignity, respect and autonomy helping to define the basis for a good society and the framework for policy.

What is wrong with social exclusion?

Before turning to some specific reasons why psychiatrists and other mental health professionals should be concerned with social exclusion in relation to people with mental health problems and learning disability, we should examine the overarching question, 'What is wrong with social exclusion?' The concept of social justice provides two main responses to this question, as argued by Barry (2002): first, social exclusion violates the value of social justice, and second, it violates the value of social solidarity.

Considering the first answer, Barry (2002) equates social justice with equality of opportunity, that is, the substantive opportunity that a person has to have the life they value and choose, and have reasons to value and choose (see Chapter 3). Social exclusion may be associated with loss of substantive freedom by, for example, leading to unequal educational and employment opportunities. But it may also lead to a direct denial of the basic human rights that were considered in Chapter 4 (Box 4.1). For example, for those on low incomes the opportunity to a fair trial (an unconditional right) may be closed, as in the absence of legal aid, they may be unable to afford the necessary legal representation. Barry (2002) also considers the inability to engage in political activity to be an aspect of social exclusion. Here political engagement is seen to go beyond voting in elections and includes, for example, taking part in political parties, lobbying and neighbourhood politics. Generally, for the individual, it involves having a voice, choice and control. In this sense it becomes clear that social exclusion is in itself a form of social injustice as it involves a denial of opportunities that should be open to all.

The concept of social justice used by Barry (2002) is sensitive to individual choices since making a voluntary separation from others or restricting opportunities through choice may not involve a denial of social justice. In other words, social isolation and social exclusion do not necessarily both represent examples of social injustice. In turn, this brings us to the matter of social exclusion as a violation of the value of social solidarity. By social solidarity, Barry means the sense of fellow feeling that extends beyond people with whom one is in direct contact and which depends on common institutions and generally shared experiences. He assumes that social solidarity is *intrinsically* valuable, as human lives tend to be enhanced in a society whose members share some kind of existence. This is understandable as it relates to matters such as cooperation, mutuality and support, and links with the value of social networks, matters familiar to us all. He also suggests that social solidarity is *instrumentally* valuable as social justice is more likely to be realised through politics in societies where there is a higher level of social solidarity. This point includes the supposition that not only might the socially excluded individual be excluded from politics, but that the socially isolated group may also be debarred, thus reducing their collective voice such that their interests are neglected and their political influence reduced. Here Barry is highlighting some of the realities of liberal democracies: the politics of self-interest, and the means of maintaining political power by splitting the electorate and identifying with the majority. The lack of empathy between the majority and the socially isolated minority makes it easier for minorities to be stigmatised or even dehumanised. Importantly, and what makes social exclusion more pernicious, is that the processes that lead to exclusion are often the same as those that lead to this stigmatisation. Barry is concerned with what he refers to as 'stratified social exclusion' and the way in which both low and high incomes can, under some conditions, lead to social isolation and exclusion. For low-income groups this may be obvious as their poverty prevents participation in mainstream institutions, but for those on high incomes this may work through these groups insulating themselves from the common fate and buying their way out of common institutions. This stratification along socioeconomic lines drives politicians to compete for the 'middle ground' and the concerns of the 'median voter'. It also points to the importance of social solidarity for an inclusive society, as:

> the more attenuated the bonds of social solidarity become, the less inclusive the concerns of the median voter will be. The socially excluded will thus be failed by democratic politics. To the extent that the median voter pays attention to those below the lower threshold of social exclusion it is liable to be in their threats to his or her prosperity and personal safety (Barry, 2002: p. 26).

Notwithstanding the human distress associated with social exclusion, these two concerns, social justice and social solidarity, highlight the fundamental argument as to the wrongs of social exclusion. They, again, emphasise the many-faceted nature of exclusion. Many of the concepts raised such as stigma, isolation, choice, involvement are familiar to mental health professionals. The effects of politics on the status of people with mental health problems are familiar to us, through the portrayal of such people as dangerous and a threat, or as weak and feckless, or with the divisive portrayal of community mental health services as failing. In addition, we may recognise the way in which some aspects of public policy over the past 30 years have undermined solidarity through the emphasis on competition rather than cooperation.

The particular importance of social exclusion for psychiatry

In Part 2 we shall see the ways in which people with mental health problems, and particularly those with severe and enduring problems, including those with learning disability, are among the most excluded in our society. The particular reasons why this is important for professionals and others working in, managing and planning mental health services are summarised in Box 5.1 and dealt with in detail below.

Social disadvantage, poverty and health

There are strong associations between poverty, disadvantage, deprivation, exclusion and mental ill health. Social exclusion and its indicators, for example joblessness, homelessness and poverty, are associated with mental and physical ill health (Willkinson, 2005, 2006). In short, social exclusion is bad for your health. We should be aware that mental health problems are both a cause and a consequence of exclusion. There are often complex and multidimensional relationships between disadvantage, mental illness and the position of people with mental ill health in society, which maintain and compound mental health problems and the negative consequences of exclusion in a circular manner.

Box 5.1   Why should psychiatry be concerned with social exclusion?

- Social disadvantage, poverty and health
  - exclusion and its indicators (e.g. joblessness, homelessness, poverty) are associated with mental and physical ill health
  - social disadvantage, poverty and mental health problems tend to go together
- Dynamic nature of exclusion
  - poverty and exclusion are not fixed states
- Transactional nature of exclusion
  - exclusion is brought about by someone or something
- Relativity
  - exclusion affects everyone
- Multiple deprivation
  - people who are excluded often suffer from multiple disadvantages
- Inter-generational aspects
  - exclusion affects families and can pass from generation to generation
- Area deprivation
  - some areas of the country are more deprived than others
- Subjective dimensions
  - exclusion is a profoundly negative experience for the individual
- The place of social quality
  - social exclusion is costly – to individuals, families, communities, the economy
- Service user views
  - people want to participate

Social disadvantage, poverty and mental health problems tend to go together. It is important to tackle poverty and exclusion if individuals are to thrive. Poverty is harmful to individuals and to society; it is a waste of human resources and a measure of the failure of our welfare state. The evidence for the contention that reducing poverty and increasing opportunity improves health is harder to establish than the overwhelming evidence of an association between disadvantage and ill health. Nevertheless, reducing exclusion is more difficult where there are larger disparities in income and accumulated wealth (Jackson & Segal, 2004; Esping-Anderson, 2005; Wilkinson & Pickett, 2009).

Dynamic nature of exclusion

Poverty and exclusion are not inevitably fixed states. Their impact will vary over time: they may be transient, recurrent or long-term experiences. People will move in and out of the conditions that lead to exclusion (poverty, unemployment, ill health); similarly, mental health problems themselves are often fluctuating, with periods of relapse followed by periods of remission. At some points in the development and course of their problems people with mental ill health and learning disability may be particularly vulnerable to experiencing loss of income, job, home, family and support, but these risks may be reduced by, for example, the adequate and timely treatment of their mental health problems and with due attention paid to their financial, employment and other social problems that may exacerbate their exclusion.

Transactional nature of exclusion

Exclusion involves reciprocal interactions between individuals and groups and wider social structures (Schneider & Bramley, 2008). Exclusion cannot exist without someone or something bringing it about, for example, through the functioning of the system (such as financial bureaucracies, institutional racism) or discrimination by individuals. The transactional nature of exclusion emphasises the multilevel causes of exclusion, which include the individual, household, community and institutions. Thus remedies cannot be found solely at the level of the individual – for psychiatry as a whole this means setting our sights widely. This may mean engaging with politics, as individuals and through our professional institutions, to represent mental health service users and lobbying and campaigning against policies that may discriminate against, or put at a disadvantage, people with mental health problems. Mental health professionals may play a role in public education (which may also be aimed at health service workers), for example, to reduce the ignorance and prejudice associated with mental ill health. It also means examining what happens in our own back yard: the culture of mental health services, the functioning of these services and our own individual practice to make mental health services more recovery-oriented and socially inclusive (see Part 3).

Relativity

Exclusion affects everyone, and the relative nature of exclusion means that the same general contemporary social forces act upon all people in the population, which includes those with mental health problems. Reducing the differences between those with mental health problems and others, be it because of income, employment, choice or control, will have a beneficial effect on individuals with mental health problems. Some of the resultant actions may be directly relevant to mental health services, such as improving access to benefits, employment, training, education, the use of direct payments, all of which are oriented towards recovery. Improving participation and the sense of control that people have over their lives may have a direct effect on mental health (Wilkinson, 2005).

Multiple deprivation

People who are excluded often suffer from multiple disadvantages and the causes of these disadvantages can be located at several different and interacting levels. This implies that the response must be multifactorial, for example aimed at the individual and wider structures, by using a range of public sector agencies (health, social care, employment, education, housing). People working in mental health services are familiar with the fact that these services are provided by a range of health, social and independent sector agencies and are aware of the importance of working with multiple social and health agencies. This multiagency approach is of central significance to the future of recovery-oriented services and there is a need to improve the partnership between these local providers.

Inter-generational aspects

Disadvantage and exclusion affect families, can be passed from generation to generation and affect a person's life chances. This implies the need to employ early intervention, prevention and promotion. Some aspects of mental health services are explicitly designed to work in a socially inclusive manner: home treatment services may help to reduce the fractured relationships that an in-patient stay can herald; intervening early in a psychotic illness may buffer against the social handicaps that accrue in a chronic relapsing condition; and assertive outreach can be a recovery-oriented, patient-centred and socially inclusive means of engaging and assisting an otherwise disenfranchised group (Killaspy et al, 2009). Some interventions, for example those aimed at parenting in families with a child with conduct disorder, may mitigate against the effects of early childhood disadvantage on adult outcomes (Scott et al, 2001a). A socially inclusive approach involves paying attention to the types of outcomes that we wish to achieve and promoting social and clinical outcomes.

Area deprivation

Social exclusion is not only bad for your health, but it also affects the physical and social environment that you live in. Indicators of inequality and exclusion are associated with a range of negative social outcomes such as higher rates of violent crime and lower levels of interpersonal trust (Hsieh & Pugh, 1993; Kawachi *et al*, 1997; Wilkinson & Pickett, 2009). The causes and consequences of social exclusion cluster in particular geographical areas, with some areas having the highest levels of disadvantage across a number of indicators of deprivation such as unemployment, poor housing, high crime rates and poor access to healthcare. Areas with high levels of deprivation have high levels of people with mental health problems and the factors associated with social exclusion and deprivation compound individuals' mental health problems and social exclusion in a circular fashion. The situation is exacerbated by the social migration of people with severe and enduring mental health problems to areas of social disadvantage through a downward social spiral. These deprived areas are the environments in which mental health professionals are likely to work and it is important to avoid replication of poor environments in the local services and the potential to hold low expectations for better social outcomes in these areas. Services need to be responsive to the nature of the local area served. They need to adapt and focus their resources and ethos accordingly.

Subjective dimensions

Exclusion is a profoundly negative experience for the individual and the processes of exclusion and agency are important. Exclusion may be viewed as subjective states of belonging and involvement in local communities which are determined by the actions of others (Sayce, 2000; Repper & Perkins, 2003; Morgan *et al*, 2007). This emphasises the lived experiences of people with mental health problems and how society's responses contribute to excluding such people from social activities and social spaces. It also reinforces the importance of a recovery-oriented approach and the role that professionals may play in advocating the rights of service users.

The place of social quality

The concept of social quality was raised in Chapter 3 and may be seen as a summary term referring to the concepts of social inclusion, socioeconomic security, social cohesion and empowerment. It reflects people's participation in the social and economic life of their communities, which may improve their well-being and individual potential (Beck *et al*, 1997; Huxley & Thornicroft, 2003). These forms of participation are absent from, or reduced in, the lives of many people with mental health problems and learning disability. Psychiatrists and other mental health workers can make significant contributions to improving social quality, through advocating improvements in services and by enhancing their understanding of service users' experiences of exclusion and thereby improving their own relationships with service users.

What are the benefits of working in a socially inclusive way?

Wider economic and social benefits

Economic benefits

Social exclusion is not only unjust, it is also extremely costly – both to the health and well-being of individuals and their families and to society as a whole. The overall cost of mental health problems in England has been estimated at £77 billion in 2002/2003, including costs of care, economic losses and reduced quality of life (Sainsbury Centre for Mental Health, 2003).

Being out of work is one dimension of social exclusion. A significant number of people with mental health problems are not in work – in 2008 there were about 1 million such people who were out of work and in receipt of incapacity benefit. Worklessness is particularly high among those with severe and long-term mental health problems. The economic costs of this form of exclusion are substantial. For example, a study published by the King's Fund has estimated that the economic losses resulting from below-average employment among all people with mental health problems currently amount to around £26 billion a year (McCrone *et al*, 2008). This looks to be very much in line with a broader estimate of £63 billion a year for the costs of worklessness resulting from all forms of ill health (physical as well as mental), as given in the review of the health of Britain's working age population (Black, 2008). Given that people with mental health problems account for 40% of the Incapacity Benefit caseload (Sainsbury Centre for Mental Health, 2007), this implies a cost of worklessness specifically attributable to mental ill health of around £25 billion a year – very similar to the King's Fund estimate.

Reducing exclusion by improving employment opportunities for people with mental health problems may therefore yield substantial economic benefits. In part these benefits would accrue to the individuals themselves in the form of higher income, but there would also be gains for the wider community. For example, government revenues (and hence the scope for public spending) would increase because of income tax and National Insurance contributions, and there would also be savings in social security spending as people move from benefits into work. In addition, there would be savings in the costs of care for those whose mental (and physical) health improves as a result of gaining employment.

There are also potential economic benefits to breaking the cycle of deprivation that affects the long-term outcome of individuals and families. Giving attention to impaired relationships in early life helps to address the potentially destructive long-term effect of stressful attachment (Howe, 2006). Conduct disorder, for instance, carries a huge cost for society, yet it is primarily a treatable disorder (Scott *et al*, 2001a). This will require a new political imperative before NHS funding can be confidently directed towards realising much longer-term social benefits (Scott *et al*, 2001*b*).

Social benefits

Greater inclusion at a micro-level, through individual social networks and support, offers some protection from the incidence, and continued prevalence, of mental health problems (Chapter 3). Lower levels of objective and subjective social capital are associated with higher levels of symptoms in both adults and children (De Silva *et al*, 2005; Wilkinson, 2005). It would appear that access to a well-developed social network may have benefits for the individual over and above improving their subjective sense of 'belonging'. This may be particularly true for people with psychotic symptoms where the poverty of social networks may give rise to specific problems of support in times of crisis and hence increase the likelihood of mental health service contact and admission.

These networks may also facilitate access to economic, cultural and information resources which then benefit the individual. It is insufficient to think in terms of simply enhancing social inclusion (employment rates, access to stable housing, etc.) without thinking of the wider social context in which such interventions will operate (friends, family, the wider public). Falzer (2007) refers to these wider social benefits as a 'strategic surplus' and suggests that they transcend the achievement of therapeutic goals.

At a macro-level, there is also the view that social capital is a characteristic of communities (De Silva *et al*, 2005). It is a 'community stock' which strengthens the fabric of society and promotes values such as citizenship, reciprocity and diversity. These benefits then cascade downwards through the community, improving its collective health and thereby the health of its individual members. There is less research to support this view, but it does have plausibility and there is some supporting evidence in relation to reduced levels of suicide and improved outcomes in schizophrenia where social capital is higher (De Silva *et al*, 2005).

In Chapter 3 we saw how some people have talked about community efficacy – the ability of communities to come together to fight for a common cause – which is a reflection of the social solidarity referred to earlier and is a important facet of macro-level social capital. Creating stronger service users' organisations that have a coherent voice and respect in their communities, will, if the associated prejudice and discrimination is addressed, allow people with mental health problems and learning disability a greater say and access to legitimate forms of power.

There may be obvious economic benefits to preventing service users from becoming institutionalised and dependent on health and social services and instead promoting their involvement in the labour market, but the benefits for society also depend on how it views people with mental health problems, and how this view has changed over time. In the 19th century, exclusion was associated with the exponential rise of the asylums. In the 1960s and 1970s, UK society promoted social inclusion of this group, believing that their social exclusion was morally wrong. In more recent times, society's view has been that community care has failed and that mental health service users are dangerous. This allows society to abrogate responsibility for social inclusion of those with mental health problems. This societal emphasis on avoidance of risk exacerbates all aspects of social exclusion on an everyday basis for service users, with obvious disincentives for them to reveal their mental health history to others. This effective silencing in turn means that those around them are not necessarily aware of the kinds of support they might find helpful to engage in society. The emphasis on public safety also creates a tension for mental health practitioners to facilitate their clients' autonomy and inclusion while attempting to ensure they cannot be criticised for their practice. The recovery and social inclusion agenda specifically encourages practitioners to focus on these areas of tension.

An additional important challenge to consider here is the degree to which service users' social exclusion can be compounded by mental health professionals' low expectations of their clients' potential to regain skills and fulfil their potential (Office of the Deputy Prime Minister, 2004). Often, inadvertently, mental health professionals (as well as the culture of the services within which they work) can represent a significant risk to service users in creating dependency and undermining service users' confidence rather than supporting them to achieve their aspirations. Socially inclusive services value what is important to patients (their family, friends, leisure activities, work and social roles). Services oriented towards recovery value involvement in life over attachment to services and services that are hard for users to leave can impede recovery. Additionally, services that create dependency are not always healthy for staff to work in, with professional demoralisation being particularly unhelpful for patients. A useful concept is of the professional being available when required ('on tap') rather than rigidly authoritarian at worst or needlessly paternalistic at best ('on top') (Repper & Perkins, 2003; Shepherd *et al*, 2008). In addition, a strong professional/patient alliance may be an especially powerful combination when advocating better services.

Benefits to service users and carers

Exclusion is pertinent to the experience of service users, for whom a major priority is the reduction of poverty, but also a desire for social roles, more friends and relationships, acceptance by neighbours, employers and family, and more opportunities to be part of mainstream groups and communities (Repper & Perkins, 2003; Slade, 2009). In short, people want to participate, and in concerning ourselves with social exclusion we are responding to the direct wishes of service users. Perhaps the most compelling reason for adopting socially inclusive principles is that this is what service users want. People do better in services that embrace social inclusion and with mental health professionals who facilitate social functioning with subsequent opportunities for improved relationships, employment and housing stability.

Working in a socially inclusive and recovery-oriented manner implies an emphasis on a collaborative partnership between service users (and where appropriate, families and carers) and psychiatrists. Working in a more collaborative way with service users in a role that goes beyond the traditional medical role and resembles more that of a coach who supports recovery and social inclusion may be a goal for all mental health professionals (Perkins & Repper, 1999; Slade, 2009). Delivery of care, through socially inclusive and recovery approaches, in line with service users' preferences and choice, is likely to lead to better outcomes for service users. Working with their preferences and choice, as far as possible, is more likely to enable them to live the lives they want to lead. This approach is also likely to promote greater levels of engagement with mental health services (Sainsbury Centre for Mental Health, 1998).

It must be recognised, however, that this ideal may not be achieved and might not be realistic for all service users. Physical safety is critical – if a person harms themselves or other people, or is vulnerable to abuse from others, then this severely restricts their possibilities for rebuilding a meaningful and valued life. Additionally, it should be recognised that the situation for most patients is a dynamic one, in which individuals may become more or less capable of collaboration according to the stage or severity of their illness. However, a relapse need not be considered a 'failure', but a part of the process of learning that can enable a person to move beyond their limitations and identify additional support and adjustments that they, or the people around them, may need to successfully pursue their ambitions.

Informal carers can be seriously affected by their own perceptions and experiences of stigma in relation to their relative's mental health problems. Relationships within the family and informal support networks can be strained beyond repair during periods of relapse or secondary to the high burden associated with care giving. Interventions from mental health services to assist and support carers and families (such as family psychoeducation) have been shown to be effective but difficult to implement. However, they are key in sustaining service users' social support networks, the importance of which cannot be overstated in minimising factors likely to exacerbate social exclusion.

The losses and exclusion that can accompany chronic relapsing psychiatric conditions are said to occur in a stepwise manner and at critical periods in the course of the condition. For example, it is often the second episode of illness (especially if this involves hospitalisation and/or significant behavioural disturbance) that disrupts relationships and domestic life, and can make a return to work harder to negotiate. Mapping a patient's journey through illness and through services and professional contacts can be a helpful way of identifying the critical stages and necessary interventions. The aim should be a 'better journey'.

The value of work

Being in work and having increased social networks and relationships provides direct health gain in terms of better mental and physical health and well-being (Berkman, 1995; Boardman, 2003; Waddell & Burton, 2006). Improved access to work opportunities is generally associated with higher living standards and quality of life, since employment provides not only a monetary reward but also has 'latent benefits', or non-financial gains, to the worker. Some of these additional benefits are: social identity and status; social contacts and support; a means of structuring and occupying time; activity and involvement; and a sense of personal achievement (Warr, 1987; Boardman, 2003). Work tells us who we are and enables us to tell others who we are; 'What do you do?' is typically the second question we ask when we meet someone.

Employment may be considered overall as beneficial to people's mental and physical health and well-being but the social gradient in health and mortality acts as a confounder and probably outweighs other work characteristics that influence health (Waddell & Burton, 2006). Job insecurity adversely affects health (Dooley, 2003). Evidence for the health benefits of employment comes mainly from examining its corollary, unemployment. Unemployment is associated with increased rates of overall mortality and illnesses such as cardiovascular disease and lung cancer, suicide, poor physical health and mental health, higher rates of consultation and hospitalisation. Unemployment can contribute or aggravate most adverse health outcomes.

There is a particularly strong relationship between unemployment and mental health difficulties. Work is particularly crucial for people with mental health problems as they are especially sensitive to the negative effects of unemployment and the associated loss of structure, purpose and identity (Bennett, 1970). Already socially excluded as a result of their mental health problems, this exclusion is aggravated by unemployment. In addition, there is a consensus from a range of stakeholders, including service users, that work and employment are beneficial in some form. Although the direction of causality is not clear, studies of schemes to get people with severe mental illness into work suggest that it is related to a reduction in symptoms and hospitalisations and a better quality of life and self-esteem (Cook & Razzano, 2000; Marwaha & Johnson, 2004). In addition, work may reduce depression and suicidal thinking in people with psychosis, which may be a consequence of the loss of social roles and goals associated with worklessness (Birchwood et al, 2000).

In addition to the social and health benefits outlined above, work may therefore be regarded as therapeutic and should feature in efforts to promote recovery and social inclusion. However, not all service users wish to return to open employment, for a variety of reasons, some of which may be fear of experiencing stigma in the workplace, fear of the stress of employment precipitating relapse, and concerns about the impact of employment on their social benefits and finances. Although skilled mental health professionals, vocational rehabilitation workers and supported employment schemes can successfully address many of these issues, other opportunities for meaningful occupation should be available to all service users. Mental health services therefore need to provide and link with other providers to ensure that a range of vocational and occupational opportunities are available.

Conclusion

Many aspects of inclusion will require attention to be paid to structural changes in society and broader policy initiatives such as taxation, welfare reform and immigration, but psychiatrists, other mental health professionals and mental health services also have a significant role. However, if social inclusion for people with mental illness is to be given greater impetus in mental health policy and practice, then leadership is required from mental health professionals as well as the user movement.

The time is now right for concerted service developments that contribute to inclusion and psychiatry has every reason to support these and to contribute to opportunities for service users to work, engage in education, and to participate in society. These matters go to the heart of social inclusion and beyond providing treatment or care alone. Recovery and social inclusion must be identified as specific goals, practice and services should be adapted to help achieve these, and opportunity should be taken to work for a reduction of discrimination and improvement of the rights of people with mental illness. Working in a socially inclusive manner can build on what has been developed in mental health services over the past 10–15 years, but it is also an opportunity to contribute to what develops in the years to come. The complementary concepts of inclusion and recovery and their application to mental health practice provides a significant basis for common ground between psychiatrists, other mental health professionals and service users.

Summary

Psychiatry should be concerned about social exclusion for several reasons that relate to its toxic effect on people with mental health problems and learning difficulties and its key relevance to psychiatric practice. Recovery ideas are integral to socially inclusive practice; recovery-oriented practice and services should form some of the key approaches to socially inclusive practice.

The benefits to broader society of a socially inclusive approach to people with mental health problems and learning difficulties are economic and social. There are many benefits to psychiatric professionals and service users in adopting socially-inclusive and recovery-oriented approaches which partly accrue from the potential to develop more collaborative relationships. Additional advantages include the latent benefits of work and employment and the attainment (and re-attainment) of valued social outcomes.

References

Barry, B. (2002) Social exclusion, social isolation, and the distribution of income. In *Understanding Social Exclusion* (eds J. Hills, J. Le Grand & D. Piachaud). Oxford University Press.

Beck, W., van der Maesen, L. & Walker, A. (1997) *The Social Quality of Europe*. Kluwer Law International.

Bennett, D. (1970) The value of work in psychiatric rehabilitation. *Social Psychiatry*, **5**, 224–230.

Berkman, L. F. (1995) The role of social relations in health promotion. *Psychosomatic Medicine*, **57**, 245–254.

Birchwood, M., Iqbal, Z., Chadwick, P., *et al* (2000) Cognitive approach to depression and suicidal thinking in psychosis: I. *Ontogeny of post-psychotic depression. British Journal of Psychiatry*, **177**, 516–528.

Black, C. (2008) *Working for a Healthier Tomorrow*. TSO (The Stationery Office).

Boardman, J. (2003) Work, employment and psychiatric disability. *Advances in Psychiatric Treatment*, **9**, 327–334.

Cook, A. & Razzano, L. (2000) Vocational rehabilitation for persons with schizophrenia: recent research and implications for practice. *Schizophrenia Bulletin*, **26**, 87–103.

De Silva, M. J., McKenzie, K., Harpham, T., *et al* (2005) Social capital and mental illness: a systematic review. *Journal Epidemiology and Community Health*, **59**, 619–627.

Dooley, D. (2003) Unemployment, underemployment and mental health: conceptualizing employment status as a continuum. *American Journal of Community Psychology*, **32**, 9–16.

Esping-Anderson, G. (2005) Inequality of incomes and opportunities. In *The New Egalitarianism* (eds A. Giddens & P. Diamonds). Policy Network.

Falzer, P. R. (2007) Developing and using social capital in public mental health. *Mental Health Review Journal*, **12**, 34–42.

Howe, D. (2006) Disabled children, maltreatment and attachment. *British Journal of Social Work*, **36**, 743–760.

Hsieh, C. & Pugh, M. (1993) Poverty, income inequality and violent crime: a meta-analysis of recent aggregate data studies. *Criminal Justice Review*, **18**, 182–202.

Huxley, P. & Thornicroft, G. (2003) Social inclusion, social quality and mental illness. *British Journal of Psychiatry*, **182**, 289–290.

Jackson, B., & Segal, P. (2004) *Why Inequality Matters* (Catalyst Working Paper). Catalyst.

Kawachi, I., Kennedy, B., Lochner, K., *et al* (1997) Social capital, income inequality and mortality. *American Journal of Public Health*, **87**, 1491–1498.

Killaspy, H., Johnson, S., Pierce, B., *et al* (2009) A mixed methods analysis of interventions delivered by assertive community treatment and community mental health teams in the REACT trial. *Social Psychiatry and Psychiatric Epidemiology*, **44**, 532–540.

Marwaha, S. & Johnson, S. (2004) Schizophrenia and employment. *Social Psychiatry and Psychiatric Epidemiology*, **39**, 337–349.

McCrone, P., Dhanasiri, S., Patel, A., *et al* (2008) *Paying the Price: The Cost of Mental Health in England to 2026*. King's Fund.

Morgan, C., Burns, T., Fitzpatrick, R., *et al* (2007) Social exclusion and mental health: conceptual and methodological review. *British Journal of Psychiatry*, **191**, 477–483.

Office of the Deputy Prime Minister (2004) *Mental Health and Social Exclusion*. ODPM.

Perkins, R. & Repper, J. (1999) Compliance or informed choice. *Journal of Mental Health*, **8**, 117–129.

Repper, J. & Perkins, R. (2003) *Social Inclusion and Recovery*. Ballière Tindall.

Sainsbury Centre for Mental Health (1998) *Keys to Engagement: Review of Care for People with Severe Mental Illness Who are Hard to Engage with Services*. Sainsbury Centre for Mental Health.

Sainsbury Centre for Mental Health (2003) *The Economic and Social Costs of Mental Illness (Policy Paper 3)*. Sainsbury Centre for Mental Health.

Sainsbury Centre for Mental Health (2007) *Mental Health at Work: Developing the Business Care*. Sainsbury Centre for Mental Health.

Sayce, L. (2000) *From Psychiatric Patient to Citizen: Overcoming Discrimination and Social Exclusion*. Macmillan.

Schneider, J. & Bramley, C. J. (2008) Towards social inclusion in mental health? *Advances in Psychiatric Treatment*, **14**, 131–138.

Scott, S., Spender, Q., Doolan, M., *et al* (2001*a*) Multicentre controlled trail of parenting groups for child antisocial behaviour in clinical practice. *BMJ*, **323**, 194–197.

Scott, S., Knapp, M., Henderson, J., *et al* (2001*b*) Financial cost of social exclusion: follow up study of antisocial children into adulthood. *BMJ*, **323**, 191–194.

Shepherd, G., Boardman, J. & Slade, M. (2008) *Making Recovery a Reality*. Sainsbury Centre for Mental Health.

Slade, M. (2009) *Personal Recovery and Mental Illness*. Cambridge University Press.

Waddell, G. & Burton, A. K. (2006) *Is Work Good for Your Health and Well-Being?* TSO (The Stationery Office).

Warr, P. (1987) *Work, Unemployment and Mental Health*. Oxford University Press.

Wilkinson, R. (2005) *The Impact of Inequality: How to Make Sick Societies Healthier*. The New Press.

Wilkinson, R. (2006) Income inequality and health: a review of the evidence. *Social Science and Medicine*, **62**, 1768–1784.

Wilkinson, R. & Pickett, K. (2009) *The Spirit Level: Why More Equal Societies Almost Always Do Better*. Penguin.

CHAPTER 6

Socially inclusive working across the psychiatric subspecialties

Helen Killaspy, Gillian Mezey, Jed Boardman and Alan Currie

In Chapter 5 we made the general case for why psychiatry should be concerned about social exclusion and the need to pay attention to its drivers and effects. In this chapter we will take the main subspecialties and examine in what way social exclusion is relevant to them and what social exclusion and inclusion may mean to their practice. For our discussion we have chosen psychiatric subspecialties represented by the Faculties of the Royal College of Psychiatrists (with the exception of the general and community psychiatry, discussed in Chapter 5): Rehabilitation and Social Psychiatry, Forensic Psychiatry, Liaison Psychiatry, Psychotherapy, Child and Adolescent Psychiatry, Psychiatry of Old Age, Addictions Psychiatry and Psychiatry of Learning Disability.

Rehabilitation and social psychiatry

Since rehabilitation services focus on individuals with the most complex needs and greatest levels of functional impairment, by definition they also work with one of the most socially excluded groups of mental health service users. In addition, large numbers of service users with high support needs are placed in community residential and nursing homes that are a long way from their local area of origin and family, thus further exacerbating their social dislocation.

Two key areas underpin much of the focus of contemporary rehabilitation services: promotion of community living and engagement in meaningful occupation. The benefits of these have been well evidenced through national and international studies and are, in short, related to the promotion of recovery, the avoidance or minimisation of institutionalisation and the promotion of social inclusion.

Markers of recovery

Rehabilitation services increasingly adopt a recovery orientation and use 'markers of recovery' to assess outcomes that have a great deal of overlap with aspects of social inclusion. These include having access to mainstream leisure, education and work, self-management of finances, positive family relationships, an enjoyable social life, and civic integration including taking part in local mainstream community groups and voting (Liberman & Kopelowicz, 2002). The specific interventions of rehabilitative psychiatry promote service users' mental health and their skills and confidence in managing everyday activities, and gradually facilitate them to hold increasing responsibility for their self-management. As this process progresses, more complex activities and a fuller daytime structure develop, leading ultimately to mainstream community participation.

For some users of rehabilitation services, some markers of recovery may remain aspirational because of the degree of functional impairment. It is therefore necessary to ensure that a variety of community resources are available to support service users' social inclusion through different stages of their recovery. Adequate facilities for 'meaningful occupation' might include: those based within services, such as courses and activities that take place in a community-based mental health setting, such as a day or resource centre run by statutory or voluntary services; supported activities within mainstream settings, such as classes for people with mental health problems held at a local college or leisure centre, or supported employment; as well as non-supported mainstream activities, such as open employment or a regular further education course open to all. Links with community resources that promote and provide these activities and facilities are therefore essential for rehabilitation services; occupational therapists are often the local leads in developing these relationships.

How not to disempower through care

The risk of disempowering service users through over-support and dependency-inducing services has already been mentioned in Chapter 5. Rehabilitation services and community services therefore have to be mindful of the need to review and adjust care plans that encourage service users to continue to gain skills, confidence and independence. However, some systems that have developed to promote independence can inadvertently impair social stability and inclusion. For example, service users may be required to move through a system of increasingly less supported accommodation every few years as they gain more independent living skills. Although this 'move-on' ethos supports the expectation of recovery and reduces institutional practices, it disadvantages service users by failing to provide permanent housing, which impedes the opportunities for civic integration. Some rehabilitation services are attempting to find alternatives to these systems. One example is the provision of highly supported flats with move on to permanent independent tenancies with outreach support, and agreements with local housing providers to reduce the chance of service users losing tenancies because of their mental health problems in the first place.

Social dislocation and the psychiatrist's role

Strategic planning between commissioners, clinicians and housing providers to review and relocate people who have been placed in nursing or residential settings away from their local area and to minimise the use of such settings is increasingly encouraged and addresses the social dislocation associated with these 'out of area' placements. A whole-system approach involving all stakeholders is required to successfully reinvest the associated financial flows into local supported tenancies, often developed and managed by third sector providers. As well as avoiding further social dislocation, these approaches ensure that appropriate local facilities are developed that specifically meet the support needs of the local mental health service user population. The participation of rehabilitation psychiatrists as members of local 'placement' panels that agree and review all placements funded by the local authority and the NHS for people with complex mental health problems facilitates this process and is strongly recommended by the Royal College of Psychiatrists' Rehabilitation and Social Psychiatry Faculty.

In summary, partnerships between mental health professionals working in rehabilitation services, commissioners and providers of statutory and third sector services, local community education and leisure resources, and employers are needed, to provide an adequately flexible system that can support people with complex mental health needs to live in their local community and strengthen their opportunities for civic, social, economic and interpersonal integration.

Forensic psychiatry

Forensic psychiatrists generally accept the basic premise that social exclusion can both cause and arise as a consequence of mental health problems. Efforts to counteract social exclusion and to promote socially inclusive practice are necessary and beneficial both to the individual user of mental health services and to the wider society. Social exclusion is the hallmark of many of the individuals who end up in forensic psychiatric services and forensic patients are doubly disadvantaged as a result of severe mental illness and an offending history.

However, social inclusion and participation may be more difficult to achieve in forensic psychiatric practice, both because of the individual patient characteristics (socio-demographic, criminological and clinical) and because of the socio-political climate within which forensic services operate. Most forensic patients have been socially excluded from an early age, tend to have little by way of educational or vocational experience, little social support or social relationships, and are predominately young men with histories of previous violent or antisocial behaviour and institutionalisation.

Do forensic patients deserve to be socially included?

It could be argued that mentally disordered offenders have not only forfeited their right to social inclusion (at least temporarily) but also require some degree of social exclusion because of their crime and because of the need to manage and reduce risk to members of the public. Individuals enter and remain under forensic psychiatric care because of concern about their level of risk (often physical or sexual violence and arson) and antisocial behaviour. Part of the clinical management of that risk will necessitate excluding them from situations and opportunities to reoffend or cause further harm, including restrictions to aspects of their home life and family relationships, leisure and employment opportunities.

Although exclusion from opportunities to participate in economic, social, vocational and familial activities may be restored as and when clinical and risk factors justify it, in reality, forensic psychiatrists are only one of a number of groups and agencies working with, and taking decisions about, the social reintegration of mentally disordered offenders. Others include multi-agency public protection panels, the Ministry of Justice, the police and the probation service. There is also a high level of concern expressed about this group by the media, by politicians and by society as a whole. Even if the individual patient and their care team may consider that social inclusion and social integration is 'low risk' and is likely to benefit the mental health of the service user, this view may not be shared by other agencies.

The fact that there may be difficulties in achieving social inclusion for this group of service users is not to suggest that forensic psychiatrists can simply give up on the social inclusion agenda. Indeed, there is an argument that forensic psychiatric patients, because of their high levels of disadvantage, deprivation and stigma, may have most to gain from socially inclusive practices, particularly those that increase their opportunities for education and work (Office of the Deputy Prime Minister, 2002). For example, educational courses have been identified as the single most effective intervention in reducing shame and depression and increasing self-esteem in prisoners (Gilligan, 1999).

Juvenile and women mentally disordered offenders

With juvenile mentally disordered offenders the prospect of reversing social exclusion and alienation may be more realistic than in the adult (male) population (Bailey & Dolan, 2004). Equally, the evidence for women mentally disordered offenders suggests that they are more likely to have relatively intact social networks and be more connected to family than their male counterparts and they are less likely to be detained under a restriction order (Home Office, 2007a). Therefore, pursuing socially inclusive practices may be more realistic in terms of risk management and more feasible in those two patient groups.

The role of the forensic psychiatrist in fostering social inclusion

The key challenge, therefore, facing forensic psychiatrists is how to reconcile the rhetoric of socially inclusive practice with the reality of managing patients who are almost exclusively detained and treated against their wishes under the terms of the Mental Health Act, as much for the protection of others as for the benefits to their own health and safety. Their admission to services, continuing detention in hospital and retention in treatment after discharge generally involves an imposed and coercive arrangement (at least as perceived by the patient). Within this context it can be difficult to achieve the ideal promoted by the General Medical Council and implied by the ideas of recovery of a true 'partnership' between patient and professional, where treatment decisions are driven by the patient, as opposed to the clinician (General Medical Council, 2006). Having said this, some useful examples of recovery-oriented approaches with detained patients have been published (Dorkins *et al*, 2008; Roberts *et al*, 2008). These emphasise the importance of trying to establish a collaborative relationship, even within the restrictions and power imbalances that apply in forensic settings. The idea of the 'therapeutic use of security' reframes the restrictions placed on patients as security to enable them to engage with rehabilitation and recovery, thereby reducing the risk of reoffending. However, the fact that most forensic psychiatric patients are unwilling participants in a system of treatment that they feel is imposed on them is one that is hard to ignore or to comfortably reconcile with socially inclusive practice.

Possible areas for improvement include:

- the identification and assessment of social deficits or impairments
- explicitly addressing these deficits with targeted interventions where they contribute to social exclusion
- the evaluation of specific interventions aimed at reducing social exclusion in mentally disordered offenders
- multi-agency work and partnership which aims to improve identification and facilitation of social inclusion opportunities should be routinely incorporated into care planning.

Liaison psychiatry

The publication of the British Medical Association's *Disability Equality within Healthcare: The Role of Healthcare Professionals* (British Medical Association Equal Opportunities Committee and Patient Liaison Group, 2007) makes this an opportune moment for the development of socially inclusive practice in liaison psychiatry.

Liaison psychiatrists work in general hospitals and assess and treat diverse groups of patients: patients who self-harm; patients with primary psychiatric disorder who have developed an unrelated physical illness; patients with psychiatric disorder (including the addictions) who have developed a medical disorder (secondary to the illness or its treatment);

patients with anxiety and affective disorders with physical symptoms of uncertain attribution; patients with organic psychiatric disorders; and patients with medically unexplained symptoms.

A key barrier to the social inclusion of patients with psychiatric disorders in the general hospital is stigma and associated impediments to access appropriate medical assessment and treatment. Healthcare professionals have among the highest levels of stigmatising attitudes towards people with mental health problems (Crisp, 2004). This can lead to discrimination and hostility as a consequence of the professionals' fear and anxiety, resulting in inadequate assessment of medical symptoms and difficulties for the patient in accessing appropriate care. A further difficulty experienced by people with both mental health problems and physical illness or disability is that their comorbidity can exclude them from initiatives targeted solely at people with either mental health problems or physical health problems.

The role of the liaison psychiatrist

Liaison psychiatrists therefore have an important role in tackling stigma and discrimination in educating other health professionals about mental illness and the determinants of social exclusion and mental illness. Potential outputs from advocating for people with mental health problems in this way include increasing appropriate access to physical healthcare services for this group and increasing the identification of psychological and psychiatric symptoms manifesting physically. Both will potentially improve clinical outcomes and reduce social exclusion.

Psychotherapy

In primary care the government's initiative to develop treatment centres offering cognitive therapy to people with mild to moderate mental health problems has been spurred onwards by its appreciation of the national economic advantages of returning individuals to work as quickly and as appropriately as possible (Department of Health, 2007). These general advantages are mirrored in advantages to individuals who, if they are unable to work for any great length of time, risk social exclusion and a downward spiral of interconnected mental health and social well-being problems. Therapies that concentrate on reversing internal barriers to social inclusion, such as depression, anxiety, agoraphobia or social phobia, are critically important in helping patients to retain or regain their place in social networks and in the workplace.

Psychotherapists are increasingly aware of the need to engage socially disadvantaged groups and have developed culturally sensitive models of delivering psychotherapy. Psychotherapists working in secondary care have also focused on patients with personality disorders, who are often marginalised both in mental health services and in the wider society (Department of Health, 2003).

91

The role of the psychotherapist

Challenges for psychotherapy services remain in dealing with socially disadvantaged groups. The standard contract of many psychotherapeutic treatments involves regular (often weekly) attendance and either formal or informal reflection time between appointments. For individuals with chaotic lives, problems with transport, financial difficulty or previous experiences of services that were unreliable this treatment format may prove unattainable, feel irrelevant, or seem inappropriately demanding. For this reason promoting a psychotherapeutic stance in all mental health workers as well as developing adapted forms of psychotherapy are important tasks for psychotherapists.

More generally, a psychotherapeutic approach that values the creativity and resilience of the human spirit without minimising or denying disadvantage and disability is central to the success of the recovery model. The routes to social inclusion and personal well-being taken by individuals whose past or present experience is that of discrimination, disadvantage or exclusion may not follow the standard or socially conventional pattern. People find creative but idiosyncratic ways to rebuild their lives and the psychotherapeutic attitude in mental healthcare services can help in valuing and supporting them on what can sometimes be very individual journeys.

Child and adolescent psychiatry

Much of the work of child and adolescent psychiatrists is in the understanding of complex presentations and in explaining these to the adults involved with the child as well as the child him- or herself. If child and adolescent psychiatrists aim to help vulnerable children becomes 'mainstream', they must design services to reflect the strengths of existing social agencies and develop collaborations. In many areas, children's health services are organisationally linked to social and education services with this very aim in mind (Mackinnon *et al*, 2008). Child and adolescent mental health services need to be aware of the potential of some interventions at their disposal that have the capability of reducing the likelihood of later adult exclusion as well as improving clinical outcomes (Scott *et al*, 2001a,b), and of the need to foster resilience in children during early development.

Contextual approach

This work cannot be done well without having a keen sense of the child's context. Children whose problems are considered to be 'treatment resistant' may represent an inappropriate draw into treatment that can potentially exacerbate the child's social exclusion by inappropriate 'pathologisation' of their behaviours and presentation. It is imperative that the contextual aspects of the child's existence are taken into account before considering whether an intervention is appropriate. Therefore, inclusive practice is a core skill for child and adolescent mental health service professionals to acquire in order to ensure that therapeutic initiatives do not founder.

The role of the child and adolescent psychiatrist

Child and adolescent mental health professionals have a responsibility to ensure that disadvantaged young patients and their families receive the attention that they require at any age or stage of development. For such efforts to flourish, child and adolescent psychiatrists must be mindful of their patients' position in society and learn to value this information in forming plans for assessment and treatment. Given the inadequacy of current service provision for excluded groups, they might also adopt a useful campaigning role within their organisation.

The mental health of children and young people is recognised as a major public health issue that has a profound effect on the functioning of the individual, the family and the broader society. Unfortunately, despite the existence of effective treatments, it has not been demonstrated that psychiatric services have an impact on reducing the overwhelming amount of childhood psychiatric disorder in our communities. Substantial progress may not be made until service provision for children and young people is revised to include all the relevant social agencies and there is new thinking about the nature of successful outcomes. Good practice in mental health is by definition socially inclusive and will aim to address the needs of children and adolescents close to where they live.

Psychiatry and older adults

Old age psychiatrists aim to enable the older person to continue to live their life as they wish, maintaining a maximum degree of independence despite any functional impairment consequent on their mental health problem and/or cognitive decline. For older people social exclusion is compounded by: age discrimination (the prevailing belief that older people have little to contribute and are a burden on their kinfolk in particular and society in general); deteriorating physical health and physical impairment; loss of roles following retirement; reduced social networks and social isolation (including death of partner and friends). Therefore, professionals working for the mental health of older people have a particular challenge in maximising the social inclusion of their clients.

Older patients and community resources

When older people present to mental health services, this offers an opportunity not only for a comprehensive assessment of their mental and physical health, leading on to appropriate treatments, but for reviewing with them aspects of their life situation and lifestyle that they might consider modifying in the wider interests of their long-term health. Old age psychiatrists and the teams they work with have knowledge and experience of local community resources that can be used by older people with potential benefit to their health and general well-being. It is important that people are encouraged and supported to use local resources where possible, rather than becoming dependent on mental health facilities. To do this sensitively necessitates a flexible, person-centred, family-friendly approach. Psychiatrists will have a lead role in establishing and maintaining this philosophy and encouraging collaborative links with, and knowledge of, local community resources for their patients.

Socially inclusive practice involves supporting older people with mental health problems to continue to contribute to society as citizens in their own way, to remain as independent as possible, and supporting their family and carers to support them.

Everybody's Business, the government's guide to the development of integrated mental health services for older people, is also concerned with recovery and social inclusion for this group (Department of Health & Care Services Improvement Partnership, 2005):

> Staying mentally and physically active gives a sense of purpose and personal worth, as well as enabling people to make an effective contribution to their communities. Participating in valued activities can also provide opportunity for social contact. Hobbies and leisure activities, lifelong learning, as well as volunteering, employment, and engagement in the development or delivery of local services should all be supported (p. 13).

The document stresses the importance of:
- respect and dignity
- purpose and meaning in life
- a person-centred approach
- improving quality of life
- social networks and combating social isolation
- ensuring financial security
- access to adequate housing
- providing people with the integrated support and assistive technologies they need to live independently at home in so far as is possible, and
- care in residential settings that promotes social inclusion.

The role of the old age psychiatrist in supporting people with dementia

For people with dementia the challenge is to facilitate that person living as valued and meaningful a life as possible for as long as possible. This involves considering the person to be living with, not dying from, dementia. Services should help them to do the things they value for as long as possible, preserving a sense of personhood even as their cognitive faculties deteriorate and celebrating the person's achievements in life and their legacy for future generations. Advance directives can assist carers to adhere to the person's preferences if they are unable at a later stage of their illness to state these for themselves. There is also a need to help the family to discover new sources of value and meaning for themselves, in their loved one and in their relationship with them. Services should be oriented to support the person to remain living in their home for as long as possible in order to maintain their local support networks, familiar surroundings and community participation. This may well involve providing tailored and innovative care packages. If a move to a more supported setting becomes necessary, its distance from the person's social support network should be taken into account as well as its provision of appropriate clinical care.

Addictions

It is generally accepted that people with serious substance misuse problems also suffer significant social exclusion, and that facilitating their social inclusion is a key component of successful management. Medical treatment of alcohol dependence probably contributes about a third towards eventual outcomes, the rest being attributable to self-help and social change (Raistrick *et al*, 2006). One of the key indices of success in methadone maintenance treatment for opiate dependence is duration of treatment (Simeons *et al*, 2002). The treatment provides a relatively safe setting against which patients can achieve over time some degree of social reintegration, through employment, housing and re-establishing of family relationships.

Government's guidelines and the role of the addiction psychiatrist

The UK drug strategy document (Department of Health, 1998) outlines four principle aims that could increase social inclusion:

1   preventing drug use among young people
2   safeguarding communities
3   providing treatment
4   reducing availability of drugs.

These are to be achieved through education, prevention programmes, expanded treatment and legal sanctions. The strategy was updated in 2002 with an increased emphasis on reducing the use of class A drugs (Department of Health, 2002). The Audit Commission (2004) assessed the local impact of the drug strategy and recommended that although treatment has improved, organisations responsible for providing housing, social care and other support services need to ensure that their services are appropriate and help the individual become employed, housed and more self-sufficient. It is therefore clear that addiction psychiatrists need to work in collaboration with multiple agencies (including the police, probation and judicial services, Social Services, local pharmacies, GPs, and statutory and third sector providers of housing and employment programmes) in order to improve the social inclusion of their service users.

The Audit Commission (2004) report suggests that those locally responsible for such services must do more to deliver coherent and tailored services but that they face short-term funding and a disjointed regulatory framework. The underlying assumption behind these recommendations is that social inclusion is a critical component of the recovery process.

Examples of initiatives that are relevant to socially inclusive work with people with addictions include Supporting People (Sullivan, 2004), which aims to improve access to housing for vulnerable individuals, and Progress2work (Dorset *et al*, 2007), aimed at helping drug users find employment. Various criminal justice measures, such as arrest referral workers and drug and alcohol rehabilitation requirement orders (Home Office, 2007*b*) aim to keep people in the community and to encourage reintegration. All these measures have been shown to have some positive effect.

Learning disabilities

A strong values base related to social inclusion has underpinned service development for people with learning disabilities over the past 30 years. More recently, the *Valuing People* strategy (Department of Health, 2001) set out aspirational values for the future lives and service delivery for all people with learning difficulties, stressing the need for socially inclusive practice. Their rights as citizens, inclusion in local communities, choices in daily life and real chances for independence were highlighted. In addition, the strategy detailed that access to appropriate mainstream primary and secondary physical and mental healthcare, social care and other services should be determined through principles and approaches that are needs-led and patient-centred, in a multi-professional and inter-agency manner.

The role of the psychiatrist of learning disability

In some localities, people with learning disabilities and mental health needs access mainstream and specialist mental health services that have varying degrees of social and service inclusion planning, facilitation or joint working with learning disability services. That may be true for service users with borderline or mild learning disabilities, limited verbal communication skills and comorbidities such as severe mental health problems, Asperger's syndrome, attention-deficit hyperactivity disorder, alcohol and substance misuse, personality disorders, autism, dementia, and complex genetic or neuropsychiatric disorders including epilepsy, with or without challenging or offending behaviours. However, such individuals require access to specialist, community-based, out-patient, in-patient and secure learning disability services.

The psychiatry of learning disability has become a discipline in which there is improved credibility and job satisfaction associated with recovery-based practice and service models. There are strong drivers for inter-agency social inclusion initiatives in which a broad range of individuals work together as multi-professional teams championing socially inclusive practices.

Further, local and national whole-systems delivery of the *Valuing People* strategy should include supporting social inclusion and appropriate access to specialist and mainstream services for people with learning disabilities. The person-centred planning assessment, frameworks and processes for review that are currently facilitated mainly by learning disability services, paid carers, advocates and families should also embrace the principles of social inclusion.

Conclusion

There are specific challenges for the subspecialties of psychiatry in promoting social inclusion for their clients, but there are complementary strengths among these specialties to do so. These derive from the wealth of experience in understanding the factors and systems associated with service users, families and carers, services, policies and wider society that influence social exclusion for specific disadvantaged and particularly socially excluded service user groups. This expertise can, and in many cases already does, manipulate these systems and addresses these factors to increase awareness of socially inclusive practices, often in collaboration with multiple other agencies. The ongoing challenge is to build socially inclusive practice into routine mental healthcare.

Summary

Socially inclusive approaches raise a number of different issues for each of the main subspecialties of psychiatry. The overarching theme for all the patient groups is the stigma associated with the presence of mental health problems plus the low levels of understanding, tolerance and awareness in society, which leads to these groups being excluded. There are challenges and rewards for all the subspecialty areas in adopting recovery and socially inclusive practices.

References

Audit Commission (2004) *Drug Misuse 2004: Reducing the Local Impact*. Audit Commission.

Bailey, S. & Dolan, M. (2004) *Adolescent Forensic Psychiatry*. Hodder Arnold.

British Medical Association Equal Opportunities Committee and Patient Liaison Group (2007) *Disability Equality within Healthcare: The Role of Healthcare Professionals*. BMA.

Crisp, A. H. (2004) *Every Family in the Land: Understanding Prejudice and Discrimination against People with Mental Illness*. Royal Society of Medicine Press.

Department of Health (1998) *Tackling Drugs to Build a Better Britain*. TSO (The Stationery Office).

Department of Health (2001) *Valuing People: A New Strategy for Learning Disability for the 21st Century – Long Report* (White Paper). HMSO.

Department of Health (2002) *Updated Drugs Strategy*. TSO (The Stationery Office).

Department of Health (2003) *Personality Disorder: No Londer a Diagnosis of Exclusion. Policy Implementation Guidance for the Development of Services for People with Personality Disorder*. Department of Health.

Department of Health (2007) *Improving Access to Psychological Therapies: Specification for the Commissioner-Led Pathfinder Programme*. Department of Health.

Department of Health & Care Services Improvement Partnership (2005) *Everybody's Business: Integrated Mental Health Service for Older Adults. A Service Development Guide*. Department of Health.

Dorkins, E., Roberts, G., Wooldridge, J., *et al* (2008) Detained – what's my choice? Part 2: Conclusions and recommendations. *Advances in Psychiatric Treatment*, **14**, 184–186.

Dorset, R., Hudson, M. & McKinnon, K. (2007) *Progress2work and Progress2work-LinkUP: An Exploratory Study to Assess Evaluation Possibilities*. Department for Work and Pensions.

General Medical Council (2006) *Good Medical Practice*. General Medical Council.

Gilligan, J. (1999) *Violence: Reflections on Our Deadliest Epidemic*. Jessica Kingsley Publishers.

Home Office (2007a) *The Corston Report: A Review of Women with Particular Vulnerabilities in the Criminal Justice System*. Home Office.

Home Office (2007b) *Working Together to Cut Crime and Deliver Justice: A Strategic Plan for 2008–2011*. Home Office.

Liberman, R. P. & Kopelowicz, A. (2002) Recovery from schizophrenia: a challenge for the 21st century. *International Review of Psychiatry*, **14**, 245–255.

Mackinnon, J., Pate, J. & Fischbacher, M. (2008) *Managing Partnerships for Improving Health and Well-Being: Research Summary for East CHCP Children's Services. Case Study 2: The Child and Adolescent Mental Health Team*. Greater Glasgow and Clyde NHS (http://library.nhsggc.org.uk/mediaAssets/CHP%20East%20Glasgow/6%20CAMHs%20Case%20Study%20Report%202008.pdf).

Office of the Deputy Prime Minister (2002) *Reducing Re-Offending by Ex-Prisoners. Report by the Social Exclusion Unit*. Office of the Deputy Prime Minister.

Raistrick D., Heather N. and Godfrey C. (2006) *Review of the Effectiveness of Treatment for Alcohol Problems*. National Treatment Agency.

Roberts, G., Dorkins, E., Wooldridge, J., *et al* (2008) Detained – what's my choice? Part 1: Discussion. *Advances in Psychiatric Treatment*, **14**, 172–180.

Scott, S., Spender, Q., Doolan, M., *et al* (2001a) Multicentre controlled trail of parenting groups for child antisocial behaviour in clinical practice. *BMJ*, **323**, 194–197.

Scott, S., Knapp, M., Henderson, J., *et al* (2001b) Financial cost of social exclusion: follow up study of antisocial children into adulthood. *BMJ*, **323**, 191–194.

Simeons S., Matheson C., Inkster K., *et al* (2002) *The Effectiveness of Treatment for Opiate Dependent Drug Users: An International Systematic Review of the Evidence*. Effective Interventions Unit, Scottish Executive Drug Misuse Research Programme.

Sullivan, E. (2004) *Review of the Supporting People Programme*. Office of the Deputy Prime Minister.

Part 2

Social exclusion:
the scope of the problem

CHAPTER 7

The extent of disadvantage, poverty and social exclusion in the UK

Jed Boardman and Kwame McKenzie

Poverty and disadvantage matter as they are costly to individuals, communities, society and the economy. Importantly, their effects can be passed across generations, producing a future stream of disadvantaged individuals. The areas of peoples' lives that are affected include those of prime importance to health and social services: physical and mental health, well-being, education, employment, antisocial and self-destructive behaviour, material hardship, abusive family and personal relationships, social isolation, stigma, lack of control, shame and low self-esteem. Poverty and disadvantage result in poor health, just as poor health can result in poverty and disadvantage. Conditions of poverty and disadvantage also provide the context in which mental health services operate and can limit the success of health and social interventions. In this chapter we will begin to paint a picture of disadvantage, poverty, and social exclusion in the UK at the beginning of the 21st century, before going on in the subsequent chapters to examine how people with mental health problems and learning disabilities sketch on to this canvas. We will examine some of the objective measures of exclusion and the extent to which the population of the UK is disadvantaged as well as the changes that have occurred over the past 20 or more years. Levels of disadvantage in Black and minority ethnic groups are highlighted.

The extent of disadvantage, poverty and social exclusion in the UK

Recent changes in the UK

During the 20th century there were huge changes in the quality of life for most people in the UK and we now experience better standards of living, health, education and housing than we did in 1900. Although the great giants of 'Disease, Ignorance, Squalor, and Idleness' described by Beveridge (Timmins, 1995: p. 23) have been reduced in the UK, they are still highly relevant for a proportion of the population. The patterns of poverty, disadvantage and equality changed drastically in the 1980s, producing levels of poverty and inequality unprecedented in the post-war years (Stewart *et al*,

2009). On average the British people became richer during the 1980s and 1990s: between 1983 and 1998/1999 the average income rose by 51% (after housing costs), from £9932 per year (£191 per week) to £15028 per year (£289 per week) (at February 2000 prices) (Gordon *et al*, 2000). Regrettably, not everyone has shared the benefits of improvement and prosperity; for example, the incomes and wealth of the richest people in the UK increased considerably over the 1980s and early to mid-1990s, while the incomes and wealth of the poorest declined in real terms after accounting for inflation and housing costs (Department of Social Security, 2000). Between 1979 and 1996, the share of the total national income taken by the bottom 10% dropped from 4% to 2%, whereas the share taken by those at the top 10% rose from 21% to 28% (Pantazis *et al*, 2006). These changes are reflected in dramatic increases in the Gini coefficient, a measure of income inequality, from 1980 onwards, despite there being little change seen in this in the 1960s and a gradual fall seen in the 1970s. Internationally, the UK and the USA had the largest rises in income inequality during the 1980s and 1990s. These UK rises in income inequality and poverty may be partly explained by rises in unemployment, large differences in rises in earnings between rich and poor, and changes in government policy (Stewart *et al*, 2009).

Since 1997/1998 there have been variable changes in poverty and disadvantage, with some indices improving and others remaining stationary or declining (Hills *et al*, 2009). Notably, these changes were greater in the 5 years after 1997 and many of these initial improvements have slowed since 2002 (Hills *et al*, 2009). In general we have seen the first sustained rise in living standards across all groups since the 1960s or 1970s (Hills *et al*, 2009). This contrasts to the 1980s, when most rises were seen in higher income groups and income growth at the bottom was very slow. However, some care is required when examining the rise in incomes since 1997, as the results of the analysis depend on the actual percentiles into which the income distribution is divided (Sefton *et al*, 2009). For example, between 1997 and 2006/2007 if the population is divided into income groups of fractions of 20%, then the growth in incomes across these groups has been relatively flat, at or around 2%, suggesting that everyone has benefited. Notably, most of this rise was seen between 1996/1997 and 2001/2002 (about 3%) and has been less than 1% since that time, with most growth in the middle income groups.

On the other hand, if the more extreme ends of the income spectrum are examined over the same period, then greater inequalities of income are seen. For example, the share of income going to the richest 10% of the population has grown by 3%, with no changes in the poorest 10%. These differences in wealth in the population are most starkly seen between the bottom 2%, whose wealth has not changed, and the top 2%, who have seen large increases in their wealth (Palmer *et al*, 2003, 2007). For the income groups in the top 10% there have been continued rises since 1997 at a rate much faster than those experienced by the rest of the population – the top 1% experienced still faster growth and the top 0.1% the fastest of all (Sefton *et al*, 2009).

These unequal distributions of income are not evenly spread across the country. For example, the proportions of the richest fifth and the poorest fifth living in various parts of Britain vary, with the east and south-east of England and outer London having the highest proportion of the richest fifth. Inner London is deeply divided, having the highest proportion of people on a low income, but also one of the highest proportions of those on high income (Palmer *et al*, 2003, 2007).

These findings are reinforced in a report from the National Equality Panel which was commissioned by the British government (Hills *et al*, 2010). Although the Panel found systematic differences in economic outcomes between social groups (men and women, ethnic groups, social classes, disadvantaged and other areas, London and other parts of the country), the differences in outcomes between the more and less advantaged within each social group are much greater than differences between groups. This suggests that even if the differences between groups disappeared, the country would remain almost as unequal overall.

Poverty

The official UK government indicator of poverty is low income and this is a relative measure of poverty. Low income is considered to be the household income that is 60% or less of the average (median) household income for that year. What this means in monetary terms will depend on the year in question, the family size and other adjustments. For example, the incomes shown in Fig. 7.1 are measured after income tax, council tax and housing costs have been deducted, where housing costs include rents, mortgage interest (but not the repayment of principal), buildings insurance and water charges. This means that they represent what the household has available to spend on everything else it needs, from food and heating to travel and entertainment. In 2007/2008, the 60% threshold was worth: £115 per week for a single adult with no dependent children; £199 per week for a couple with no dependent children; £195 per week for a single adult with two dependent children under 14; and £279 per week for a couple with two dependent children under 14 (see www.poverty.org.uk).

Poverty in the UK, as measured in this way, reached a historic high in the 1990s. In 1979 there were 7 million poor people in Britain, but by 1997 this had risen to 13.8 million. Figures monitored by the Joseph Rowntree Trust (www.poverty.org.uk) show that the number of people below the poverty income threshold fell between 1998/1999 and 2004/2005 to 11.4 million, with the first rise occurring in 2005/2006 and 2006/2007 (Fig. 7.1). In 2007/2008 there were 13.4 million people in the UK (just over 22% of the population) living in poverty. If a 50% threshold of median income is used, a similar pattern is seen, with increases in the three most recent years following decreases throughout the previous 8 years. In 2007/2008, 9.3 million people or 15% of the population living in households at or below this income level (Fig. 7.1). However, a different picture is seen for those

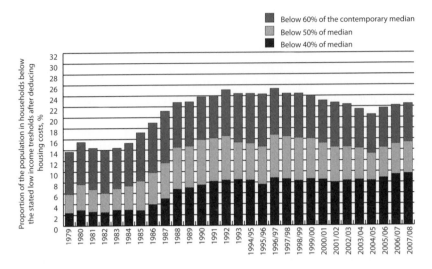

Below 60% of the contemporary median

Below 50% of median

Below 40% of median

Fig. 7.1 Households in poverty in the UK, 1979–2008. Source: Joseph Rowntree Foundation, The Poverty Site Key Facts.

on even lower income levels (40% of median income). These levels varied only slightly throughout the 1990s and have risen in the three most recent years; they are now the highest since records began in 1979 – 5.7 million people were living in households on these very low incomes in 2007/2008. The number of people on low income is still lower than it was in the early 1990s, but much greater than in the early 1980s. For some this is a long-term experience with around 20% of the population (over 10 million people) experience poverty for at least 2 years in 3 and 10% experience this over 3 consecutive years (Palmer *et al*, 2003, 2007).

Over the 10 years up to 2007 the proportion of children and pensioners living in poverty fell, while the proportion of working age adults in poverty remained almost unchanged until 2006/2007, when child, pensioner and overall poverty rates rose (see Figs 7.1–7.3). The UK has a higher proportion of the population with a relative low income than most other EU countries – only five of the 27 EU states have a higher proportion than the UK (Hirsch, 2006*a*). Poverty is related to other forms of disadvantage, some of which are illustrated in Box 7.1. Poverty as a measure of poor material circumstances has a direct effect on health (Townsend & Davidson, 1982). Older calculations show the healthy living minimum income to be £131.86 per week (range £106.47–163.86) UK April 1999 prices, higher than the UK minimum wage after statutory deductions or the basic benefit rates (Morris *et al*, 2000; Deeming, 2005).

Trends in child poverty

The UK government has highlighted the problem of child poverty and has set targets for its reduction and eradication (Hills & Stewart, 2005; Joseph

Box 7.1 Disadvantage in the UK (2005/2006 and 2007/2008)

- In 2007/2008 13.4 million people (22% of the population) in the UK were living in poverty. Poverty had risen during the 1980s and 1990s but began to fall after 1990, only to begin to rise again after 2005
- 3.8 million children lived in poverty in 2005/2006. Since 1998/1999 this has fallen by 600 000, leaving 500 000 above the government's 2004/2005 target. In 2007/2008 this figure rose to 4 million
- Half of these children are in jobless families and two-fifths live with lone parents
- In 2007/2008, 2.1 million children lived in low-income households where at least one adult works – the highest it has ever been
- 1.5 million young adults aged 16–24 years lived in poverty in 2005/2006
- The rate of poverty in adults who are disabled is 30%, twice the rate among those not disabled; this gap has increased over the past 10 years
- Unemployment in adults aged over 25 years fell from 1.6 million in 1996 to 0.9 million in 2006, with large falls in long-term unemployment. The rate for young adults (19–24 years) was 11.5% in 2006, a rise since 2004 (9.5%) and three times the rate of unemployment in older workers
- In 2009 the number of people unemployed or othewise wanting work was the highest since 1997. Unemployment among 16- to 24-year-olds was higher than at any point since 1993. These increases did not begin with the recession: unemployment has been rising since 2005, and the young adult unemployment rate stopped falling in 2001
- In 2005/2006, 11% of 16-year-olds obtained fewer than five General Certificates of Secondary Education (GCSEs), the same as in 1999/2000
- About 25% of 19-year-olds have not been qualified at National Vocational Qualifications (NVQ) level 2 or above over the past 10 years. If people do not reach NVQ2 by age 19 years, they are unlikely to do so in the next few years
- However, by 2008 the proportion of 11-year-olds not meeting basic standards in mathematics and English had fallen every year since the late 1990s. The number of 16-year-olds getting fewer than 5 GCSEs was lower than at any point in the previous 10 years
- In 2006, 15% of men and 20% of women lived in a household with no car. Households without a car are more likely to report difficulties accessing local services than those with one
- In 2005/2006, 25% of women aged over 60 years reported feeling very unsafe walking alone at night (four times the rate for men). In lower-income households, 30% of women and 10% of men reported feeling very unsafe walking alone at night. Overall, by 2009 about 15% of adults in England and Wales said they were very worried about being a victim of violent crime and about 10% said they were very worried about being burgled – half the levels of a decade earlier
- The proportion of households without a bank account in 2005/2006 was 6% for the poorest fifth and 3% for households with average incomes, a reduction over recent years
- Half of households in the poorest fifth lack home contents insurance, nearly three times the level for households with average incomes and the same as a decade ago.

Source: Palmer *et al* (2007); MacInnes *et al* (2009).

Rowntree Foundation, 2005). In 1999 the government announced their intention to wipe out child poverty in a generation, aiming to halve it between 1998/1999 and 2010/2011 and to eradicate it by 2020 (Hirsch, 2006*b*); eradication of child poverty also has international significance (UNICEF, 2007).

A key feature of the changes in levels of poverty over the past 30 years is that children have replaced pensioners as the group most at risk of poverty. Of the 11.4 million poor in 2004/2005, children and their parents made up 6 million. In 1970, nearly half of the poor were pensioners, though this has now fallen to one in six (Fig. 7.2). Still, many single and older pensioners remain susceptible to poverty as they often live just above the poverty threshold (Sefton *et al*, 2009).

As with the overall level of poverty, the number of children living in poor households rose between the 1970s and mid-1990s. In 1968, about 55% of children would have been defined as living in poverty by recent standards (living in households below half of average 1995/1996 income, adjusted for inflation). This fell to 36% by 1979 and remained at this level in 1995/1996, although the general standards of living rose over this 16-year period (Gregg *et al*, 1999).

Since the late 1990s the number of children living in poverty has gradually fallen, from 4.4 million in 1998/1999 to 3.8 million in 2005/2006. Yet this fall was lower than the government target of 3.1 million (www.poverty.org. uk) (Fig. 7.3). In 2007/2008, 4.0 million children in the UK were living in low-income households (after deducting housing costs) – this is 0.4 million (10%) less than in 1998/1999, but back up to the levels of 2001/2002. Despite a general lowering of the levels of child poverty, children are still much more likely to live in low-income households than the population as a whole – 31% v. 22%. In 2004/2005 bout a fifth of children lived in households with incomes 50% below the median income. This figure showed only a small reduction since 1998/1999 (Hirsch, 2006*b*) (Fig. 7.4).

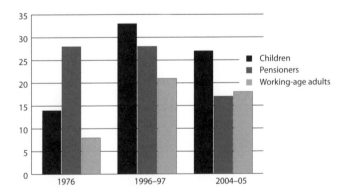

Fig. 7.2 In the past generation, children have become the group most at risk from poverty. Source: Hisch (2006*b*: p. 14); Department for Work and Pensions (2006).

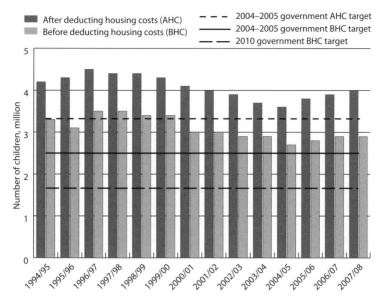

Fig. 7.3 Number of children in households below 60% of median income. Source: Joseph Rowntree Foundation, The Poverty Site Key Facts.

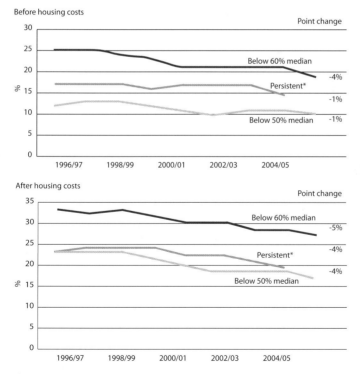

Fig. 7.4 Child poverty rates since 1996/97 showing severe and persistent rates. *Below 60% median in at least 3 of past 4 years. Source: Hirsch (2006*b*: p. 18).

107

Some poor children experience only temporary adversity, but others remain poor over several years. In 2004/2005, 16% of children had lived in persistent poverty (below 60% median income) for at least 3 of the past 4 years (Hirsch, 2006b), a reduction from 24% since 1998/1999 (Fig. 7.4).

The changes to child poverty are linked to changes in the number of families living without work. Between 1968 and 1995/1996, the proportion of all children with no working parent rose from 2% to 10% of those in two-parent families and from 30% to 58% of the children of lone parents. In 1968 workless families accounted for a third of all poor children, but by 1995/1996 that figure had risen to account for 54%. Over the same period the proportion of poor children living in lone-parent families rose from 19% to 43% (Gregg et al, 1999). Ten years later, 42% of poor children were in lone families. Half of lone parents are on low incomes, compared to one in five working age couples with children. The risk of low income for a child varies according to how much paid work the family does, and unless all adults are working (and at least one full time) the risks of being in poverty are high: 90% for unemployed families, 75% for other workless families and 35% for those where the adults are working part-time. A total of 78% of lone parents in low-income households are not working, compared with 26% of couple families with low income (www.poverty.org.uk). In the mid-1990s the majority of poor children were in workless families, but this pattern has changed. For children in low-income families, the number who are in working families is higher than in the mid-1990s; more than half (56%) of all poor children now live in families where at least one of the adults is in paid work. This changing pattern is due to increased rates of low income among working families and a decreased number of children in workless families. Now most of the children in low-income households are either in couple families where someone is in paid work or in workless lone-parent families (www.poverty.org.uk).

Extending poverty to encompass other associated disadvantages, the Social Exclusion Task Force (HM Government, 2006; Cabinet Office, 2007) has focused attention on families who experience multiple problems. About 2% of families experience problems in five or more of the following domains: no parent in work; living in poor-quality or overcrowded housing; no parent with a qualification; mother with health problems; parent with long-standing limiting illness; disability or infirmity; low income (less than 60% of median household income); cannot afford some essential items. These families are likely to be living in social housing, have a mother whose main language is not English, be a lone parent or have a young mother. Compared with families who do not experience multiple problems the children are likely to be experiencing difficulties at school (poor performance, school suspension), poor social networks outside the home and problems with the police (Cabinet Office, 2007).

Rates of child poverty are similar in England, Scotland and Wales, but may be higher in Northern Ireland (Hirsch, 2006b). Inner London has a far higher proportion of children in low-income families than any other part of Britain. Half of all children in inner London are in low-income households compared with a third in the next worst affected region (outer London) (www.poverty.org.uk).

There are stark differences in the rates of children in households receiving benefits across the 10061 electoral wards in Britain. In all, 56% of children are in such households in the 100 most socially disadvantaged wards, half of which are in Glasgow, Liverpool, London and Manchester. In 300 wards at the other end of the spectrum fewer than 10 children per ward are in benefit-receiving households. The remainder of wards are 'average', with 21% of children in this situation (Hirsch, 2006b). The Families and Children Study in 2005 showed that there is a greater concentration of families with multiple problems in deprived areas of England (Cabinet Office, 2007) (Fig. 7.5).

The UK's experience of a large rise in child poverty since 1980 to well above the adult rate is not a universal problem. Compared with other countries in the EU, the UK has high rates of child poverty (60% below the median income), with only Italy, Portugal and Slovakia having higher rates (Hirsch, 2006b). In a comparison of material well-being (using indices of the proportion of families below 50% median income, households without jobs, and reported deprivation) for children in 21 nations in the industrial world (Organisation for Economic Co-operation and Development countries), the UK was fourth from the bottom (UNICEF, 2007). These differences between the UK and other countries may be due to the relatively large proportion of children living in households without work, pay inequality affecting parents who do work, and a less redistributive tax and benefits system than in other countries (Hirsch, 2006b).

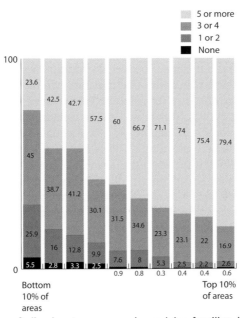

Fig. 7.5 Number of disadvantages experienced by families in England. Source: Cabinet Office (2007), data from the Families and Children Study (2005).

Longitudinal views of poverty and exclusion

The figures presented above provide a relatively up-to-date report on the state of disadvantage in the UK today. However, what would be useful is information that combines both measures of poverty and other measures of social exclusion and provides us with a clear longitudinal view of how states of exclusion may change or remain persistent for people. Several national surveys can be used for these purposes (Levitas *et al*, 2007) and two in particular will be used here as they offer an analysis of poverty and exclusion at several points in time: the Poverty and Social Exclusion (PSE) Survey in Britain (Gordon *et al*, 2000; Pantazis *et al*, 2006) and the British Household Panel Survey (BHPS) (Barnes, 2005).

Poverty and Social Exclusion Survey

This is the most comprehensive survey of poverty and social exclusion carried out in Britain, giving a view of poverty over the 1980s and 1990s. It was designed to replicate two previous national surveys (the 'Breadline Britain' surveys) carried out in 1983 and 1990. The survey was carried out in 1999 and included a follow-up survey of a subsample of respondents to the 1998/1999 General Household Survey. Its measure of poverty was based on socially perceived necessities and a systematic definition of deprivation. It also measured subjectively assessed poverty and several dimensions of social exclusion. The survey was concerned with the impact of poverty and lack of paid work on the quality of life of the population and social relations.

Poverty

Thirty-five items were considered by 50% or more of the population to be necessary for an acceptable standard of living in Britain at the end of the 20th century. These included: beds and bedding for everyone, heating to living areas of the home, damp-free housing, two meals a day, medicines prescribed by the doctor, a refrigerator. Taking these necessary items and using a poverty threshold that was set at lacking two or more of these necessities due to lack of income, 58.1% of people lacked no necessities, 14.2% lacked one necessity and 27.7% lacked two or more necessities.

When the person's income was taken into consideration 25.6% were considered as poor. In addition, 10.3% were considered vulnerable to poverty and 1.8% had risen out of poverty. Thus, about 14 million people were living in poverty in Britain in 1999; the chief characteristics of this group are summarised in Box 7.2.

Similar figures were found for subjective poverty. When asked whether their income was below the level necessary to keep them out of general poverty (£219 per week after tax) and absolute poverty (£178 per week after tax), 20% of households considered themselves to be in general poverty and 17% in absolute poverty. Lone parents, single pensioners and single adults were all highly represented in these poverty groups.

For older people, there appear to be two groups that vary in the degree that they experience poverty and social exclusion: a better-off group made up of younger pensioners living in households with their spouse, and a worse-off group, often women living alone, who experience much higher levels of poverty and exclusion (Patsios, 2006). Other studies have suggested that poverty rates are especially pronounced in socially deprived urban communities and among key minority ethnic groups (Scharf *et al*, 2002). Further data on older people can be found in the English Longitudinal Study of Aging (Barnes *et al*, 2006) and in Scharf *et al* (2002).

Child poverty

Child poverty was studied separately. Children were considered in poverty if they lacked two or more items or activities from an agreed list, including toys, three meals a day, out-of-school activities, adequate clothing; 18% were poor in this way (34% if lacking one or more item was considered). The characteristics of the families of these necessity-deprived children are shown in Box 7.2.

Box 7.2   Poverty in adults and children in Britain

Groups making up a high proportion of those living in poverty:

- non-retired people who are not working because they are unemployed or sick and disabled
- those on income support
- lone parents
- local authority tenants, housing association tenants
- divorced or separated
- those with three or more children
- those with youngest child 0–4 years old or 5–11 years old
- households with one adult
- younger people: 16–24 years old or 25–34 years old
- those finishing education before age 16 years
- geographical distribution was not even across the country: highest rates in Wales, London and the Midlands.

Characteristics of necessities-deprived children:

- live in jobless households
- one or more in the household works part-time
- lone parents
- three or more children in the household
- parents with long-standing illness
- live in local authority housing
- on income support or job seeker's allowance
- families with lower incomes.

Source: Poverty and Social Exclusion Survey (Gordon *et al*, 2000)

Growth of poverty in Britain

Comparison of the three PSE surveys in 1983, 1990 and 1999 showed that the proportion of households that could not afford one item did not change overall between 1990 and 1999 and changed only by 0.5% between 1983 and 1999. If lacking three or more items is considered to define poverty, then between 1983 and 1990 the number of households who are poor increased by about a half, from 14% to 21%, and that rose to 24% by 1999.

Long-term poverty

The long-term poor were defined as households who had deprivation scores of three or more (lacking three or more items) (objective poverty), who considered themselves to be generally 'poor all the time' (subjective poverty), and who had lived in poverty in the past either 'often' or 'most of the time'. Altogether, 4% of households were long-term poor in 1990 and this fell to 2.5% in 1999.

Social exclusion

In addition to poverty, three other areas of social exclusion were recorded:

1   exclusion from the labour market
2   service exclusion: utility services (gas, electric, water, telephone), public services (e.g. hospitals, libraries, post offices) and private services (e.g. corner shops, banks, pubs), and
3   social relations: visiting friends, relatives, schools, celebrations; isolation; support; civic engagement (voting, helping fund raising, member of club or society).

The main findings from the PSE survey of exclusion in these areas are shown in Box 7.3.

It is worth trying to summarise the numbers of people excluded using the figures shown in Box 7.3. Levitas (2006) did this by taking eight of the dimensions (poverty, lack of paid work, living in jobless households, service exclusion, non-participation in social activities, social isolation, poor social support, civil and political disengagement). She found that 22% of the population were excluded in four or more of these dimensions. Joblessness is very common among these and may be better considered as a risk factor for exclusion rather than a direct indicator of exclusion. In general, individuals in work have lower poverty rates than those not in work and full-time workers have lower rates than part-time workers (Bailey, 2006). The main obstacle to using services was lack of availability and unsuitability, rather than affordability, but poorer households face poorer quality services and poverty reinforces constraints on service usage. Further, the use of services was only weakly related to participating in social and civic activities, but was more strongly related to being in a poor or jobless household. For example, 22% of people in jobless households and 25% of those with low incomes were excluded from three or more services (Fisher & Bramley, 2006).

Box 7.3   Social exclusion in Britain

Labour market:

- 43% of the population have no paid work
- many of these people are retired, others are sick or disabled or engaged in domestic or caring activities
- 3% are unemployed
- one in three of the population live in a jobless household (pensioner household 21%, jobless non-pensioner household 13%).

Service exclusion:

- 6% experienced disconnection of gas, water, electricity or telephone
- 11% used less than they needed as they were unable to afford more ('restricted consumption')
- 24% were excluded from two or more services as they were either unaffordable or unavailable
- only 54% had access to a full range of services
- lack of availability (33%) rather than lack of affordability is the main barrier to use (10%)
- older people tended to be more at risk of lack of access (52% one or more services, 29% two or more).

Those at risk were:

- households with children (7% had disconnections, 15% restricted consumption)
- people with long-standing illness were more likely to have restricted consumption (17%)
- non-pensioner jobless (14% had disconnections, 31% restricted consumption)
- unemployed (20% had disconnections, 33% restricted consumption).

Of those people with long-standing illness and disability:

- one in three had difficulty using services such as cinema, museums, shops, restaurants
- one in six had problems arranging accommodation or insurance or using banks, building societies and telephones.

Social relations:

- only 63% can afford a full range of social activities
- 1 in 120 were excluded by lack of money in five or more activities (20% three or more, 27% two or more activities)
- holidays, going out, eating out are activities most likely to be curtailed by lack of money
- especially affected are the unemployed, jobless non-pensioner households, households with children, young adults aged 16–34 years, people over 65, poorer families.

Isolation:

- 41% do not have at least one non-household family member with whom they speak on a daily basis and 9% have no family member whom they speak to weekly
- 1% have no effective family contact outside the household (no family member they speak to at least once a year)

Box 7.3   *(contd)*

- 28% have no friend with whom they are in contact with on a daily basis, 8% have no friend with whom they are in contact with at least weekly, 3% have no friend they speak to at least yearly
- just over 1% of respondents (all men) have neither a family member nor friend with whom they are in contact at least weekly
- lack of contact is more common in jobless or pensioner households.

Lack of support:

- 54% of the population expected to be able to call on 'some' or 'a lot of' support in all seven categories of practical and emotional support listed in the survey
- 23% lacked support in at least four out of the seven categories
- 10% had no support or support in only one category.

Social participation/disengagement:

- 17% had not engaged in any civic activities in the past 3 years
- the most common type of civic engagement was voting (65–73%)
- 41% were not presently a member of any form of civic engagement
- members of sports clubs (18%) or religious groups (12%) were most common
- altogether, 88% were engaged in some way but 12% were not – but if voting is removed then this figure rises to 30%.

Source: Poverty and Social Exclusion Survey (Gordon *et al*, 2000; Pantazis *et al*, 2006).

Poverty inhibited participation in social activities. Although high proportions of people claimed that they were not participating because they did not want to, rather than because they could not afford to, those below 60% of median household income were three times more likely not to participate in seven or more activities than those with higher incomes. Low income may restrict participation progressively and may reinforce not wanting to participate or produce disinterest (Levitas, 2006). Social networks did not differ radically between rich and poor, although contacts were biased towards the family for the poor and friends for the non-poor. However, poor people had weaker practical and emotional supports than others; inferior support was experienced by working age jobless households and pensioner households and the lowest levels were reported by those living alone.

British Household Panel Survey

Similar figures for exclusion were found using different survey material from the British Household Panel Survey (BHPS). This national survey of adults has been conducted since 1991. It contains information collected on the same individuals annually for the repeated waves of the study. Barnes (2005) chose seven indicators of social exclusion in his analysis of the BHPS for the nine waves of data from 1991 to 1999 on adults of working age (Box 7.4). He examined cross-sectional measures of disadvantage from the 1996 wave and longer-term measures using all nine waves from 1991 to 1999.

Box 7.4   Main findings of the British Household Panel Survey 1991 to 1999 (Barnes, 2005)

Single indices of disadvantage (1996 survey)

Proportion of population having disadvantage in any one of the areas:

- financial situation – individual lived in a household with income below the 'absolute poverty' threshold (as in the PSE survey), 16%
- material possessions – individual lived in a household disadvantaged on material possessions (television, freezer, washing machine), 9%
- housing circumstance – individual lived in a household with disadvantaged housing circumstances (heating, overcrowding), 11%
- neighbourhood perception – individual wanted to move because of neighbourhood-related problems (isolation, traffic, safety, noise), 12%
- social relations – individual lacked social support (someone to listen, crisis help, someone to comfort), 9%
- physical health – individual had physical health problems or disabilities (in past 12 months), 15%
- mental health – individual had mental health problems (scores seven or more on the GHQ–12), 10%

Multiple indices of disadvantage (1996 survey)

0 areas	49%
1 area	30%
2 areas	14%
3 areas	5%
4 or more areas	3%

- Being below the disadvantage threshold on any one of the seven indicators leads to an increased likelihood of being disadvantaged according to at least one of the other six
- Those who experienced disadvantage in three or more areas were particularly likely to have mental health problems
- People experiencing one form of disadvantage had a greater likelihood of experiencing another form of disadvantage.

Long-term persistent disadvantage (all nine waves of BHPS, 1991 to 1999)

Disadvantage in seven or more of the waves:

Financial situation	6%
Material possessions	4%
Housing circumstance	6%
Neighbourhood perception	2%
Social relations	3%
Physical health	6%
Mental health	1%

Long-term persistent and multiple disadvantage (all nine waves of BHPS, 1991 to 1999)

1 area	16%
2 areas	4%
3 areas	1%
4 or more areas	0.5%

GHQ, General Health Questionnaire; PSE, Poverty and Social Exclusion.

As with the PSE survey, providing summary indicators of exclusion can be difficult, but from the data used in the BHPS, three main summary domains of social inclusion were derived using a factor analysis of the cross-sectional and longitudinal data:

1   household economic deprivation (elements were: financial situation, material possessions, housing circumstance)

2   personal civic exclusion (elements were: neighbourhood perception and social relations), and

3   personal health exclusion (elements were: physical and mental health).

In 1996, 16% of people were excluded through household economic deprivation (5% on all three elements), 19% through personal civic exclusion (2% in both elements) and 21% through personal health exclusion (3% in both elements). As with the PSE survey, these domains of exclusion were linked. Those with household economic deprivation were likely to be out of work and to live in households where no one worked. An experience of personal civic exclusion was linked to being unemployed, a lone parent with dependent children and being physically ill or disabled. Personal health exclusion was more likely to be experienced by those who had a poor income ('income-poor') and minimal education.

A small but significant number of people had persistent (over 9 years) and multiple disadvantage. For example, for household economic deprivation, 4% were persistent in both financial and material deprivation, whereas 5% were persistent in financial plus housing. For personal civic and personal health exclusion, 3% and 4% respectively were persistent on both elements.

Exclusion in specific groups: rural communities and women

A significant minority of households live in poverty in the British countryside (Milbourne, 2006). For example, in 1980/1981, 25% of households in five areas of rural England were living in, or on the margins of, poverty (McLaughlin, 1986) and by 1990/1991, 23% of households in 12 areas of rural England (including the five studied in 1980/1981) were living thus (Cloke *et al*, 1994). In rural Wales in 1991/1992, 27% of households were living in poverty (Cloke *et al*, 1997) and in 2004, 25% of households had incomes less than 60% of the median income level (Milbourne & Hughes, 2005). In rural Scotland in 1995 65% of households had incomes below the Low Pay Unit's low pay threshold (Shucksmith *et al*, 1996).

These rural populations also showed evidence of exclusion (Milbourne, 2006): 33% had no central heating, 21% had no washing machine, 23% had no telephone. When access to services was considered, 23% (38% in poor households) had limited mobility resulting from long-term illness and 11% (32% in poor households) had no access to private vehicles.

In rural Wales in 2004, nine out of ten rural communities had no access to local support services for the unemployed, homeless, people with drug problems or women experiencing domestic violence. However, most people, including the poor, identified high levels of social and community capital (Milbourne & Hughes, 2005).

Overall, women are more likely to experience poverty than men; the 1999/2000 Family Resources Survey showed 25% of the female population in Britain were living in households with an equivalent income less than 60% of the median (compared with 22% of men) and lone mothers and older single women are most likely to experience poverty (Bradshaw et al, 2003). There is a gender pay gap, with most jobs done by women tending to be low-paid, women tending to work part-time and to have their employment interrupted by child birth and caring responsibilities (especially those with low educational qualifications). Women are paid 21% less in terms of median hourly pay than men and, allowing for shorter working hours, the weekly earnings of women in full-time employment are 22% less than those of men (Hills et al, 2010). Women's disadvantage in the labour market continues to have an impact after retirement (Bradshaw et al, 2003). There has been some improvement in the pay gap over the past 15 years; for example, the median net individual income for women rose from 53% of that for men in 1995–1997 to 64% in 2006–2008 (Hills et al, 2010).

Social exclusion and poverty

The above findings suggest that a considerable number of people in the British population were in poverty and were excluded at some time during the 1990s, some of them on multiple indices, and that this picture had not changed significantly since the early 1980s despite increases in overall prosperity. What is clear is that these disadvantages are not randomly distributed among the population and that some groups are overrepresented, for example women, the jobless, older people, single parents, people with long-term sickness and those who are disabled. Poverty and lack of employment do seem to contribute significantly to social exclusion. It is difficult to come up with definitive figures for the numbers of people excluded as the assessments of disadvantage and associations between the different dimensions are sensitive to the actual definitions and thresholds used (Burchardt, 2000). It does appear that exclusion is not a single entity and is better seen according to the different dimensions or elements outlined above.

For many households the experience of poverty is unpleasant but relatively brief and there are relatively few people who experience persistent and multiple disadvantages and are cut off from the principal activities of mainstream society for an extended period of time (Burchardt, 2000; Levitas et al, 2007). This suggests that social exclusion is more of a process than a state and that it may be a transient, recurrent or more long-term experience. But the figures may hide some of the repeated instances of poverty and exclusion experienced by people. In a separate analysis of the first five waves (1991–1995) of the BHPS, Burchardt (2000) found no evidence for significant long-term exclusion, but she did show that many more people suffered exclusion over time than did in any single year and that there was a continuum on each of the exclusion dimensions between those experiencing exclusion in a single year and those excluded for 2, 3, 4 or 5 years. In addition, long-term exclusion on a single dimension was associated with a greater risk of multiple exclusion. People with low incomes at each of the first four waves were 3.5 times more likely to be excluded on one dimension by wave five than those who had never been poor.

People with multiple disadvantages do seem to be at most risk of exclusion. For example, the likelihood of being out of work increases with the number of disadvantages experienced by an individual: more than half of those with three or more labour market disadvantages were out of work compared with only 3% of those with no disadvantages (Berthoud, 2003).

The studies quoted above are all household surveys which may omit some people who are at most risk of social exclusion, such as those living in institutions, those in prison, children in local authority care or young offenders institutions, some disabled people, older adults living in residential homes, asylum seekers and the homeless. In addition, the surveys, although otherwise comprehensive and extensive, do have relatively small samples which do not allow sufficient subgroup analysis (for example, of some minority ethnic groups). This may account for the lack of evidence for long-term and severe (or 'deep') exclusion in the household surveys such as the BHPS (Burchardt, 2000; Levitas et al, 2007). Specific focused surveys are required to examine the smaller groups and the groups that are omitted from larger surveys.

From the examples given above, the overlap of poverty and ill health is apparent and those defined as poor had significantly higher scores on the 12-item General Health Questionnaire than those who were not (PSE survey). Occurrences of physical ill health appear to increase the likelihood of mental ill health: 29% of those who had persistent physical ill health also had mental ill health and this was four times higher than those who experienced no physical health disadvantage (Barnes, 2005).

The profile of the poor and excluded outlined above presents a familiar picture to those working with people who have long-term mental illness or people working in specialist teams such as those for the homeless or refugees or asylum seekers, many of whom have the demographic characteristics of the poor. Those working with children and families and older people will also find the characteristics familiar.

People at risk of exclusion

The focus of the Social Exclusion Task Force (HM Government, 2006; Cabinet Office, 2007) has been on a relatively small group of people at high risk of exclusion, but there are larger numbers of people who face problems that could be reasonably described as exclusion.

Kenway & Palmer (2006) identify three groups with two different but overlapping kinds of problems. The first type of problem is for people in incomplete transition: those who have failed to reach the minimum educational standards at ages 16 and 19 and beyond and who as a consequence face higher risks of low income, unemployment and worklessness. The other group with these problems is those who are unable to find affordable housing, only some of whom are homeless. The second type of problem is insecurity: a core set of problems for people who live alone, are disabled (including those with mental disorders) and live in workless households, all of whom are dependent on support from family and friends who do not live with them.

In the government's drive on tackling poverty and social exclusion the reduction of child poverty has been set as a national target. There are no targets for working age poverty, older people's poverty, for the population as a whole or for overall inequality (Joseph Rowntree Foundation, 2005).

There is often a conflict between raising standards for all and reducing differences between disadvantaged groups and others, and so overall improvements in health and educational achievements have sometimes left the most disadvantaged even further behind.

Disadvantage matters: future outcomes and future generations

The UNICEF (2007) report not only ranked the UK as having one of the highest rates of child poverty among the major industrialised nations, but also one of the lowest rates of child well-being (Black & Jeffery, 2007). These poor rates of well-being are correlated with income inequality across the 23 rich countries (Pickett & Wilkinson, 2007). The evidence is that poverty and other forms of disadvantage in early life increase the likelihood of disadvantage in later life and that these disadvantages may be transmitted across generations. People who have grown up poor are more likely to face adverse social and economic circumstances well into adulthood. Even before children reach school, the effects of class differences are already apparent, differences that may be hard to break later (Feinstein & Bynner, 2004; Sinclair, 2007).

Poverty itself is associated with worklessness, financial problems and debt, which may lead to housing problems, relationship conflict and breakdown, and ill health caused by stress (Kempson et al, 2004; Pleasence et al, 2007). Lack of education and skills increases the chances of being unemployed and having a poor earning capacity (HM Treasury, 2006; Cabinet Office, 2007). Poor housing is associated with ill health (Vostanis & Cumella, 1999), family and school disruption (Mitchell et al, 2004) and increased risk of being on the Child Protection Register. These may reinforce barriers to children getting ahead in later life and contribute to experiences of worklessness, offending behaviour, mental health problems or institutionalisation. Children born into the particularly disadvantaged households identified by the Social Exclusion Task Force (Cabinet Office,

2007) may be at particularly high risk of these problems. In a study in New Zealand (Fergusson *et al*, 1994), 22% of children born to the 5% most disadvantaged families had multiple problems at age 15, compared with 0.2% of children born to the 50% most advantaged families.

The consequences of harm caused by poverty to children's development seem to be growing in the long term. Successive cohort studies indicate an exacerbating effect on people's life chances. The relative impact on adult outcomes of experiencing poverty as a teenager doubled between the cohort who were children in the 1970s (now in their 40s) and those ten years younger (now in their 30s) – the latter became adult in a riskier world. There is a strong association between parental income and the child's subsequent earnings as an adult (Ermisch *et al*, 2001). Gregg *et al* (1999), using the 1958 cohort of the National Child Development Survey, showed that young adults who as children had lived in poor households, were in trouble with the law or played truant had significantly greater than average chances of earning low wages, being unemployed, spending time in prison (men) or becoming a lone parent (women). Whereas education was thought to be important as a 'transmission medium', the disadvantages identified had a significant impact over and above their effect on education. Of the family-based measures of childhood disadvantage, poverty was found to be the most important factor linking childhood development with subsequent social and economic outcomes. For example, being brought up in a lone parent family does not seem to matter in the absence of family poverty. The link between a person's social class and birth and the probability of multiple deprivations by age 30 years has also been shown in the 1970 cohort (Fig. 7.6).

The National Child Development Survey also suggested an intergenerational link in the cycle of family disadvantage. In situations where parents had themselves grown up in socially disadvantaged situations, the average cognitive ability of their children was lower than those whose parents were more advantaged. This link may spill over to affect the subsequent economic fortunes of the children of disadvantaged individuals. A similar effect on cognitive outcomes has been clearly demonstrated by

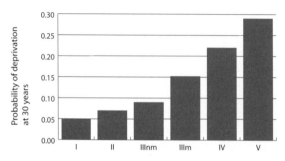

Fig. 7.6 Probability of multiple deprivation at 30 years, by birth socioeconomic status (1970 cohort study). Source: Feinstein (2008).

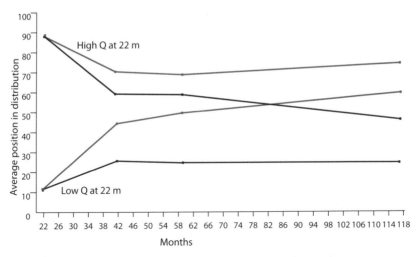

Fig. 7.7 Relative cognitive shifts in children, from 22-month-old to 10-year-old. Source: Feinstein (2008).

Feinstein (2003) using the 1970 birth cohort (Fig. 7.7), showing that poor cognitive performance at 22 months can improve in children born into more privileged families, but not in those from disadvantaged families, and indeed cognitive functioning of more able children in these families at 22 months may decline by the time children are 10 years old.

Health inequalities

Health inequalities are a central concern of this book and are associated with factors of deprivation discussed earlier, including socioeconomic status, gender and geographic location. These inequalities are pervasive and have not been reduced over the past three decades (Sassi, 2009). Some current examples are shown in Box 7.5.

The problem of social inequality in health is not confined to the poorest members of society; rather, there is a social gradient of mortality and morbidity across the whole of society (Siegrist & Marmot, 2006). In general, the gradient varies across the life course (steepest in early childhood and mid-life) and between men and women (generally steeper among men). The size of the inequality varies across countries and according to the measure of social status adopted. The differences between social groups are most pronounced for highly prevalent chronic disorders (e.g. cardiovascular disease, type 2 diabetes, respiratory disorders) and less pronounced for neurological disorders, some cancers and gastrointestinal diseases. Some disorders (e.g. breast cancer and asthma) follow the opposite gradient and rise with social status.

One important shift in the approach to health inequalities over the past 20 years has been the increasing realisation that although poverty is directly

---

Box 7.5   Inequalities in health – some examples in the UK

- In 2005, the infant death rate in England and Wales was 5.4 per 1000 live births from manual social backgrounds and 3.8 per 1000 in those from non-manual social backgrounds. The rates have fallen slightly since 1996 but the gradient has remained
- In 2005, children from manual social backgrounds in England and Wales were 1.5 times more likely to be of low birth weight (8.5%) than those from non-manual backgrounds (6.5%). The rates in both groups have not substantially changed over the past decade.
- Babies of lone parents are more likely to be of low birth weight (10%) than babies born to couples (7%)
- Rates of premature death (death before age 65) is twice as high in men as in women
- Premature death is much higher in Scotland than anywhere else in the UK, particularly among men
- The two single most common causes of death in people aged 55–64 years are heart disease and lung cancer; rates of these are much higher among people from manual than non-manual social backgrounds. This is the case for both men and women.

Source: Joseph Rowntree Foundation, Poverty Site Key Facts.

---

related to poor health, in rich countries it is the inequalities of income that are most strongly related to life expectancy and levels of morbidity, mortality and well-being, with average income level having a much weaker relationship to ill health (Wilkinson, 1996; 2005; 2006; Wilkinson & Pickett, 2009).

> Mortality rates in the developed world are no longer related to per capita economic growth, but are related instead to the scale of income inequality in each society. This represents a transition from the primacy of material constraints to social constraint as the limiting condition on the quality of human life (Wilkinson, 1994: p. 61).

This implies a limit to the effects of improving overall income level beyond which they have little impact on health and suggests that just raising the living standards of the poorest will not reduce these inequalities in the absence of attempts to reduce the inequalities in wealth. This is particularly pertinent in the UK with its unprecedented increases in income inequality since the 1970s and may explain the failure to improve health inequalities over that period.

Inequalities in health in the UK widened during the 1980s and 1990s (Shaw *et al*, 2005) and have not decreased over the past 15 years (Sassi, 2009). Inequalities in life expectancy between poor and rich areas of the UK widened in the first years of the 21st century (Shaw *et al*, 2005) and have exposed some stark disparities: for example, in the Calton area of Glasgow the life expectancy at birth for men is 54 years, whereas in Lenzie only a few kilometres away it is 82 years (WHO, 2008).

This approach to health inequalities has focused attention on the social inequalities of health and the effects of psychosocial factors such as anxiety and depression, self-determinacy, insecurity, control, and social affiliations and hierarchies in explaining these health gradients. The WHO Commission on the Social Determinants of Health has examined the link between health and social stratification. It highlighted the inequalities in health and their relation to social justice as well as the harmful effects of gender inequality, discrimination and social exclusion on health (Davey-Smith & Krieger, 2008; WHO, 2008). The Commission acknowledges the limits of economic growth and dependence on markets as means of improving health and instead recommends improving the daily living conditions of people through attention to children's early development, providing healthy living conditions, decent work and employment, social protection through the lifespan and universal healthcare. It also recommends tackling the inequitable distribution of power, money and resources and improving basic data systems to assist policy and programmes to improve the education and training of professionals. All these recommendations are consistent with attempts to improve social inclusion.

There are social inequalities in mental ill health, which we will return to in the next chapter, and the relationship between ill health and income inequality also applies to mental health problems (Pickett *et al*, 2006). Although social class may be an inconsistent marker for common mental disorders, there are more consistent associations with unemployment, low education levels, and low income or material standard of living (Fryers *et al*, 2003). Disadvantaged adult socioeconomic position has been shown to be related to depression and anxiety in longitudinal (Rodgers, 1991; Poulton *et al*, 2002; Stansfeld *et al*, 2008) and cross-sectional studies (Lewis *et al*, 1998; Muntaner *et al*, 1998). Functional psychoses are unequally distributed by social position, a consistent finding in many studies (Foster at al, 1996; Murray *et al*, 2003; Morgan *et al*, 2007).

Social exclusion of Black and minority ethnic groups

In this section we examine the available data on the social exclusion of Black and minority ethnic groups. Their exclusion in a mental health context will be covered in Chapter 9.

The Black and minority ethnic population of the UK numbered 4.6 million (7.9% of total population) at the last national census in April 2001. Detailed information on these groups can be found in a series of reports from the Office of National Statistics, *Focus on Ethnicity and Identity* (2004) which are summarised in Box 7.6. People of Indian origin represent the largest group, followed by those of Pakistani origin, those of mixed ethnic backgrounds, Black Caribbeans, Black Africans and Bangladeshis. The remaining minority ethnic groups each account for less than 1.5% of the UK population.

The Black and minority ethnic population in the UK is diverse; the different groups have different histories, age structures and socioeconomic

Box 7.6   Black and minority ethnic groups in the UK – main sociodemographic characteristics

Population size: 7.9% of the UK population are from a Black and minority ethnic group

Age/gender distribution: Black and minority ethnic groups are younger

Geographic distribution: 45% of Black and minority ethnic people live in London

Inter-ethnic marriage: 2% of marriages are inter-ethnic

Households: Asians have largest households

Religion: seven in ten identify as White Christian

Identity: nine in ten of mixed group identify as British

Education: Chinese pupils have best GCSE results

Labour market: Black and minority ethnic unemployment highest

Employment patterns: Pakistanis most likely to be self-employed

Health: Asians have worst self-reported health

Care: one in ten White and Indian people provide unpaid care

Smoking and drinking: Bangladeshi men have highest smoking rates

Victims of crime: highest risk for mixed-race people

Housing: Indians most likely to own their homes

Geographic diversity: Brent council, in north London, is the most ethnically diverse area in the UK

Source: Office for National Statistics (2004)

and cultural contexts. Considering age, the White Irish group have the oldest age structure, with 25% aged 65 and over, whereas perhaps not surprisingly the 'mixed' group have the youngest age structure, with 50% under the age of 16.

Any comparison between Black and minority ethnic groups and the White British group is also complicated by the fact that the former are concentrated in the large urban centres – 78% of Black Africans, 61% of Black Caribbeans and 54% of Bangladeshis live in London.

Reliable and good-quality information on these groups across the UK is difficult to find. General surveys would need large sample sizes to provide detailed analysis of each group, especially in less populous areas. Because of this targeted surveys are required but these are often not performed. For matters of policy, if you are not counted, you do not count. This lack of good information can itself exacerbate social exclusion. The general rule in evidence-based policy making is that there need to be data that quantify the problem as well as some data on what can be done about it before policy is set. An example would the suicide in Black and minority ethnic groups. Place of birth, not ethnicity, is collected on death certificates. Because at least half of the UK Black and minority ethnic population were born here, they are not in fact counted as Black and minority ethnic. This makes it difficult to estimate the rate of suicide in any Black and minority ethnic group in the UK and the problem is getting worse because year on year a greater percentage of the Black and minority ethnic population is born in the UK. The lack of easily available data undermines the building of evidence about the rates of suicide and interventions. Because of this when the UK national suicide prevention strategy was set there were no specific plans for decreasing suicide rates in Black and minority ethnic groups (McKenzie et al, 2008).

There are many reasons why people from Black and minority ethnic groups in the UK are likely to suffer social exclusion. Recent immigrants may need some time to find their feet in another country and culture, and those who speak another language face an additional barrier to inclusion. For those who have been in the UK for some time, who were born in the UK or whose parents were born in the UK the reasons for the exclusion are more complex. It is initiated and sustained at least in part by inequalities in access to education, employment and the receipt of welfare benefits and social services as well as differential treatment because of ethnic minority status.

Within Black and minority ethnic groups the problems and markers of social exclusion, unemployment, poor skills, low incomes, poor housing, high crime and family breakdown are mutually reinforcing. There is an intergenerational component in that the poor socioeconomic status or poor mental health in one generation can undermine the chances of the next. But in addition the stresses and strains of migration and acculturation may be an extra burden. Without clear opportunities to break the cycle and with external pressures of discrimination multiple disadvantages can accrue (Office for National Statistics, 2004).

The specific disadvantages experienced by particular ethnic groups vary. It would be erroneous to present the 'Black and minority ethnic experience' as if this was the same for all groups. It is, however, reasonable to assert that in general, UK citizens from Black and minority ethnic groups are under significant socioeconomic strain – 70% live in the 88 most deprived local authority wards (Office of the Deputy Prime Minister, 2004).

Resources

There is little information available on economic resources by ethnic group. Economic resources reflect the resources of the country of origin, the social cohesion of the group and the educational achievements of the group. One index is home ownership (measured by whether a person in the census was living in a home which was owned by them or their family) and the figures vary widely.

Most minority ethnic groups are less likely to own their own home than the White British, with Black Africans the least likely group to own their own home. Those of Indian and Pakistani origin have the same level of home ownership as the White British (over 70%) but this may not reflect a similar level of resources in the different communities because the households of these South Asian origin groups are on average larger than other households in the UK. Overcrowding is an important issue. At the last census the rate of overcrowding in the Bangladeshi and Black African households was seven times as high as that of White British households. Levels of overcrowding are not explained by household size alone. They may be related to poverty, the need to rent and the availability of suitable housing in different parts of the country (Office for National Statistics, 2004).

It is generally accepted that access to public services and the standards of care received are different for different ethnic groups. The Race Relations Amendment Act 2000 gives public services formal duties to produce equitable services and to promote good race relations. The concept of institutional racism has been used to help public services understand how their unintentional actions can lead to disparities. In healthcare, disparities in access and equity of efficacy are well documented. The annual UK patient survey gives some insight into the experience of Black and minority ethnic groups in the NHS: the 2008 and 2009 reports are similar (Department of Health, 2009).

There are areas where the experience of Black and minority ethnic groups is more positive than White British groups but in general where differences exist the former are more likely to have a negative experience. Different groups have different levels of satisfaction in various healthcare settings but in general Black and minority ethnic individuals were less positive about questions relating to 'access and waiting' or to 'better information and more choice' in most healthcare settings, with the starkest differences in the primary care survey (Department of Health, 2009). In psychiatry we have considered the impact of institutional racism (see Chapter 9) on mental healthcare and have made great strides. It is of note that the patient survey singles out the community mental health survey as a place where differences between ethnic groups was least evident.

Education

Culture, education and skills also offer some information on disparities, but the picture is again complex (Office for National Statistics, 2004). Both Chinese boys and girls achieve the highest GCSE grades in the UK. They are followed by pupils of Indian origin, those of Irish origin and then White British. The lowest attainment is by Black Caribbean boys and girls. School exclusions are a particular problem. Children from the 'Other' Black and Black Caribbean groups are over three times more likely to be excluded from school than White children; Indian pupils are four times less likely to be excluded than Whites. The permanent exclusion rates for pupils from the other Black, Black Caribbean and mixed White and Black Caribbean groups were 42 pupils per 10000, 41 per 10000 and 37 per 10000 respectively. These were up to three times the rate for White pupils (14 per 10000).

Chinese and Indian pupils had the lowest exclusion rates, at 2 or fewer pupils excluded per 10 000.

There are significant differences in the educational levels of different groups in the workforce. These are complex. For instance, although the Chinese group are most likely to have a degree (31%), a relatively high proportion have no qualifications (20% v. 27% and 15% respectively for White British (Office for National Statistics, 2004; Department for Education and Skills, 2006).

Employment

More information is available on the economic participation of Black and minority ethnic individuals (Office for National Statistics, 2004). The picture is mixed but essentially they are less likely to be economically active, more likely to be unemployed and are paid less than the White British. Unemployment is a problem for Black and minority ethnic groups (Hills et al, 2010). The rates of unemployment in the latter are generally higher than for White individuals in all but Indian men, who have a similar level of unemployment to White men. Women are particularly at risk, with an unemployment rate three to five times that of the White British group, topped by Pakistani women, who have the highest unemployment rate in the UK. For men, Black Caribbean, Black African, Bangladeshi and mixed ethnic groups have the highest unemployment rates, around three times the rates for White British men.

Another area where differences between ethnic groups arise is economic activity. People of working age from Black and minority ethnic groups are less likely to be available for work or looking for work (economically inactive). Reasons for this could include being a student, disabled or a carer. The balance of reasons for economic inactivity is different for different groups and between genders. They may reflect cultural practices, with up to 75% of Bangladeshi and Pakistani women classed as economically inactive, mainly looking after their family or home, compared with say 25% inactivity in White British women (Office for National Statistics, 2004). Further, although Chinese men are twice as likely to be economically inactive as White British men, this reflects the fact that the former are more likely to be students. There is, however, evidence of prejudicial practice in employment, where people with apparently Asian or Caribbean names are less likely to be offered a job or be invited to an interview than those with other names even if the rest of their CV is the same (Hills et al, 2010).

Employment itself is concentrated in particular industries. For instance, 60% of Bangladeshi men and nearly 50% of Chinese men work in the distribution, hotel and restaurant industry compared with just over 15% of White British men. Pakistani men are concentrated in the transport and communication industry or are self-employed and White Irish men nearly twice as likely work in the construction industry than others. About 10% of Black African women and one in seven of 'other' Asian (as defined in the

Office for National Statistics document) women work as nurses, compared with around 1 in 30 White British women. This may reflect the availability of work at the time of migration or a selection bias towards those who are able to travel or who have certain occupational skills (Office for National Statistics, 2004).

The level of occupation varies by ethnic group and mirrors in part the shape of educational attainment. Some ethnic groups are more likely to be employed in managerial or professional occupations (Chinese, Indian, White Irish and other non-British White groups) than British White people and others are less likely (Black Caribbean, Black Africans and Bangladeshis).

Social support

Social support varies significantly between ethnic groups. People of Caribbean origin are most likely to live alone and have lower levels of social support than other groups, whereas people of South Asian and East Asian origin have the highest levels of social support. Although refugee and asylum seeker groups have low levels of social support, recent permanent migrant groups such as those of Bangladeshi origin have high levels of social support.

Health and well-being

People from certain Black and minority ethnic groups are more likely to report poor health (Office for National Statistics, 2004). This is not accounted for simply by socioeconomic factors. The reasons for poorer health in any particular group are complex. They are an interaction between vulnerabilities to specific illnesses, the context in which people live and prevailing access to health promotion and prevention. Cultural practices and diet may be important in some instances but they are generally unlikely to be as important as an increased exposure to risk factors which are known to have an impact on all groups. The poorer and more recently migrant South Asian individuals (Pakistani and Bangladeshi) reported the highest rates of 'not good' health in the last census. The importance of this statistic is that people who report poor health are more likely to use health services and have a higher mortality rate. These groups had the highest rates of disability, at around 1.5 times higher than their White British counterparts.

The information that we have on the comparative health of Black and minority ethnic groups and the reasons for this is growing. However, problems with data and with the tools we use to assess health and well-being are a concern. One reason is that methods of measuring quality of life are often ethnocentric and do not address the challenges of understanding what a fulfilling life means across cultural groups (Collinge et al, 2002).

Different ethnic groups have different lifestyles. Some of these are built into their culture but most are an interaction between their socioeconomic and migrant group status. Bangladeshi, White Irish and Black Caribbean men are more likely to smoke cigarettes than the general population (Office for National Statistics, 2004), yet for all but the Black Caribbean group, women from Black and minority ethnic populations smoke less than the general population. On the other hand, chewing tobacco is particularly prevalent in Bangladeshi women. Smoking is strongly related to a person's socioeconomic status, with lower social classes being more likely to smoke.

Fifty eight per cent of men and 37% of women from a White Irish background in the UK drink in excess of the government recommended guidelines (Office for National Statistics, 2004). Traditionally, alcohol is not considered a problem for Black and minority ethnic groups, but more detailed analyses find that there are sub-populations within particular groups (e.g. Sikh men in London) where alcohol use is problematic.

Crime, harm and criminalisation

Crime, harm and criminalisation are matters that are often highlighted because of the reporting of crime figures by ethnic group. However, these data only tell part of the story (Office for National Statistics, 2004). People in the 'mixed' ethnic group are more likely to be victims of crime even when their socioeconomic status, age and area they live in are taken into account. Black Caribbeans and Black Africans are disproportionately represented in the prison population. It is of note that the White population is less likely to be worried about violent crime and less likely to experience it. Racially aggravated crime is a growing problem. Each year about 1% of the White population are victims of a crime they think may be racially aggravated, but this figure rises to 4% in some ethnic groups.

Racism and migrant status

Racism is a complex concept that is best considered as a mixture of discrimination by colour or perceived ethnic or national origin and power. It can occur at multiple levels – cognitive, interpersonal, between groups, in the receipt of services and in law.

Interpersonal perceived racism is the type that is usually measured. On national surveys 14% of ethnic minorities say that they have experienced serious verbal abuse or a racist attack in the previous 12 months. There are over 50 000 racially motivated crimes reported each year. Between 25% and 40% of White people in UK surveys say they would discriminate against someone who was Chinese, Asian or Black. Not surprisingly then over 60% of those from ethnic minorities believe that employers discriminate.

Racism has a number of effects on health and the determinants of health. Not only does it change personality and cognitive development, but it changes the possible trajectory of life through its impact on career progression. Socioeconomic and educational effects are reflected in the inability of some Black and minority ethnic groups to move out of multiple deprivations and poverty. Apart from the determinants of health, the effects of racism on the hypothalamic–pituitary–adrenal axis have all of the long-term effects of stress. The process has been termed 'weathering' in the US literature because African Americans seem to get most illnesses earlier (McKenzie, 2006).

Migration also has impacts on health. The reasons for migration, the process itself and the response of the host country are all important in defining the migrant experience and health status. For refugee and asylum seekers we often concentrate on pre-migration issues such as war and link these to post-traumatic stress disorder, but post-migration problems, such as being denied the right to work or being housed in a detention centre, have a greater impact on this group, with depression being by far the most common mental disorder. Acculturation, adaptation and dual cultural heritage are all significant stressors (McColl *et al*, 2008; McKenzie, 2008).

Some of the problems faced by ethnic minorities are the direct result of racism; some of them are exacerbated by racism (McKenzie, 2003). Racism and migration stress offer specific extra burdens on ethnic minority groups which lead to social exclusion.

Conclusion

Social exclusion is a reality for a considerable number of people in the UK in the 21st century. Providing exact figures for the numbers who are excluded can be difficult, not least because of the dynamic and multidimensional nature of the problem. It would, however, be reasonable to say that at least 20% of the population are excluded at any one time and up to 5% are excluded persistently and in multiple ways, as measured by the proportion of people who are unable to afford socially defined necessities. Relative poverty forms a good overall indicator of exclusion, and lack of income and material means are strong drivers of exclusion. The pervasive nature of exclusion is seen through its effects on all age groups and on the likelihood that the life chances of people brought up in excluded households are curtailed. It is also clear that it has a damaging and lethal effect on people's health and illness. Poverty and exclusion is not randomly distributed and there are deep-rooted and systematic differences between social groups. The figures emphasise matters of equality, rights, fairness and justice as exclusion shuts people off from opportunities, choices and options in life that many others in society take for granted. It causes disruption and distress to individuals and families and to the community around them, and is costly to society not least because of the waste of people's potential. These inequalities are cumulative over an individual's lifetime and are carried from one generation to the next.

Although poverty and exclusion have always been with us, the existence of absolute poverty has become rarer in the UK during the 20th century. The modern context in which poverty exists has changed and the final two decades of the last century saw a greater and increasing gap emerge between the rich and poor, with the incomes of a small number of people accelerating away in an unprecedented manner. Along with this we have seen a hardening of public attitudes towards the poor and to the tackling of poverty (Sefton, 2009), a reduction in public sympathy for poverty, an acceptance of high income inequality and little support for redistribution, along with a hardening of attitudes to recipients of benefits.

Summary

There have been improvements in the quality of life for most people in the UK and in the standards of living, health, education and housing during the 20th century. Nonetheless, there remains an unequal distribution of incomes, an increasing income gap between the richest and poorest fifth of the population and inequities across the UK.

Poverty, as measured by income levels, reached a historic high in the 1990s, and although there has been some reduction since, there remains a high proportion of children living in poor families.

For many people the experience of poverty is unpleasant, but relatively brief. Still, about 2–4% live in persistent poverty and for others poverty may be a recurrent experience. People with multiple disadvantages are most at risk of poverty and poverty is related to social exclusion. Certain people (the jobless, older people, single parents, the long-term sick and the disabled) are overrepresented in the disadvantaged groups. Disadvantage in early life increases the likelihood of disadvantage in later life and this may be transmitted across generations.

Social disadvantages are related to health inequalities for physical and mental health problems.

People from Black and minority ethnic groups in the UK are more likely to suffer social exclusion, especially if recently migrant or linguistically and culturally isolated.

References

Bailey, N. (2006) Does work pay? Employment, poverty and exclusion from social relations. In *Poverty and Social Exclusion in Britain* (eds P. Pantzalis, D. Gordon & R. Levitas). Policy Press.

Barnes, M. (2005) *Social Exclusion in Great Britain: An Empirical Investigation and Comparison with the EU*. Ashgate.

Barnes, M., Blom, A., Cox, K., *et al* (2006) *The Social Exclusion of Older People: Evidence from the First Wave of the English Longitudinal Study of Aging (ELSA). Final Report*. Social Exclusion Unit/Office of the Deputy Prime Minister.

Berthoud, R. (2003) *Multiple Disadvantage in Employment: A Quantitative Analysis*. Joseph Rowntree Foundation.

Black, M. E. & Jeffery, H. E. (2007) Child wellbeing and inequalities in rich countries. *BMJ*, **335**, 1054–1055.

Bradshaw, J., Finch, N., Kemp, P. A., *et al* (2003) *Gender and Poverty in Britain* (Working Paper Series no. 6). Equal Opportunities Commission.

Burchardt, T. (2000) Social exclusion: concepts and evidence. In *Breadline Europe: The Measurement of Poverty* (eds D. Gordon & P. Towsend). Policy Press.

Cabinet Office (2007) *Reaching Out: Think Family*. Cabinet Office.

Cloke, P., Milbourne, P. & Thomas, C. (1994) *Lifestyles in Rural England*. Rural Development Commission.

Cloke, P., Goodwin, M. & Milbourne, P. (1997) *Rural Wales: Community and Marginalisation*. University of Wales Press.

Collinge, A., Rudell, K. & Bhui, K. (2002) Quality of life assessment in non-Western cultures. *International Review of Psychiatry*, **14**, 212–218.

Davey-Smith, G. & Krieger, N. (2008) Tackling global inequalities. *BMJ*, **337**, 529–530.

Deeming, C. (2005) Keeping healthy on a minimum wage. *BMJ*, **331**, 857–858.

Department for Education and Skills (2006) *National Curriculum Assessment, GCSE and Equivalent Attainment and Post-16 Attainment by Pupil Characteristics in England 2005*. Department for Education and Skills.

Department of Health (2009) *Report on the Self-Reported Experience of Patients from Black and Minority Ethnic Groups*. Department of Health.

Department of Social Security (2000) *Households Below Average Income 1998/9*. Corporate Document Services.

Department for Work and Pensions (2006) *Households below average income 1994/5–2004/5*. TSO (The Stationery Office).

Ermisch, J., Francesconi, M. & Pevalin, D. J. (2001) *The Outcomes for Children of Poverty* (Research report 158). Department for Work and Pensions.

Feinstein, L. (2003) Inequality in the early cognitive development of British children in the 1970 cohort. *Economica*, **70**, 73–97.

Feinstein, L. (2008) *Life Chances and Reform of the Primary Curriculum*. Institute of Education (http://www.cabinetoffice.gov.uk/media/cabinetoffice/strategy/assets/seminars/life_chances/leon_feinstein_presentation.pdf).

Feinstein, L. & Bynner, J. (2004) The importance of cognitive development in middle childhood for adult socioeconomic status, mental health, and problem behaviour. *Child Development*, **75**, 1329–1339.

Fergusson, D. M., Horwood, L. J. & Lynskey, M. (1994) The Childhoods of Multiple Problem Adolescents: a 15-year longitudinal study. *Journal of Child Psychology and Psychiatry*, **35**, 1123–1140.

Fisher, T. & Bramley, G. (2006) Social exclusion and local services. In *Poverty and Social Exclusion in Britain* (eds P. Pantzalis, D. Gordon & R. Levitas). Policy Press.

Foster, K., Meltzer, H., Gill, B., et al (1996) *Adults with a Psychotic Disorder Living in the Community. OPCS Surveys of Psychiatric Morbidity in Great Britain. Report 8*. HMSO.

Fryers, T., Melzer, D. & Jenkins, R. (2003) Social inequalities and the common mental disorders. *Social Psychiatry and Psychiatric Epidemiology*, **38**, 229–237.

Gordon, D., Adelman, L., Ashworth, K., et al (2000) *Poverty and Social Exclusion in Britain*. Joseph Rowntree Foundation.

Gregg, P., Harkness, S. & Machin, S. (1999) *Child Development and Family Income*. Joseph Rowntree Foundation.

Hills, J. & Stewart, K. (2005) *A More Equal Society? New Labour, Inequality and Exclusion*. Policy Press.

Hills, J., Sefton, T. & Stewart, K. (2009) *Towards a More Equal Society? Poverty, Inequality and Policy since 1997*. Policy Press.

Hills, J., Brewer, M., Jenkins, S., et al (2010) *An Anatomy of Economic Inequality in the UK: Report of the National Equality Panel*. Government Equalities Office.

Hirsch, D. (2006a) *Where Poverty Intersects with Social Exclusion*. Joseph Rowntree Foundation.

Hirsch, D. (2006b) *What will It Take to End Child Poverty: Firing on All Cylinders*. Joseph Rowntree Foundation.

HM Government (2006) *Reaching Out: An Action Plan on Social Exclusion*. Cabinet Office.

HM Treasury (2006) *The Leitch Review of Skills: Prosperity for All in the Global Economy, World Class Skills*. HM Treasury.

Joseph Rowntree Foundation (2005) *Policies towards Poverty, Inequality and Exclusion since 1997*. Joseph Rowntree Foundation.

Kempson, E., McKay, S. & Willets, M. (2004) *Characteristics of Families in Debt and the Nature of Indebtedness. Research Report 21*. Department for Work and Pensions.

Kenway, P. & Palmer, G. (2006) *Social Exclusion: Some Possible Broader Areas of Concern*. Joseph Rowntree Foundation.

Levitas, R. (2006) The concept and measurement of social exclusion. In *Poverty and Social Exclusion in Britain* (eds P. Pantazis, D. Gordon & R. Levitas). Policy Press.

Levitas, R., Pantazis, C., Fahmy, E., *et al* (2007) *The Multidimensional Analysis of Social Exclusion: A Research Report for the Social Exclusion Task Force*. Cabinet Office.

Lewis, G., Bebbington, P., Brughra, T., *et al* (1998) Socioeconomic status, standard of living and neurotic disorder. *Lancet*, **352**, 605–609.

MacInnes, T., Kenway, P., Parekh, A. (2009) *Monitoring Poverty and Social Exclusion*. Joseph Rowntree Foundation.

McColl, H., McKenzie, K. & Bhui, K. (2008) Mental healthcare of asylum-seekers and refugees. *Advances in Psychiatric Treatment*, **14**, 452–459.

McKenzie, K. (2003) Racism and health. *BMJ*, **326**, 65–66.

McKenzie, K. (2006) Racial discrimination and mental health. *Psychiatry*, **5**, 383–387.

McKenzie, K. (2008) Improving mental healthcare for ethnic minorities. *Advances in Psychiatric Treatment*, **14**, 285–291.

McKenzie, K., Bhui, K., Nanchahal, K., *et al* (2008) Suicide rates in people of South Asian origin in England and Wales: 1993–2003. *British Journal of Psychiatry*, **193**, 406–409.

McLaughlin, B. (1986) The rhetoric and reality of rural deprivation. *Journal of Rural Studies*, **2**, 291–307.

Milbourne, P. (2006) *Poverty, Social Exclusion and Welfare in Rural Britain*. Institute for Public Policy Research.

Milbourne, P. & Hughes, R. (2005) *Poverty and Social Exclusion in Rural Wales*. Wales Rural Observatory.

Mitchell, F., Neuberger, J., Radebe, D., *et al* (2004) *Living in Limbo: Survey of Homeless Households Living in Temporary Accommodation*. Shelter.

Morgan, C., Burns, T., Fitzpatrick, R., *et al* (2007) Social exclusion and mental health: conceptual and methodological review. *British Journal of Psychiatry*, **191**, 477–483.

Morris, J. N., Donkin, A. J. M., Wonderling, D., *et al* (2000) A minimum wage for healthy living. *Journal of Epidemiology and Community Health*, **54**, 885–889.

Muntaner, C., Eaton, W. W., Diala, C., *et al* (1998) Social class, assets, organizational control and the prevalence of common groups of psychiatric disorders. *Social Science and Medicine*, **47**, 2043–2053.

Murray, R. M., Jonews, P. B., Susser, E., *et al* (2003) *The Epidemiology of Schizophrenia*. Cambridge University Press.

Office of the Deputy Prime Minister (2004) *Mental Health and Social Exclusion – Social Exclusion Unit Report*. ODPM.

Office for National Statistics (2004) *Focus on Ethnicity and Identity*. ONS (http://www.statistics.gov.uk/focuson/ethnicity/).

Palmer, G., North, J., Carr, J., *et al* (2003) *Monitoring Poverty and Social Exclusion 2003*. Joseph Rowntree Foundation.

Palmer, G., MacInnes, T. & Kenway, P. (2007) *Monitoring Poverty and Social Exclusion 2007*. Joseph Rowntree Foundation.

Pantazis, P., Gordon, D. & Levitas, R. (2006) *Poverty and Social Exclusion in Britain*. Policy Press.

Patsios, D. (2006) Pensioners, poverty and social exclusion. In *Poverty and Social Exclusion in Britain* (eds P. Pantzalis, D. Gordon & R. Levitas). Policy Press.

Pickett, K. E., James, O. W. & Wilkinson, R. G. (2006) Income inequality and the prevalence of mental illness: a preliminary international analysis. *Journal of Epidemiology and Community Health*, **60**, 646–647.

Pickett, K. E. & Wilkinson, R. G. (2007) Child wellbeing and income inequality in rich societies: ecological cross sectional study. *BMJ*, **335**, 1080–1087.

Pleasence, P., Buck, A., Balmer, N., *et al* (2007) *A Helping Hand: The Impact of Debt Advice on People's Lives*. LSRC Research Paper No. 15. Legal Services Commission.

Poulton, R., Caspi, A., Milne, B. J., *et al* (2002) Association between children's experience of socioeconomic disadvantage and adult health: a life-course study. *Lancet*, **360**, 1640–1645.

Rodgers, B. (1991) Socio-economic status, employment and neurosis. *Social Psychiatry and Psychiatric Epidemiology*, **26**, 104–114.

Sassi, F. (2009) Health inequalities: a persistent problem. In *Towards a More Equal Society? Poverty, Inequality and Policy since 1997* (eds J. Hills, T. Sefton & K. Stewart). Policy Press.

Scharf, T., Phillipson, C., Smith, A., *et al* (2002) *Growing Older in Socially Deprived Areas*. Help the Aged.

Sefton, T. (2009) Moving in the right direction? Public attitudes to poverty, inequality and redistribution In *Towards a More Equal Society? Poverty, Inequality and Policy since 1997* (eds J. Hills, T. Sefton & K. Stewart). Policy Press.

Sefton, T., Hills, J. & Sutherland, H. (2009) Poverty, inequality and redistribution. In *Towards a More Equal Society? Poverty, Inequality and Policy since 1997* (eds J. Hills, T. Sefton & K. Stewart). Policy Press.

Shaw, M., Davey-Smith, G. & Dorling, D. (2005) Health inequalities and New Labour: how the promises compare with the real progress. *BMJ*, **330**, 1016–1021.

Shucksmith, M., Chapman, P. & Clark, G. (1996) *Rural Scotland Today: The Best of Both Worlds*. Avebury.

Siegrist, J. & Marmot, M. (2006) *Social Inequalities in Health: New Evidence and Policy Implications*. Oxford University Press.

Sinclair, A. (2007) *0–5: How Small Children Make a Big Difference*. The Work Foundation.

Stansfeld, S. A., Clark, C., Rodgers, B., *et al* (2008) Childhood and adult socio-economic position and midlife depressive and anxiety disorders. *British Journal of Psychiatry*, **192**, 152–153.

Stewart, K., Sefton, T. & Hills, J. (2009) Introduction. In *Towards a More Equal Society? Poverty, Inequality and Policy since 1997* (eds J. Hills, T. Sefton & K. Stewart). Policy Press.

Timmins, N. (1995) *The Five Giants: A Biography of the Welfare State*. HarperCollins.

Townsend, P. & Davidson, N. (eds) *(1982) Inequalities in Health: The Black Report*. Penguin.

UNICEF (2007) *Child Poverty in Perspective: An Overview of Child Well-Being in Rich Countries*. Innocenti Report Card 7. UNICEF Innocenti Research Centre.

Vostanis, P. & Cumella, S. (1999) *Homeless Children: Problems and Needs*. Jessica Kingsley.

Wilkinson, R. G. (1994) The epidemiological transition: from material scarcity to social disadvantage. *Daedalus*, **123**, 61–77.

Wilkinson, R. G. (1996) *Unhealthy Societies: The Afflictions of Inequality*. Routledge.

Wilkinson, R. (2005) *The Impact of Inequality: How to Make Sick Societies Healthier*. The New Press.

Wilkinson, R. (2006) Income inequality and health: a review of the evidence. *Social Science and Medicine*, **62**, 1768–1784.

Wilkinson, R. & Pickett, K. (2009) *The Spirit Level: Why More Equal Societies Almost Always Do Better*. Penguin.

World Health Organization Commission on Social Determinants of Health (2008) *Closing the Gap in a Generation: Health Equity through Action on the Social Determinants of Health*. Final Report of the Commission on Social Determinants of Health. World Health Organization.

CHAPTER 8

How are people with mental health problems excluded?

Jed Boardman

From the evidence presented in Chapter 6 we can readily see that many people with mental health problems and those with learning disability are likely to be represented in the areas of disadvantage illustrated. In this chapter we will examine this further across all age groups and types of mental health problems and detail the ways in which exclusion may take place. Exclusion is described across the five general areas of participation described in Chapter 3: consumption (exclusion from material resources), production (exclusion from socially valued productive activity), social interaction (exclusion from social relations and neighbourhoods), political engagement (exclusion from civic participation), health and health service engagement (service exclusion). People with mental health problems may be excluded in any one, or more, of these areas and, not surprisingly, there are associations between the factors that act as indicators of exclusion.

We are all aware that people with mental health problems are not a homogeneous group but have a range of incapacities and have varying risks and experiences of exclusion. Notwithstanding individual differences, it is generally clear that some groups are particularly at risk of exclusion, especially those who experience psychoses and those whose problems fall into multiple diagnostic categories. In this chapter I have attempted to differentiate the evidence for exclusion in people with psychoses or other severe mental health problems from those with disorders that are more prevalent in the general population, often termed the 'common mental health problems'.

In trying to find evidence for the ways in which people with mental health problems and with learning disability are excluded, a range of publications has been quoted, including both the research literature and the 'grey' literature. It is often difficult to find evidence for associations between mental health problems and material disadvantage or inequality, particularly at the population level, not because the evidence suggests that there is no association, but because there is a lack of published evidence. In the UK this has been partly remedied by the British national surveys of psychiatric morbidity (Melzer *et al*, 2004). In Chapter 7 it was noted that the gap between the rich and the poor in UK society measured by income inequality or the Gini coefficient had risen significantly since the 1970s. Such income inequality has been linked to levels of physical morbidity, mortality and social phenomena such as violence (Wilkinson & Pickett, 2009), but there has been less available evidence to link it to mental health problems. However, there is no reason to expect this not to be so. A preliminary analysis (Pickett *et al*, 2006) of the association between national income inequality and the prevalence of mental health problems, using data from national surveys of diagnosable disorder in eight developed countries across the world (WHO World Mental Health Survey Consortium, 2004), showed strong linear correlations between income inequality and any mental health problems ($\rho = 0.73$) and serious mental health problems ($\rho = 0.74$). Those countries with high income inequality (e.g. the USA) had higher levels of mental health problems than those with low inequality (e.g. Japan). Data from other national surveys in Europe, North America and Australia all show strong associations between common mental health problems and indicators of socioeconomic disadvantage, including poor education, material disadvantage and unemployment (Fryers *et al*, 2005). There is thus international evidence to link mental health problems with disadvantage.

Areas of exclusion for people with mental health problems

Consumption

Social inequalities are associated with all forms of mental health problems (see Chapter 7). People with severe mental health problems are more likely to be from lower socioeconomic classes – for example, almost 70% of people with functional psychoses are in manual occupation (Meltzer *et al*, 1995a). This is less consistently found in people with common mental disorders, but there are more consistent associations with unemployment, low education levels, low income or material standard of living (Fryers *et al*, 2003; Melzer *et al*, 2004). There is a social class gradient, with an increase in incidence and mortality in severe learning disability in lower social class groups. It is unclear whether there is a true increase in incidence of mild learning disabilities in lower social classes or if the additional social problems lead to more people with mild learning disabilities from lower social classes presenting to services (Fryers & Russell, 2003).

Poverty, income and finance

People with severe mental illness often live in material poverty; they have less income and more debt and financial hardship than those without mental health problems (Dunn, 1999; Jenkins *et al*, 2008). In Britain about 90% of people with psychoses have control of their own finances (Foster *et al*, 1996) and in 1993 the median gross weekly income of people with psychoses who had control of their own finances was £60–79, compared with £80–99 for people with common mental disorders and £140–159 for the general population (Foster *et al*, 1996). The percentage of people with psychosis rises significantly as gross weekly household income decreases (Jenkins *et al*, 2008). Although these actual income levels will have now changed, there is no reason to expect the relative income levels to have reduced as most people with psychoses get their income from welfare benefits, with only about 17% receiving it from earned income (Foster *et al*, 1996). However, those with an earned income do have a higher median weekly income (£120–139) than those on benefits (£60–79) (Foster *et al*, 1996). In addition, many of those with severe mental health problems who are on benefits may not be receiving the full range of benefits to which they are entitled. For example, in a survey of individuals in contact with community mental health services in England that was true for about half the sample (Slade *et al*, 1995; McCrone & Thornicroft, 1997). Access to welfare benefits for which people are eligible can be significantly improved by the provision of specialist benefit workers in community mental health teams (CMHTs) (Frost-Gaskin *et al*, 2003).

The low incomes of this group of people with mental health problems places many of them firmly in the relative poverty bands of those described in Chapter 7 and means that they are not able to afford many of the basic necessities such as those outlined in the *Poverty and Social Exclusion Survey* (Gordon *et al*, 2000; Pantazis *et al*, 2006), including healthy food, clothes, domestic appliances and holidays or usual social activities (Bird, 2001; Blenkiron & Hammill, 2003) (Box 8.1). They may also be in debt or be unable to afford insurance or other financial services (Read & Baker, 1996). People with schizophrenia who have low income are also very likely to be disadvantaged on multiple measures of exclusion (Morgan *et al*, 2008).

People with common mental health problems are less likely to receive benefits than those with psychoses and generally have higher incomes, but compared with the general population they are twice as likely to be receiving income support and four to five times as likely to receive invalidity benefit; they are also less likely to have an earned income (47% *v.* 58% in the general population) (Meltzer *et al*, 1995*b*). As with psychoses, the proportion of people with common mental health problems rises significantly as gross weekly household income decreases; the prevalence of substance dependency is not associated with low income, although debt is (Jenkins *et al*, 2008). The risk of common mental disorders is high among the poor – several studies have found an association between poor mental health and the experience of poverty (e.g. Weich & Lewis, 1998*a,b*; Whitley *et al*, 1999). Here poverty can be seen as a trigger to poor mental health, a factor in maintaining common mental disorders and as part of the key experience of poor mental health.

In the *Poverty and Social Exclusion Survey*, of the 26% of people defined as poor, half had common mental health problems, and higher rates of these problems were found among people in low-income households

Box 8.1   Lack of necessities and poor mental health as experienced by people with common mental disorders

Fresh fruit and vegetables, 71%

Warm waterproof coat, 65%

Two pairs of all weather shoes, 54%

Special outfit, 49%

Money to spend on self weekly, 46%

Money to spend to keep the home decorated, 45%

Roast joint, 45%

Replace broken electrical goods, 42%

Home insurance, 40%

Damp-free home, 37%

Appropriate clothes for job interviews, 37%

Replace worn out furniture, 35%

Regular savings, 34%

Source: Payne (2006)

– 25% of those living in households with an equivalised weekly gross income of under £100 have poor mental health compared with 12% of those in households with over £700 per week (Payne, 2006). In addition to low income, living in rented accommodation, having structural housing problems, having no access to a van or car, and not saving from an income are all associated with experiencing common mental health problems (Weich & Lewis, 1998a). If the experience of multiple indicators of poverty is used as an index of severity of disadvantage then it is clear that people with common mental health problems are more likely to suffer from severe disadvantage than those without these problems. For example, 45% of people who had a combination of five indicators of poverty as outlined earlier had common mental health problems and were two-and-a-half times as likely to experience these five problems as those without mental health problems (Weich & Lewis, 1998a). The risk of experiencing mental ill health increases with decreasing material standards of living, and poverty is associated with longer duration of common mental disorders (Weich & Lewis, 1998a). Poor mental health may not only be associated with the experience of being poor but also with the subjective experience of inequality. People on lower incomes had higher rates of mental ill health in areas of greater income equality, but the well off were also more likely to experience common mental disorders when living in areas of high income inequality (Weich et al, 2001). This supports the findings from the international data (Pickett et al, 2006).

Child poverty

The trends in child poverty in the UK were outlined in Chapter 7 and it is now well established that poor children are much more likely to experience mental health problems than those living in more affluent strata of society (Meltzer *et al*, 2000; Green *et al*, 2005). The likelihood of having a diagnosable mental health problem is three times higher for children in the lowest income household than in the highest earning group (Fig. 8.1). Children living in households where an adult is in receipt of state benefit payments are 2.5 times more likely to have a mental health problem than is the average child (Meltzer *et al*, 2000). Diagnosable mental health problems in children are highly associated with physical illness, accidental injury and neurological problems, all of which occur more commonly in economically disadvantaged groups (Meltzer *et al*, 2000). Many of the parents of these children have a background of adversity in their own childhood which may also be reflected in previous generations, the so-called 'cycle of deprivation'. The concept of a self-perpetuating cultural group defined by poverty and relationship difficulties has become familiar to those working with these populations and may give rise to low expectations of advancement.

Poverty and older people

Less information exists as to the financial status of older people with mental health problems, but it may be similar to that for working age adults, although there is some evidence that poverty may affect a larger proportion of older people with mental health problems (Chapter 7) (Help the Aged, 2008). Older people from Black and minority ethnic groups are particularly likely to live in low-income households and to experience

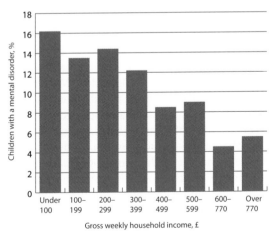

Fig. 8.1 Prevalence of mental disorders by gross weekly household income in Great Britain, 2004. Source: Green *et al* (2005)

139

multiple deprivations (Age Concern, 2002). Older women have lower incomes than men (Bunt & McAndrew, 2005).

The consequences of having a low income

Having a low income has consequences for people's access to material necessities, capital resources, their ability to save and their access to social outlets. In the Poverty and Social Exclusion survey 'list of necessities' (see Box 8.1), some items were more closely associated with poor mental health than others and more than a third of those who need, but are unable to afford, these necessities experience poor mental health (Payne, 2006). Almost 60% of people with mental health problems describe themselves as 'feeling poor all the time' (Payne, 2006). The low income of people with mental health problems means that many are not able to afford basic necessities, such as adequate heating. Domestic appliances, holidays and common social activities may be seen by them as luxuries. The low income may restrict their travel opportunities as most will not be able to afford a car or discretionary transport. This reinforces isolation and may also affect access to services. They may also be discriminated against in the financial sphere – a quarter of people with mental health problems said they had been refused insurance or other financial services (Read & Baker, 1996). They are unlikely to have any significant savings or capital and often do not have a bank account. They may also be in debt. People who borrow money from other sources have poorer mental health than those with access to better rates of credit: a total of 40% of people who borrowed from their family, and 50% of those who borrowed from friends, in order to pay for day-to-day needs, had common mental disorders (Payne, 2006). This financial insecurity is not helped by largely unintended disincentives related to welfare benefits, the so-called 'benefits trap', which make people feel insecure about changes to their circumstances (Seebohn & Scott, 2004).

Debt

The experience of debt is a particular problem for people with mental ill health (Nettleton & Burrows, 1998; Fitch *et al* 2007). They are three times as likely to be in debt and twice as often have problems managing their money compared with the general population (Melzer *et al*, 2002). This high proportion of people in debt applies to individuals with any type of mental health problem; for example, a quarter of people with common mental health problems, a third of those with a diagnosis of psychosis, a quarter of those with alcohol dependency and over a third with drug dependency had debts, compared with 8% of the general population (Jenkins *et al*, 2008). People with mental health problems are often in debt to utility services – over half of those who owed money on their telephone bill had mental health problems and of those with mortgage arrears, 80% had mental health problems (Payne, 2006; Jenkins *et al*, 2008).

It is often difficult to establish whether debt is a determinant or consequence of a mental health problem, but in a longitudinal study of

UK families, Reading & Reynolds (2001) reported an association between debt and the development of postnatal depression. Debt may exacerbate the person's mental health difficulties. It is associated with feelings of anxiety, depression and stress, and with raised likelihood of visiting the GP for help with these symptoms (Edwards, 2003). Mental well-being is worse among people who fall into housing payment arrears, especially if these problems persist (Taylor *et al*, 2007), and people with mortgage debt have significantly poorer mental health scores (on the General Health Questionnaire) than those with no mortgage problems. Debt has also been linked to suicidal ideas and self-harm (Hatcher, 1994; Taylor, 1994; Hintikka *et al*, 1998). However, it is the consequences of debt that seem to be important, especially when the debt cannot be repaid. The resulting 'debt spiral' (Fitch *et al*, 2007) where there are missed payments and penalties, the attempts to juggle personal finances or borrow additional money, the increasing pressure from creditors, the attempts to make unrealistic arrangements to repay the debts and the threat or occurrence of legal proceedings, lead to an entrenchment of the problems and to the eventual loss of important resources such as accommodation. These matters are not only associated with feelings of worry, anxiety and low mood, but also feelings of shame, social embarrassment and a sense of personal failure (Hayes, 2000).

Mental health problems may act as a pathway into debt and this may be compounded by people's experiences of the irresponsible practices of the financial services industry (Edwards, 2003). Debt, or the threat of it, leads to borrowing money. In a survey of over 1800 people in England and Wales with mental health problems of a range of diagnoses, 72% had borrowed money over the previous 12 months, over half of whom borrowed more than £2500 and 60% owed money on a credit or store card (Mind, 2008). Just over half had been two or more consecutive payments behind with a bill in the past 12 months (defined as having 'problem debt'). Of these people with problem debt: 50% lived on household incomes of less than £200 per week, 78% had been threatened with legal or court action, 51% had been contacted by bailiffs or debt collectors, and 25% had received a County Court Judgment to repay the debt. Their mental health problems, living on low income and difficulties in managing money were key reasons given for being in problem debt.

Neighbourhoods

Personal poverty and deprived neighbourhoods tend to go together and are associated with mental health problems. The Poverty and Social Exclusion Survey found a clear relationship between living in a poor area and individual poverty – those who are poor are likely to live in neighbourhoods with problems. Higher than average rates of poor mental health are found among those respondents who live in a poor environment: a third of people who had problems with noisy neighbours had mental health problems, compared with 10% who did not; 38% of men and 35% of women who were dissatisfied with the area they lived in had mental health problems (Payne, 2006). Several studies have found an association between deprived neighbourhoods and contact with mental health services for people diagnosed with psychoses and those with common mental health problems, and for suicide (Thornicroft, 1991; Boardman *et al*, 1997; Lewis *et al*, 1998; Whitley *et al*, 1999; Croudace *et al*, 2000). Some of the reasons for this may be downward mobility and the impact of poor areas: poor social ties, social space which discourages the formation of friendships, and wider urban processes which promote divisions and inequalities. Rates of criminal victimisation are higher, which lead to increased fear of crime, social withdrawal and mental health problems among both direct victims and non-victimised residents (Brewin *et al*, 1999). Poor housing is often an obvious feature of these neighbourhoods.

The problems of substance misuse also feed into poor neighbourhoods. Drug misuse is much more common in deprived districts, reflected, for example, in drug-related hospital emergencies, which are 30 times more common in deprived than in affluent districts (Lupton *et al*, 2002). In these deprived areas substance misuse is linked to unemployment and low income, housing conditions, levels of education and opportunities, health, discrimination, and integration into the local community (*ibid*). This exclusion is also seen in the criminal justice system where drug-related offences are common (see Chapter 9).

Housing

Only a small proportion of people with mental health problems live in sheltered or residential housing schemes and most live in mainstream housing. This is true of almost all people with common mental health problems. Four out of five people with severe mental health problems live in mainstream housing, with the rest living in supported housing or other specialist accommodation, and half of those with their own home or tenancy live alone (Weich & Lewis, 1998*a,b*; Davis, 2003). Good-quality housing represents not only shelter, but also the stability of a home and relates to mental health through its physical design, meaning and control, social support and financial security (Dunn, 2008). It is also of developmental importance to children.

Most people with severe mental health problems live in social housing (owned by local authorities or registered social landlords). Compared with the general population, people with common mental health problems are one-and-a-half times more likely to live in rented housing – with higher uncertainty about how long they will remain in their current home (Meltzer *et al*, 2002). They are twice as likely to say that they are very dissatisfied with their accommodation or that the state of repair is poor, and four times more likely to say that their health has been made worse by their housing (Meltzer *et al*, 2002).

Along with the growth of owner occupancy since the 1960s, the quality and nature of social housing has changed and it now houses a higher proportion of disadvantaged groups than in the past (Feinstein *et al*, 2007).

In 2004, a third of people living in social housing had incomes within the poorest fifth of the income distribution (Hills, 2007). Examining data from the 1946, 1958 and 1970 birth cohorts, Feinstein *et al* (2007) found that the strength of the relationship between living in social housing and multiple forms of disadvantage and deprivation had increased between the 1946 and 1970 cohorts. When people from the 1970 cohort reached 30 years of age, those living in social housing were nine times more likely to be 'not in employment, education or training' than the rest of the cohort and over twice as likely to have depression or other mental health problems, low self-efficacy and to be dissatisfied with life. Poor adult outcomes were also found for those born in social housing in the 1958 and 1970 cohorts. These poor outcomes were not found in the 1946 cohort. They could not be explained away by selection factors and may be caused by the life experiences of those in social housing, which are driven by factors such as enduring poverty, debt, poor mental health, family and relationship breakdown, joblessness, stigma and discrimination.

People in social housing are more likely to experience poor mental health than those who live in owner-occupied accommodation (Meltzer *et al*, 1995b; Lewis *et al*, 1998). Poor-quality housing (e.g. damp, lack of security, noise) is associated with high levels of depression (Hyndman, 1990; Hopton & Hunt, 1996). In the Poverty and Social Exclusion Survey (Payne, 2006), 12% of people with no accommodation problems had poor mental health compared with over a third who had four or more problems (e.g. damp, wood rot, shortage of space, lack of adequate heating). Housing problems may exist alongside poverty, in isolation from it, or in combination. They may be associated with debt – one in four tenants with mental health problems has serious rent arrears and risk losing their home (Neuburger, 2003). There are higher concentrations of individuals with mental health problems in inner cities where poor housing predominates (Office of the Deputy Prime Minister, 2004).

In the UK, health authorities and local authorities are expected to provide a range of care and support services for people with severe mental disorders. Local housing authorities are responsible for assessing and meeting the needs of vulnerable people, but only in unitary authorities will the housing and social care authority be the same body. Both housing and care and support services are often achieved in collaboration with healthcare trusts, and with third sector organisations, including housing associations. Despite the importance of housing and housing support for people with mental health problems, there is little evidence as to the efficacy of housing interventions (Grove, 2008). There is some descriptive literature on joint working between housing and other agencies (National Social Inclusion Programme, 2007). Medical priority re-housing can have a particularly beneficial effect for people with mental health problems (Blackman *et al*, 2003). Neighbourhood renewal initiatives have had a mixed success, possibly because of the disruptive effects of building work (Kai *et al*, 2000; Ellaway & MacIntyre 2004). A Cochrane review (Chilvers *et al*, 2002) examined studies in which people with severe mental health problems were allocated to supported housing and that was compared with outreach support and standard care. Although 136 such studies were found, none reached the initial criteria set by the review. A US evaluation of a 'Housing First' project for people with a dual diagnosis of severe mental illness and substance misuse shows some promise (Tsemberis *et al*, 2004), as do supported schemes for homeless people with severe mental health problems (Nelson *et al*, 2007).

It is likely that the types of housing and support available for people with mental health problems are determined to a great extent by what is available at a local level. For example, in London serious inadequacies in the capital's provision of housing for people with severe mental health problems have been reported, including unavailability of move-on accommodation, weakness in planning and poor interagency working (Boyle & Jenkins, 2003; Sainsbury Centre for Mental Health, 2003). Since 2003, housing support for vulnerable people in England has been based on the Supporting People programme (Department of Environment, Transport and the Regions, 1999; Sainsbury Centre for Mental Health, 2004). The programme is locally devolved and there is a national outcome framework measuring the extent to which it meets clients' needs, although no published evaluation of the framework is yet available (www.spclientrecord.org.uk).

Transport

As most people with severe mental illness depend on welfare benefits for their basic and everyday needs, this may restrict their travel opportunities as most will not be able to afford a car or discretionary transport, and are unlikely to have holidays (Thornicroft, 2006). Other problems may arise as, for example, travel insurance may be hard to obtain (Read & Baker, 1996). In addition, access to services may be difficult. Up to one in four people have been unable to get help from mental health services owing to an inability to pay for transport (Mental Health Foundation, 2001).

Poor access to transport may contribute to isolation. Around a third of people who are isolated because of lack of transport or inability to afford transport have a mental health problem. Those reporting isolation because of lack of transport were three times more likely to have poor mental health than those who did not experience this isolation (Payne, 2006).

Production

Education

Many diagnosable mental health problems begin early in life (Kim-Cohen, 2003; Kim-Cohen *et al*, 2003) and as a consequence may have an impact on educational attainment. Population-based studies in the USA and New Zealand show that mental disorders beginning in early life or adolescence are associated with an increased risk of early termination of education (Kessler *et al*, 1995; Johnson *et al*, 1999; Meich *et al*, 1999; Fergusson &

Woodward, 2001; Woodward & Fergusson, 2001). This often results in disadvantages in acquiring skills, impairment of life chances during adulthood and loss of human capital (Lee *et al*, 2009).

In general there is an association between low levels of education and mental health problems. In a review of epidemiological studies of common mental disorder four out of five key studies showed positive associations with higher rates of common mental health problems and less education, whether measured by qualifications achieved, years of completed education or age at completion (Melzer *et al*, 2004). In the British Psychiatric Morbidity Survey (Meltzer *et al*, 1995a) those who left school before 16 years of age or had no qualifications had the highest levels of common mental disorder. These links between education and mental health problems probably reflect the other features of disadvantage outlined above, as the gradient found with education and common mental disorder disappears when other sociodemographic variables are controlled for (Lewis *et al*, 1998). People with common mental disorder may have poor literacy skills – the occurrence of depression is five times higher in women with poor literacy skills than in those with good literacy skills (Bynner *et al*, 1997). People with a diagnosis of psychosis are very likely to have low levels of education and training, as young people are particularly vulnerable to these disorders and the early stages or onset of the problems are disrupting to their education. Over half of people with psychoses have no educational qualifications (Foster *et al*, 1996).

Low education attainment in early years may be difficult to make up for later in life and adults with mental health difficulties face barriers to participating in learning, not least because of gaps in the provision of adult education. A recent survey conducted by the National Institute of Adult Continuing Education and NIMHE showed that although the amount of provision has increased in recent years, there are still gaps in provision in some areas (James, 2003). Lack of education and skills also reduce the likelihood of attaining employment (Boardman, 2003).

Employment

The poor labour market position of people with mental health problems is well known. They are, in the main, less likely to be in employment and are at more than double the risk of losing their job than people without mental health problems (Boardman, 2003; Burchardt, 2003). They have a high rate of unemployment and represent the highest number of those claiming sickness and disability benefits. Many people experience their first episode of a mental health problem in their late teens or early 20s, which can have serious consequences for their education and employment prospects (Kim-Cohen, 2003; Kim-Cohen *et al*, 2003). In an economic downturn they have a lower re-entry rate into the labour market.

Lack of employment is associated with drug misuse. Unemployed 16- to 29-year-olds have higher rates of use of most illegal drugs, including heroin (Home Office, 2001). Alcohol and drug problems have an impact on a person's ability to work productively and hold down a job. In a one-day census of 10 000 individuals receiving help for alcohol problems, 36% were unemployed (Shand & Mattick, 2002); over 75% of people in treatment for drug misuse in England and Wales are unemployed (Gossop *et al*, 1998); 17 million working days are lost a year due to alcohol, and it is estimated that lost productivity costs the country £6.4 billion per year (Prime Minister's Strategy Unit, 2003). Employment is a crucial feature of a return to mainstream life for many people who misuse drugs (Platt, 1995).

The figures for mental health problems and unemployment vary according to the type of mental health problem experienced but can be conveniently summarised by examining the findings for people with schizophrenia and other psychoses, people with long-term mental disorders and those with common mental disorders.

Schizophrenia and other psychoses

Studies in this area are often hampered by varying definitions of employment, but consistently show large variations between study centres and low employment rates compared with the general population (Box 8.2). The rate of employment for people with schizophrenia appears to have dropped over the years: studies show that between 10 and 20% are in some form of employment (Marwaha & Johnson, 2004). Before 1990, employment rates of 20–30% were reported. Several studies that have reported rates at two time points also show a decrease. For example, in Wandsworth between 1990 and 1999 the proportion of people with schizophrenia who were in work decreased from 8% to 4% (Perkins & Rinaldi, 2002).

Rates of employment for people with schizophrenia vary between and within countries. One study involving 1208 people with schizophrenia who were in contact with psychiatric services in England, Germany or France (Marwaha *et al*, 2007) used a broad employment definition of having a job that was full- or part-time open employment (working and supporting oneself with earnings only) or sheltered employment. It found broad rates

---

Box 8.2   Employment rates in people with schizophrenia in the UK

- 4–31% over the past 20 years, with most samples showing a rate of 10–20%
- 20–30% up until the 1990s
- rates from a single centre at two time points suggest a decrease in the rates of employment over time
- in studies of people with a first episode of psychosis more are employed, but these rates overlap with those of people with established schizophrenia
- poor employment outcomes are a consistent finding in research into people with first-episode psychosis

Source: Marwaha & Johnson (2004)

of employment which varied from 6.7% in London to 60% in Heilbronn, Germany. The rates of open employment were 2.7% in London and 18.3% in Hemer, Germany. The differences between London and Germany possibly reflect the greater provision of vocational services available in Germany. In the other English centre, Leicester, the broad employment rate was 19% and the open rate 15.1%. Less is known about the proportion of people with schizophrenia who have ever been in employment: 15.8% of the London sample and 0.8% of the Leicester sample had never been employed, but no details as to the length of time or whether this was before or after the onset of schizophrenia are given. In people with schizophrenia presenting to mental health services for the first time the rates of employment in the UK vary from 13 to 65% (Marwaha et al, 2004). Notably, when these groups of people are followed up, their rate of employment drops, from 52 to 25% after 1 year (Birchwood et al, 1992) and from 65 to 49% over 2 years (Johnstone et al, 1986).

Overall, most jobs that are carried out by people with schizophrenia are 'elementary', for example cleaning and labouring, or are skilled trade occupations such as plumbing or metal work. However, some people are in managerial or senior official positions. Although a diagnosis of schizo-phrenia is probably not a bar to doing any kind of job, it does make entry into certain jobs less likely. This is corroborated by experience of supported employment programmes. In south London the supported schemes for a variety of people with long-term mental health problems (Rinaldi et al, 2006) showed that people in the schemes found a wide variety of jobs, not just entry-level positions requiring low skills. However, people with a diagnosis of psychosis were less likely to get (or retain) jobs as managers or senior officers and were more likely to be employed in elementary occupations than people with a diagnosis of a non-psychotic illness.

Pre-morbid social and occupational history are the most common factors associated with employment in people with schizophrenia (Marwaha & Jonhson, 2004; Catty et al, 2008). The desire to have a job is one of the best predictors of future employment (Marwaha & Johnson, 2004). There is some evidence to suggest that some types of psychotic symptoms and the negative symptoms of schizophrenia are associated with unemployment (Marwaha & Johnson, 2004).

Long-term mental health problems

Employment rates for people with long-term disabilities are collected as part of the Labour Force Survey, a continuous household survey carried out in Great Britain (www.statistics.gov.uk). Data for people with long-term mental health problems are recorded, but there is no record of the specific diagnosis and this group is likely to contain a heterogeneous sample of people with various diagnoses. However, the survey shows low employment rates in people with long-term disabilities related to mental health problems and that people with enduring mental health problems are much less likely to be economically active than those with physical or sensory impairments

(Box 8.3). People with long-term mental health problems appear to be particularly disadvantaged in the labour market.

Common mental health problems

The Office of Population Censuses and Surveys' study of psychiatric morbidity in Great Britain found significant levels of unemployment and sickness absence in those with 'neurotic' disorders (Box 8.4). The Poverty and Social Exclusion Survey (Payne, 2006) found that mental health problems were more common in those who were not in employment: 33% of those who were unemployed had mental health problems compared with 26% of those who were permanently unable to work, 21% of those who had domestic and caring responsibilities and 16% of those who were working. General practitioners provide the main source of care for most people with mental health problems, the bulk of whom have common mental health problems. People who are unemployed consult their GPs more often than the general population and those who have been unemployed for more than 12 weeks show between four and ten times the prevalence of depression, anxiety and somatic illness (Meltzer *et al*, 1995*b*).

Social interaction

In general people with mental health problems are more likely to be socially isolated than others in the general population, to have reduced interaction with others and to have low access to opportunities and facilities in the community. This is particularly the case for people with severe mental health problems.

Children who grow up in a climate of social adversity, family dysfunction and breakdown will learn coping skills that allow them to survive in that environment, but these may not translate into a skill set appropriate for other spheres of life. Successful integration into society is also hampered by the presence of diagnosable childhood mental health problems, some

---

Box 8.3   Employment in people with long-term mental illness

- The long-term disabled with mental health problems as the main difficulty represent 8% of the long-term disabled of working age; 18% of this group were in employment in 2000
- The long-term disabled with no mental health difficulties represent 84% of the long-term disabled of working age; 52% of this group were in employment in 2000
- 30–40% are capable of holding down a job
- In 2003, 24% of people with mental health problems were in employment, compared with 49% of disabled people overall

Source: Office for National Statistics (2004).

Box 8.4   Levels of unemployment and sickness absence in those with common mental health problems

- Adults with neurotic disorder were four to five times more likely than the rest of the sample to be permanently unable to work
- Overall, 61% of men with one neurotic disorder and 46% with two disorders were working, compared with 77% of those with no disorder; the equivalent figures in women were 58%, 33% and 65%
- The lowest rates of employment among people with neurotic disorders were found in those with phobias: 43% of men and 30% of women with phobias were working
- Among the sample with any neurotic disorder who were unemployed and seeking work, 70% had been unemployed for a year or more (that is 7% of all people with a neurotic disorder)
- Compared with the general population, adults with neurosis were twice as likely to be receiving income support (19% v. 10%) and four to five times more likely to receive invalidity benefit (9% v. 2%)

Source: Meltzer et al (1995b).

types of disorder being particularly destructive in later life. Maughn et al (2004) report that children with disruptive behaviour face a number of poor outcomes: they are more likely to show poor educational attainments and drop out of school; leave their homes and families at younger ages; and have poorer early work histories with higher risks of unemployment. They are also more likely to enter romantic and sexual relationships earlier, and experience more difficulties and breakdown in those relationships; become pregnant or father children earlier than their peers; be involved in crime; and have poor general health in their early adult lives. The long-term effect of emotional difficulties in childhood is less clear, but as these are linked to educational failure and relationship problems, it is likely that adverse interpersonal effects will follow. Depressive illness in adolescence is linked with adult depression (Harrington, 2002), and attention-deficit hyperactivity disorder in children is associated with psychiatric disorder in adult life (Schachar & Tannock 2002).

Family

For most people in modern Britain the family provides the main source of contact and support. However, many people with mental health problems are isolated or estranged from their family, with many living alone or in one-parent households. Many people with a diagnosis of psychosis never marry and often live alone or in supported or residential settings: 52% of people with psychoses are single and 22% are widowed, divorced or separated; about a quarter marry (Foster et al, 1996). People with psychoses are three times more likely to be divorced than those without and less than 40% live in a family setting (Foster et al, 1996; Meltzer et al, 2002). For people

149

with common mental health problems isolation from family may be less common, but they are more likely to have an unmet desire to participate more fully in family and social activities than those with no mental health problems (Meltzer *et al*, 2002).

Over a million children are at risk owing to parental alcohol abuse, which also accounts for a third of domestic violence (Advisory Council on the Misuse of Drugs, 2003). Similar figures are found for illicit drug misuse. The Advisory Council on the Misuse of Drugs (2003) report *Hidden Harm* has highlighted the vast scope of this problem, and indicated the long-term damage suffered by these children, including the high risk of them beginning to misuse substances themselves. There is a high rate of relationship breakdown among people who misuse substances. The parents and other relatives of people with substance misuse often come under huge stress as a result of inconsistent behaviour, dishonesty and occasional violence, and they often end up caring for the person's children, with associated financial problems.

Over 60 000 children in England do not live with their families and are 'looked after' by local authorities, some of them in children's homes and about 70% in foster care (2006 figures from the Department for Education and Skills). They represent a vulnerable group of children who not only experience the stigma of being 'in care' but also had experienced a range of family problems and abuse before they entered local authority care. These children have a disproportionately high rate of mental and physical health problems (Richardson & Joughin, 2000; Meltzer *et al*, 2003; Meltzer, 2008). In a national survey of children in care aged 5–17 years (Meltzer *et al*, 2003), 45% had mental health problems (conduct disorders, anxiety and depression, hyperactivity), four time the rate of those living in private households (Green *et al*, 2005). Those with mental health problems were more likely to have factors predicting later social exclusion. For example, they had twice the rate of scholastic problems as their looked-after peers with no mental health problems: 35% were 3 or more years behind in their intellectual development, 42% had a statement of special educational needs, and over 35% had difficulties in reading, mathematics or spelling. They were also likely to have begun to use alcohol or drugs in their teens and to have suffered sexual abuse or rape (Meltzer, 2008).

Between 20 and 50% of adults using mental health services are parents (Falkov, 1998). About 28% of lone parents have mental health problems (Meltzer *et al*, 2002; Melzer, 2003). Lone mothers are three-and-a-half times more likely than women in the general population and three times more likely than supported mothers to develop depression, and more likely to be economically inactive, live in social housing and to be isolated than these other women (Targosz *et al*, 2003). Black Caribbean children have a 50% chance of being born to a lone parent, and Caribbean single mothers have higher rates of severe and enduring mental health problems than married women (but lower rates of common mental health problems) (Maher & Green, 2000; Platt, 2002).

Mental health problems have an impact on the family. Up to 420000 people in the UK care for someone with a mental health problem (Maher & Green, 2000), of which 6000–17000 are young carers (Aldridge & Becker, 2003). Carers are twice as likely to have mental health problems themselves if they provide substantial care (Singleton *et al*, 2002). One-third to two-thirds of children whose parents have mental health problems will experience difficulties themselves (Falkov, 1998) and childcare social workers estimate that 50–90% of parents on their caseloads have mental health problems, alcohol or substance misuse (Social Care Institute for Excellence, 2003).

In a survey of carers in Britain (Partners in Care, 2004), over half of whom cared for someone with a mental disorder (including learning difficulties and dementia), nearly half of them rated their health as not very good or not at all good. Poor health was especially common among those looking after people with mental illness, long-term physical illness and dementia, and this was manifest in both physical and mental complaints – nearly a third reported they suffered from depression. In addition to a diagnosed disorder, many felt drained, stressed, frustrated and slept poorly. Many families of people with mental disorders report serious concerns about the future. They worry about their capability of continuing to look after the person, including their financial capability, have specific concerns about what happens to their family member if they die, and have a lack of understanding about the condition of the person they are looking after (Partners in Care, 2004).

Carers report a lack of support from professionals in the medical and community field (less so from GPs). In particular, carers felt that they were not being sufficiently informed on what to do and how to react in certain situations. They reported getting little respite from caring – a couple of hours per week respite paid for by others and a couple of hours paid for by themselves or the person they care for. They believed that an average of an extra 7 hours' help a week would make a significant difference to their own health (Partners in Care, 2004).

People with learning disabilities may present with behaviour that causes problems to those who care for them. The term 'challenging behaviour' was developed in the USA to emphasise the challenge that is presented to carers, services and professional to find different, more appropriate, creative and robust ways of supporting the individual. This change in emphasis aimed to help people move away from behavioural and environmental approaches that focused on trying to eliminate the behaviour and often being aversive or punitive to the individual. This change in meaning has become lost over the past decade or so and people incorrectly labelled as 'having' challenging behaviour are among those who are most likely to be in receipt of restrictive, punitive or invalidating professional and service responses. This may lead to them being excluded from local resources and to an increased burden of care on family members. This can have a very negative effect on the person with learning disabilities self-esteem and lead to more problems with behaviour. Eventually they may end up in a placement away from their home area because local services cannot meet their needs and they are erroneously labelled as being 'too challenging' or 'incurable'. Such separation from their family results in their isolation and distress.

Social networks

Poor social networks have long been recognised as a risk factor for mental health problems. People with common mental health problems often have poor social networks, and those of people with severe mental health problems are often severely restricted. Adults with severe mental health problems are five times, and those with common mental health problems two times, as likely to report a personal severe lack of support as those with no illness. People with common mental health problems generally have low social support, even lower in people with psychoses (Box 8.5). People in contact with mental health services are relatively isolated and are likely to derive many of their social contacts from other service users (Box 8.5).

Leisure

Participation in leisure activities varies in people with common mental health problems. Meltzer *et al* (1995*b*) compared rates of participation in people with and without common mental health problems. In their sample people with a diagnosis of depression spend less time than others in leisure activities in and around the home (e.g. reading, listening to the radio, entertaining): 41% entertained friends or relatives, compared with 56% of those with no mental health problem. Rates of participation in leisure activities outside the home were generally lower in people with common mental health problems than in those without, especially for those with phobias. People with common mental health problems engaged in fewer leisure activities than those without: 12% engaged in up to three activities (0–3) and 29% in ten or more activities, compared with 5% and 40% respectively of people with no mental health problem. People with depressive disorders were four times as likely to participate in 0–3 activities than those with no mental health problems (21% *v*. 5%). Adults with common mental health problems are less likely to belong to a sports or social club than those without (Evans, 2004*a*). Although some of this low participation may relate to the nature of these mental health problems, it may also be caused by the poor material circumstances of these groups. For example, the mental health of people who cannot afford social activities such as holidays, eating out, trips on public transport, evenings out, is worse than those who can (Payne, 2006).

Figures for participation in leisure activities are similar for people with psychoses: 13% engage in up to three activities (0–3) and 26% in ten or more activities; 40% attend a club or day centre and 7% an adult education or training centre (Foster *et al*, 1996). However, people with schizophrenia often describe impoverished lifestyles in terms of their use of time during the day. In a study of use of time in 229 people with schizophrenia living in north London, few were engaged in work, active leisure, education or voluntary occupations (Shimitras *et al*, 2003). Compared with the

Box 8.5   Social networks and mental health problems: levels of support and isolation

Common mental health problems:

- of people with common mental health disorders, 55% report no perceived lack of social support, 28% report a moderate lack and 17% a severe lack of support (compared with 66%, 26% and 8% of those with no disorders) (Meltzer *et al*, 1995*b*)
- in people with a severe lack of perceived social support, 29% had a common mental health disorder, double that of the group with no perceived lack (14%) (Meltzer *et al*, 1995*b*)
- adults with a primary support group (close friends and relatives) of three or fewer people are most at risk of common mental health disorders (Brugha *et al*, 1987; Meltzer *et al*, 1995*b*)
- in adults without common mental health disorders, 64% have a primary support group of 9 or more people, 31% have 4–8 people, and 6% 0–3 people; lone parents and adults living with one parent have smaller primary support groups (Meltzer *et al*, 1995*b*)
- in adults with common mental health disorders, 48% have a primary support group of 9 or more people, 40% have 4–8 people and 13% 0–3 people; adults with depressive disorders have support groups of reduced size: 46% have 4–8 people and 20% 0–3 people (Meltzer *et al*, 1995*b*)
- people who reported feeling isolated and cut off from society are likely to have mental health problems (Payne, 2006); reasons given for this were: lack of transport, cost of transport, child care, lack of paid work, no friends or family.

People with psychoses (Foster *et al*, 1996):

- of people with psychoses, 39% report no lack of perceived social support, 29% report a moderate lack and 33% a severe lack of support
- 31% have a primary support group of 9 or more people, 43% have 4–8 people and 26% 0–3 people
- people with psychoses living in supported accommodation were more likely to report a severe lack of support and had smaller primary support groups than those living independently

People in contact with mental health services:

- social networks of four in ten people with mental health problems living in the community are restricted to people within mental health services (Ford *et al*, 1993)
- of people with severe mental illness in contact with support organisations, a quarter had no or limited contact with community activities (Pinfold, 2004)
- 84% of people with mental health problems have felt isolated compared with 29% of the general population (Pinfold, 2004); young people, ethnic minorities and people in rural communities were most isolated
- are four times more likely than average not to have one close friend and more than a third say they have no one to turn to for help (Meltzer *et al*, 1995*b*; Evans & Huxley, 2000).

general population surveyed in the UK National Time Use Survey (Office for National Statistics, 2002), people with schizophrenia spend longer proportions of their time on eating and personal care activities, but smaller proportions of time in domestic, work, educational and active leisure pursuits (Shimitras *et al*, 2003).

This restricted participation of people with schizophrenia in social and active leisure pursuits is found in other studies of people with severe and enduring mental health problems (Weeder, 1986; Skantze *et al*, 1992; Hayes & Halford, 1996; Trauer *et al*, 1998; Mayers, 2000). Some of these restrictions may be related to the nature of schizophrenia, but structural barriers such as lack of opportunity, limited income and discrimination also play a part. Overall, less affluent people are less likely to take part in active leisure activities than those better off (Office for National Statistics, 2002). Little detailed information is available on how frequently people with severe mental health problems access mainstream social and leisure facilities (Thornicroft, 2006), but it is likely that these opportunities are restricted (West, 1984).

Personal safety

Despite the fact that much of the literature has focused on violence by people with mental illness, it is more likely that they will be victims of violence or other crime than members of the general population (Murphy, 1991; Read & Baker, 1996; Walsh *et al*, 2003; Dinos *et al*, 2004; Teplin *et al*, 2005). About half of people treated at community mental health services in north London described experiences of verbal and physical abuse. Physical abuse was more commonly experienced by people with psychoses than other disorders (Dinos *et al*, 2004). Patients on psychiatric in-patient units may also experience violence towards them (Sainsbury Centre for Mental Health, 2002; Royal College of Psychiatrists, 2007). Some of this violence and crime may be associated with the more impoverished neighbourhoods that people with severe mental illness live in.

Older people

Older people with mental health problems may be particularly vulnerable to exclusion in all the areas of social interaction. For them, social isolation may result from life events associated with later life – bereavements, retirement from work and physical ill health – and is compounded by other social factors associated with later life such as limited income, lack of access to transport and fear of crime. The English Longitudinal Study of Ageing has reported that the more wealthy older people are, the less likely they are to report feeling lonely (Demakakos *et al*, 2006). Absence of, or restricted access to, appropriate amenities and services (shops, hospitals, banks), and availability of suitable transport, is a problem for older people (Musselwhite & Haddad, 2007). The English Longitudinal Study of Ageing found that relationships with friends and family exert a powerful influence on people's life satisfaction (Demakakos *et al*, 2006). Similarly, Scharf *et al* (2002) also found that contact with neighbours, family members and friends was important in preventing exclusion in later life. Vulnerability to crime is a major concern for older people, and the fear of crime may limit their ability to play a part in community life (Brammar, 2006).

Depression, dementia and other mental health problems in later life increase the risk of people experiencing social exclusion. The Social Exclusion Unit report (Office of the Deputy Prime Minister, 2006) *Sure Start to Later Life* notes that older people with depression are more likely to be multiply excluded. Individuals are affected by cumulative stigma and discrimination: the stigma of mental illness, plus stigma related to age, plus assumptions about cognitive function and dementia. Older adults with learning disabilities and dementia are at especially high risk of social exclusion, including exclusion from formal social relationships and civic activities (Scharf *et al*, 2002; Care Services Improvement Partnership, 2005).

Political engagement

There is a general lack of information about the involvement of people with any sort of mental health problems in local or national decision-making (having a voice, choice and control). The Poverty and Social Exclusion Survey has some data on civic participation but there was little relation between mental health and engagement in these activities, with the exception that those who have taken part in a political campaign or who have stood for civic office are much less likely to have suffered poor mental health (Payne, 2006). The list of civic activities and involvement in civic organisations used in the survey is shown in Box 8.6. For many people with severe mental health problems it is unlikely that they would have engaged in many of these activities. Although there is a lack of information about the engagement of service, there is some evidence about curtailment of citizenship and political and human rights for people with mental illness (Dunn, 1999; Sayce, 2000; Thornicroft, 2006). Scharf *et al* (2002) found that about a third of older people, in the inner city areas they investigated in Manchester, Liverpool and London, exhibited a moderate or high level of participation in civic affairs, but just under a quarter had not been involved in any type of civic activity in the previous 3 years.

One clear example is seen in relation to the central political right of voting. In England, for a psychiatric in-patient to vote they must have a non-hospital address and capacity, thus restricting this right for many detained patients. It is, however, likely that even if entitled to vote, participation of service users in elections may be marginal (Nash, 2002). Reliable figures relating to participation of people with mental health problems in voting are hard to come by, but a survey by United Response (a third-sector organisation that provides services for people with learning disability; www.unitedresponse. org.uk) found that 80% of the people with learning disability supported by the organisation were registered to vote in the 2005 election, but only 16% used their vote (overall turnout in the election was 61%) (Sayer, 2010).

Jury service is another example. In England, under the Juries Act 1974, there is a blanket exclusion of 'mentally disordered persons' who are ineligible to serve on a jury. Thus excluded is anyone who:

suffers or who has suffered from mental illness, psychopathic disorder, mental disorder, mental handicap, or severe mental handicap and because of that condition; (a) is resident in hospital or other similar institution, regularly attends treatment by a medical practitioner, or is under guardianship, or has been determined by a judge to be incapable, by reasons of mental disorder, of managing and administrating his/her property and affairs (Thornicroft, 2006: p. 74).

These conditions could apply to significant proportions of the population and restrict their civic engagement.

Apart from people who are unable to meet the age and residence requirements for jury service, or who have criminal convictions, people receiving treatment for their mental health problems are now the only group who are ineligible for jury service in the UK (Smith, 2010). There are no accurate figures, but probably about 750 people a month are being

---

Box 8.6   Civic activities included in the Poverty and Social Exclusion Survey

Civic activities undertaken in the past 3 years:

- voted in last general election
- voted in last local election
- helped on fundraising drives
- urged someone outside the family to vote
- presented views to a local councillor
- urged someone to get in touch with a local councillor
- been an officer of an organisation or club
- made a speech before an organised group
- written a letter to an editor
- taken an active part in a political campaign
- stood for civic office.

Current active involvement in civic organisations:

- sports club
- religious group or church organisation
- any other group or organisation
- trade union
- social club or working men's club
- tenants' or residents' association, neighbourhood watch
- voluntary service group
- patents' or school association
- environmental group
- other community or civic group
- women's group or organisation
- political party
- other pressure group
- Women's Institute or Townswomen's Guild.

Source: Gordon *et al* (2000)

---

disqualified from jury service on mental health grounds. This figure comes from the answer to a Parliamentary Question tabled on 14 May 2008, which resulted in the reply from the Minister Maria Eagle:

> In March and April 2008, the Jury Central Summoning Bureau summoned 62,559 people for jury service and disqualified 14,647 (23.4 per cent.). Of these, 1,524 were disqualified on grounds of mental health (2 per cent. of the total). These data are subject to the information supplied by the individual summoned (*Hansard*, 2008).

A further example of this discrimination is seen in relation to members of parliament (MPs). Under Section 141 of the Mental Health Act 1983, an MP will automatically lose their seat if they are detained under the Act for 6 months (but they would not lose their seat if they were unable to perform their duties owing to a physical illness for this period) (All-Party Parliamentary Group on Mental Health, 2008).

Health and health service engagement

One test of the health and strength of a society is how well it cares for its most vulnerable members. It is well established that access to mental health services is not equitable across the diagnostic groups and varies across different parts of the UK. For example, people with dual diagnoses (substance misuse and psychoses) (Department of Health, 2002) and personality disorders (NIMHE, 2003) are inappropriately excluded from mental health services and lack access to specialist treatment. There are inequities of access to alcohol services nationally and in some parts of the country less than 1 in a 100 dependent drinkers have access to appropriate treatment (Alcohol Needs Assessment Research Report Project, 2004). People with learning disabilities have higher than normal rates of mental health problems, psychoses and dementia (Cooper *et al*, 2007a,b; Strydom *et al*, 2007) but often have problems accessing appropriate services (Cooper *et al*, 2004).

In children's services, for every child seen in child and adolescent mental health service (CAMHS) clinics there are five times that number who do not enter clinical treatment (Green *et al*, 2005). Children from socially disadvantaged families are less likely to keep their appointments than those from the more affluent background despite their higher prevalence of mental health problems (Audit Commission, 1999). One in ten children across the social divide have a psychiatric disorder at any one time, but in most areas, child and adolescent mental health services attract only 5% of the mental health budget (Audit Commission, 1999). A workforce report in Scotland recommends an increase of 10% in CAMHS staffing per year for 10 years but there are no signs of the political will needed to realise this (Childhood Health Support Group, 2006). As children rarely refer themselves to services, they come to clinical attention because of concerns by others about aspects of their behaviour, thereby skewing the referral profile towards activity-related disorders such as conduct disorder and attention-deficit hyperactivity disorder. Children and young people who are withdrawn, anxious or depressed may be particularly hard to reach and vulnerable to exclusion from mental health service provision (Scottish Intercollegiate Guidelines Network, 2001; Callaghan & Vostanis, 2004). Children in care experience a disproportionate number of mental health and physical problems and often do not get access to the services to which all children are entitled (Richardson & Joughin, 2000; Meltzer, 2008).

There are also inequalities in service provision for older people (Age Concern, 2007). Older people's mental health services, including provision of psychotherapies, are relatively underfunded compared with those for younger adults (Evans, 2004b). In addition, institutional care for older people is characterised by a lack of basic physical care and little to stimulate or engender interest (National Audit Office, 2007). There is evidence that sedative drugs are overused in care homes (Fahey et al, 2003). Mental illnesses in later life may be unrecognised, and, when they are recognised in older adults, therapeutic nihilism and lack of resources may mean that people are less likely to be offered effective treatments. Health promotion is very limited for people with mental health problems in later life (Faculty of Old Age Psychiatry, 2006). Older people with dementia are particularly disadvantaged: there is an unwillingness and inability to hear their voice or to seek or respect their views, and they are habitually excluded from the community. There is restricted access to anti-Alzheimer's drug treatments in the UK in comparison with many other European nations (NICE, 2006a; National Audit Office, 2007) and physical health problems are often missed or untreated in people with dementia (Fahey et al, 2003).

Physical health inequalities

People with all forms of mental health problems are at increased risk of premature death, from both natural and unnatural causes (Harris & Barraclough, 1998), and a range of inequalities in physical health is seen in people with mental health problems (Box 8.7). A Disability Rights Commission general formal investigation in 2006 found that people with significant mental health problems experience a 'triple jeopardy' – they are more likely to get heart disease, diabetes and some cancers, especially when young and, once diagnosed, are more likely to die within 5 years. Generally, they experience poorer quality healthcare than people without mental health problems. People with a diagnosis of schizophrenia, bipolar disorder or depression die younger than other people; they have significantly higher rates of obesity, smoking, heart disease, hypertension, respiratory disease, diabetes, stroke and breast cancer than other citizens. The Commission also made an internationally new finding that people with schizophrenia are almost twice as likely to have bowel cancer. In addition, they are more likely than others to get illnesses like strokes and coronary heart disease before age 55 years and once they have them they are less likely to survive for 5 years. For almost all the key conditions studied the 5-year survival rates were found to be lower for people with mental health problems than other groups (Hippisley-Cox et al, 2006a).

> **Box 8.7** Inequalities in physical health in people with mental health problems
>
> - Physical ill health is a risk factor for the presence of common mental disorders: in a study by Meltzer *et al* (2004) about 7% of the sample had two or more physical illnesses, and a third of these people had a diagnosis of common mental disorder
> - People with severe mental illness are more likely to suffer from a range of physical disorders and have higher rates of death than the general population (Brown, 1997; Phelan *et al*, 2001; Osborn *et al*, 2007)
> - People with severe mental illness are more likely to die from diseases such as heart disease and respiratory disease, accidents and suicide than members of the general population
> - People with severe mental illness treated with antipsychotic medication have an excess of metabolic dysfunction and increased risk of cardiovascular disease (Macklin *et al*, 2007)
> - The UK guidelines on the management of schizophrenia (NICE, 2002) and bipolar disorder (NICE, 2006*b*) recognise the impact of physical disorders in these groups as well as the paucity of high-quality research in this field

Despite these disproportionate rates of physical disorder and death, these groups are less likely to get some of the expected evidence-based checks and treatments. People with schizophrenia are less likely to be screened or prescribed evidence-based treatments, such as statins (Hippisley-Cox *et al*, 2006*b*). Mental health service users often experience 'diagnostic overshadowing' where physical health problems are being viewed as part of the mental health problems and not fully explored or treated. Despite the fact that both mental health service users and mental health practitioners see access difficulties as the responsibility of the health service, primary care practitioners tended to see the problems – for example, not attending because of a chaotic lifestyle or not understanding the 24-hour clock – as inherent to the individual. In almost all interviews with primary care staff the researchers heard that mental health service users do not follow advice as given, cannot cope with its implications and do not attend appointments. However, there were no strategies in place to support these patients (Samele *et al*, 2006). The Disability Rights Commission (2006) investigation also identified low expectations among health service personnel, for example that people with mental health problems 'just do' die younger or 'just won't' participate in health services designed to improve physical health. It found non-adherence to Disability Discrimination Act duties to make reasonable adjustments and a lack of policy impetus and leadership to create change right through the health system.

The lifestyle of patients with personality disorders puts them at increased risk of physical health problems such as cardiovascular disease compared with the general population and they are as a result at risk of early mortality and death (Moran *et al*, 2007). Furthermore, patients with personality disorders tend to have difficulties in accessing, and may be excluded from, healthcare either because they are too chaotic to engage effectively or because behaviours that are part of their personality disorder result in exclusion from healthcare.

Physical health inequalities also exist in older people with mental health problems (Chandola *et al*, 2007) and in people with learning disabilities (van Schrojenstein Landman-de Valk & Walsh, 2008). The latter group have a higher prevalence of health problems than the general public and these are often unrecognised and unmet (Cooper *et al*, 2004). Reports from Mencap (2004, 2007) have shown indifference by health services to the physical health problems of people with learning disabilities. The Disability Rights Commission (2006) had highlighted inequalities in access to, and delivery of, appropriate treatment in primary care for people with learning disabilities. An independent national inquiry into physical healthcare for people with learning disabilities found evidence of good practice, but also appalling examples of discrimination, abuse and neglect across the range of health services (Michael, 2008).

People with multiple diagnoses

People who have more than one diagnosis may have multiple problems, present certain challenges to services and may be excluded by services as they do not reach the criteria for the individual health and social services departments. This may affect people who have combinations of diagnoses such as psychotic or non-psychotic mental illness, alcohol and/or drug dependence, learning disability, personality disorder and adult neurodevelopmental disorders (Asperger syndrome, autism, attention-deficit hyperactivity disorder). Few accurate figures exist as to the numbers of people with these multiple diagnoses ('multiple needs'), but a review by Schneider (2007) using UK surveys of these disorders found that in the UK adult population living in private households, 3.5% of individuals had two or more of the categories of disorders listed above, mostly a mental disorder in association with one of the other categories. There were high concentrations of people with multiple needs in prisons and among the homeless population (Schneider, 2007). Mental health problems (psychotic and non-psychotic illnesses) are nearly twice as common among people with learning difficulties than in the general population and affect up to half of people in prisons and those who are homeless (Schneider, 2007). Personality disorder is common among those two groups, but it does not affect a large proportion of people with learning difficulties when compared with the general population. Alcohol dependence is five times higher among the homeless and 11 times higher among prisoners than the general population. Prisoners also have a much higher rate of drug problems than the general population (Schneider, 2007).

People with multiple diagnoses are more likely to be excluded (in other ways than in prison or by being homeless) than others without these multiple needs (some of whom may also have mental health problems) (Table 8.1). In examining the variables listed in the table, Schneider (2007) looked at people with combinations of the problems listed and defined people with a combination of four or more of these problems as leading 'chaotic lifestyles'. She found that 0.9% of the general population and 6.5% of people with multiple needs have chaotic lifestyles, and 23% of people with chaotic lifestyles also have multiple needs. People with mental disorders alone account for an additional 18%, learning difficulty alone a further 10% and schizoid personality alone a further 9% of those who have chaotic lifestyles.

The report by Schneider was commissioned as part of the Cabinet Office Social Exclusion Task Force's programme on adults facing chronic exclusion. The Task Force has no set definition of adults facing chronic exclusion, but suggests they may have a range of characteristics: a history of exclusion, institutionalisation or abuse; behavioural and control difficulties; difficulties forming relationships; a lack of skills; limited economic means; poor job prospects; poor housing or homelessness; poor physical or mental health; a history of offending. People with these characteristics are familiar to mental health services and often do not fit readily into the criteria adopted by services. They may be difficult to engage or not settled in one place. In a review, also commissioned by the Task Force's programme, Bloor *et al* (2007) examined the characteristics of adults described as having 'chaotic lives and multiple needs'. This group often have 'mental health issues'

Table 8.1   Individuals with multiple needs compared with those who did not have multiple needs in the study sample (Schneider, 2007)

	Multiple needs	No multiple needs
Difficulty dealing with paperwork	27.3%	7.3%
Difficulty managing money	26.5%	3.6%
No qualifications	35.7%	26.0%
How many adults cohabiting do you feel close to?	mean=1.3	mean=1.4
How many adults generally do you feel close to?	mean=4.23	mean=5.9
How many people would you describe as good friends?	mean=4.82	mean=6.78
How many friends have you spoken to in the past week?	mean=4.55	mean=5.93
Economically inactive	37.1%	30.6%
Unemployed	7.8%	2.6%
Accommodation moves in past year	mean=2.54	mean=1.63
Lowest personal income group	35.5%	27.9%

that are ill-defined by diagnostic criteria (although they may be rejected by some as having 'personality disorders'), misuse drugs and alcohol, have difficulty sustaining tenancies, are homeless or rough sleepers, are estranged from their family and have disruptive family and social relationships, have problems managing their finances and have patchy employment histories. They present to a range of agencies including health and social services, housing and a range of third sector organisations dealing with homelessness, drug problems and those who are ex-offenders. They are challenging to services, who have no consistent response to these groups.

Conclusion

In this chapter we have examined five main areas in which people with mental ill-health can be considered to be excluded. Although the issue of the direction of causality is not resolved, there are nevertheless clear associations between poverty, exclusion and mental well-being and ill health. In general terms, mental ill health can be a cause and consequence of social exclusion. Anyone can be affected by mental ill health but people from disadvantaged backgrounds are at significantly greater risk. This cuts across all types of mental health problems and all age groups and is a phenomenon of universal significance (World Health Organization Commission on Social Determinants of Health, 2008). People with mental health problems may be excluded in any one of the five areas of exclusion discussed in this chapter, but these categories are not independent and people are more often excluded across several of the dimensions.

The excess of common mental disorders in disadvantaged people, whether measured by occupational social class, education, unemployment, income or material possessions is now well established. People with common mental disorders are not universally excluded but there are specific groups who are most disadvantaged in this context and who are marked out by combinations of factors including poor education, low income, inadequate social support and physical illness or disability (Melzer *et al*, 2004). There is a relationship between the seriousness of the mental health problems, certain broad diagnoses (in particular schizophrenia and schizoaffective disorder) and people who fall into multiple diagnostic categories and are excluded in multiple areas. These are associated with a number of related problems that interact with, and exacerbate, social exclusion: poor or abusive family background; poor social and functional skills; poverty; poor housing and homelessness; poor educational attainment and unemployment; social isolation with impoverished and non-reciprocal social networks and a high probability of lack of partner or cohabitee; lack of access to leisure activities; stigma (external and internalised) and discrimination; risk of criminality and victimisation. This multiple exclusion can be seen in the Aetiology and Ethnicity in Schizophrenia and Other Psychoses (AESOP study) of 390 people with first ever contact with mental health services for schizophrenia, who were more likely to be socially disadvantaged or isolated than matched controls as measured by a number of indicators, such as having no educational qualifications, being unemployed, living in rented accommodation and living alone (Morgan *et al*, 2008). They were between 2.7 and 3.5 times more likely to be in these circumstances than other members of the population and were more likely to experience multiple features of social disadvantage. Only 19% of those with schizophrenia did not have at least one indicator of disadvantage, compared with 54% of the general population, and 34% had four or more indicators, compared with 13% of controls.

Other groups who fall into this multiply-excluded category include those with contact with forensic services and those diagnosed as having personality disorders. People with personality disorders face a range of pervasive difficulties across a wide range of functioning. Indeed, many personality disorders are defined by difficulties with employment, personal relationships, relationships with authority and social and political structures (Skodol *et al*, 2002; Frankenburg & Zanarini, 2004). They are often seen as responsible for their own difficulties and resistant to, or undeserving of, treatment. Those people who come into contact with forensic mental health services are likely to have been socially excluded even before entering mental healthcare, independent of mental health considerations but rather related to deeply entrenched socioeconomic and cultural indicators of deprivation and disadvantage. Compared with users of general psychiatric services, mentally disordered offenders are over-represented by: young men; people from Black and minority ethnic groups; people from low socioeconomic classes; those with high rates of childhood deprivation, abuse and institutionalisation; those with low educational and vocational attainments (and with high rates of school exclusion); and people who are homeless (Farrington, 2008). In addition, many mentally disordered offender patients have no previous experience of mature, intimate and non-abusive relationships, and have already got extensive forensic histories (convictions) before entering mental healthcare (Farrington, 2008). Many male offenders are detained specifically because of their risk to women and children (Farrington, 2008).

It does seem that the more severe or complex the illness, the greater the risk of social marginalisation experienced by service users. In addition, large numbers of service users with high support needs, particularly those with learning disability or long-term schizophrenia, are placed in community residential and nursing homes which are often a long way from their local area of origin and family (so-called out-of-area treatments). This further exacerbates their social dislocation.

This multiple exclusion has economic consequences, but is of concern for more than economic reasons. There is strong evidence that health outcomes are heavily influenced by disadvantage (Chapters 7 and 10); for example, unemployment is damaging to health, whereas work is generally good for health and well-being (Waddell & Burton, 2006). There is also evidence that the great majority of people who use secondary mental health services aspire to live more fulfilling lives, including entering into paid employment (Seebohm & Secker, 2005). The barriers to achieving their ambitions are, however, significant. Active symptoms, cognitive impairment and episodic illness all present hard, but not insuperable, challenges for the individual and the clinician (Waghorn & Lloyd, 2005). Good clinical outcomes are important, if often difficult to achieve (Leff & Warner, 2006), but perhaps even more difficult to overcome are the social barriers: low expectations by clinicians and family, the effects of treatment, stigma and discrimination, and disincentives in the welfare system that put basic income at risk (Seebohm & Scott, 2004).

Summary

There is a wealth of evidence that people with mental health problems may be excluded in any one of the five areas of exclusion (consumption, production, social interaction, political engagement, and health and health service engagement). They are more often excluded across several of these areas.

People from disadvantaged backgrounds are at significantly greater risk of mental ill health, which can be a cause and consequence of social exclusion. This applies to all types of mental health problems across all age groups and is a phenomenon of universal significance.

Some groups are more likely to be excluded than others, particularly people with psychoses, learning disabilities and those whose problems can be described under multiple diagnostic categories.

References

Advisory Council on the Misuse of Drugs (2003) *Hidden Harm: Responding to the Needs of Children of Problem Drug Users*. ACMD.

Age Concern (2002) *Black and Minority Ethnic Elders' Issues*. Age Concern (www.ageconcern.org.uk/AgeConcern/Documents/Ethnic_MinorityeldersissuepppSept2002.pdf).

Age Concern (2007) *Improving Services and Support for Older People with Mental Health Problems. The Second Report from the UK Inquiry into Mental Health and Well-Being in Later Life*. Age Concern (http://www.ageconcern.org.uk/AgeConcern/Documents/full_report.pdf).

Alcohol Needs Assessment Research Project (2004) *The 2004 National Alcohol Needs Assessment for England*. Department of Health.

Aldridge, J. & Becker, S. (2003) *Children Caring for Parents with Mental Illness: Perspectives of Young Carers, Parents and Professionals*. Policy Press.

All-Party Parliamentary Group on Mental Health (2008) *Mental Health in Parliament. Report by the All-Party Parliamentary Group on Mental Health*. Mind.

Audit Commission (1999) *Children in Mind*. Audit Commission.

Birchwood, M., Cochrane, R., Macmillan, F., *et al* (1992) The influence of ethnicity and family structure on relapse in first-episode schizophrenia. A comparison of Asian, Afro-Caribbean and white patients. *British Journal of Psychiatry*, **161**, 783–790.

Bird, L. (2001) Poverty, social exclusion and mental health: a survey of people's personal experiences. *A Life in the Day*, **5**, 3.

Blackman T., Anderson, J. & Pye, P. (2003) Change in adult health following medical priority rehousing: a longitudinal study. *Journal of Public Health Medicine*, **25**, 22–28.

Blenkiron, P. & Hammill, C. A. (2003) What determines patients' satisfaction with their mental health care and quality of life. *Postgraduate Medical Journal*, **79**, 337–340.

Bloor, R., Crome, I., Astari, D., *et al* (2007) *Service Responses and Outcomes for Adults Described as Having Chaotic Lives and Multiple Needs. A Scoping Exercise*. Clinical Effectiveness Support Unit & Keele University.

Boardman, A. P., Hodgson, R. E., Lewis, M., *et al* (1997) Social indicators and the prediction of psychiatric admission in different diagnostic groups. *British Journal of Psychiatry*, **171**, 457–462.

Boardman, J. (2003) Work, employment and psychiatric disability. *Advances in Psychiatric Treatment*, **9**, 327–334.

Boyle, K. & Jenkins, C. (2003) *Housing for Londoners with Mental Health Needs*. King's Fund.

Brammar, J. (2006) *Fear of Crime and the Impact of Crime: A Consultative Report of Older People Living in Stoke on Trent*. Beth Johnson Foundation (www.bjf.org.uk/Libraries/Local/66/Docs/Fear%20of%20Crime%20Report.pdf).

Brewin, C., Andrews, B., Rose, S., *et al* (1999) Acute stress disorder and post-traumatic stress disorder in victims of violent crime. *American Journal of Psychiatry*, **156**, 360–366.

Brown, S. (1997) Excess mortality of schizophrenia. A meta-analysis. *British Journal of Psychiatry*, **182**, 502–508.

Brugha, T., Bebbington, P. E., MacCarthy, B., *et al* (1987) Social networks, social support and the type of depressive illness. *Acta Psychiatrica Scandinavica*, **76**, 664–673.

Bunt, K. & McAndrew, F. (2005) *Women's Attitudes towards Pension Reform* (Working Paper no. 38). Equal Opportunities Commission.

Burchardt, T. (2003) *Employment Retention and the Onset of Sickness or Disability: Evidence from the Labour Force Survey Longitudinal Datasets* (Report no. 109). Department for Work and Pensions.

Bynner, J., Parsons, S. & Basic Skills Agency (1997) *It Doesn't Get Any Better: The Impact of Poor Basic Skills on the Lives of 37-year-olds*. Basic Skills Agency.

Callaghan, J. & Vostanis, P. (2004) *Prevention of Mental Health Problems in Socially Excluded Children and Young People: A Model for Mental Health Provision*. Jessica Kingsley.

Care Services Improvement Partnership (2005) *Everybody's Business: Integrated Mental Health Service for Older Adults: A Service Development Guide*. Department of Health.

Catty, J., Lissouba, P., White, S., *et al* (2008) Predictors of employment for people with severe mental illness: results of an international six-centre randomised controlled trial. *British Journal of Psychiatry*, **192**, 224–231.

Chandola, T., Ferrie, J., Sacker, A., *et al* (2007) Social inequalities in self-reported health in early old age: follow up of prospective cohort study. *BMJ*, **334**, 990.

Child Health Support Group (2006) *Getting the Right Workforce, Getting the Workforce Right. A Strategic Review of the Child and Adolescent Mental Health Workforce*. NHS Scotland (http://www.sehd.scot.nhs.uk/workforcedevelopment/publications/camh_workforce_strategic_rev.pdf).

Chilvers, R., Macdonald, G. & Hayes, A. (2002) Supported housing for people with severe mental disorders. *Cochrane Database of Systematic Reviews*, **Issue 2**, doi: 10.1002/14651858.CD000453.pub2.

Cooper, S. A., Melville, C. & Morrison, J. (2004) People with intellectual disabilities. *BMJ*, **329**, 414–415.

Cooper, S. A., Smiley, E., Morrison, J., *et al* (2007a) Mental ill-health in adults with intellectual disabilities: prevalence and associated factors. *British Journal of Psychiatry*, **190**, 27–35.

Cooper, S. A., Smiley, E., Morrison, J., *et al* (2007b) Psychosis and adults with intellectual disabilities: prevalence, incidence and related factors. *Social Psychiatry and Psychiatric Epidemiology*, **42**, 530–536.

Croudace, T. J., Kayne, R., Jones, P. B., *et al* (2000) Non-linear relationship between an index of social deprivation, psychiatric admission prevalence and the incidence of psychosis. *Psychological Medicine*, **30**, 177–185.

Davis, A. (2003) *Mental Health and Personal Finances – A Literature Review*. Prepared for the Social Exclusion Unit, quoted in *Mental Health and Social Exclusion* (p. 143), Social Exclusion Unit (2004), Office of the Deputy Prime Minister.

Demakakos, P., Nunn, S. & Nazroo, J. (2006) Loneliness, relative deprivation and life satisfaction. In *Retirement, Health and Relationships of the Older Population in England: The 2004 English Longitudinal Study of Ageing (Wave 2)* (eds J. Banks, E. Breeze, C. Lessof, *et al*). Institute of Fiscal Studies (http://www.ifs.org.uk/elsa/report06/ch10.pdf).

Department of Health (2002) *Mental Health Policy Implementation Guide: Dual Diagnosis Good Practice Guide*. Department of Health.

Department of Environment, Transport and the Regions (1999) *Supporting People: A New National Policy and Funding Framework*. HMSO.

Dinos, S., Stevens, S., Serfaty, M., *et al* (2004) Stigma: the feelings and experiences of 46 people with mental illness. *Qualitative study. British Journal of Psychiatry*, **184**, 176–181.

Disability Rights Commission (2006) *Equal Treatment: Closing the Gap. A Formal Investigation into Physical Health Inequalities Experienced by People with Learning Disabilities and/or Mental Health Problems*. Disability Rights Commission.

Dunn, J. R. (2008) *Mental Capital and Wellbeing: Making the Most of Ourselves in the 21st Century*. Government Office for Science.

Dunn, S. (1999) *Creating Accepting Communities: Report of the Mind Inquiry into Social Exclusion and Mental Health Problems*. Mind.

Edwards, S. (2003) *In Too Deep: CAB Clients' Experience of Debt*. Citizens Advice.

Ellaway, M. & McIntyre, S (2004) You are where you live. *Mental Health Today*, **November**, 10–12.

Evans, S. (2004*a*) *Further Analysis of IOP Community Data*. Report prepared for the Social Exclusion unit, quoted in *Mental Health and Social Exclusion* (p. 72), Social Exclusion Unit (2004), Office of the Deputy Prime Minister.

Evans, S. (2004*b*) A survey of the provision of psychological treatments to older adults in the NHS. *Psychiatric Bulletin*, **28**, 411–414.

Evans, S. & Huxley, P. I. (2000) Quality of life measurement in mental health: some recent findings. In *Proceedings of the Third Conference of the International Society for Quality of Life Studies* (eds F. Casas & C. Saurina), pp. 271–282. Institut de Recerca sobre Qualitat de Vida, University of Girona.

Faculty of Old Age Psychiatry (2006) *Raising the Standard*. Royal College of Psychiatrists (http://www.rcpsych.ac.uk/PDF/RaisingtheStandardOAPwebsite.pdf).

Fahey, T., Montgomery, A. A., Barnes. J., *et al* (2003) Quality of care for elderly residents in nursing homes and elderly people living at home: controlled observational study. *BMJ*, **326**, 580.

Falkov, A. (1998) *Crossing Bridges: Training Resources for Working with Mentally Ill Parents and Their Children*. Department of Health & Pavillion Publishing.

Farrington, D. (2008) The psychosocial milieu of the offender. In *Forensic Psychiatry: Clinical, Legal and Ethical Issues* (eds J. Gunn & P. Taylor), pp. 252–285. Butterworth Heinemann.

Feinstein, L., Lupton, R., Hammond, C., *et al* (2007) *The Public Value of Social Housing: A Longitudinal Analysis of the Relationship of Housing and Life Chances*. Institute of Education.

Fergusson, D. M. & Woodward, L. J. (2001) Mental health, educational and social role outcomes of adolescents with depression. *Archives of General Psychiatry*, **59**, 225–231.

Fitch, C., Chaplin, R., Trend, C., *et al* (2007) Debt and mental health: the role of psychiatrists. *Advances in Psychiatric Treatment*, **13**, 194–202.

Ford, R., Beadsmore, A., Norton, P., *et al* (1993) Developing case management for the long-term mentally ill. *Psychiatric Bulletin*, **17**, 409–411.

Foster, K., Meltzer, H., Gill, B., *et al* (1996) *Economic Activity and Social Functioning of Adults with Psychiatric Disorders*. OPCS Surveys of Psychiatric Morbidity in Great Britain Report No. 8. HMSO.

Frankenburg F. R. & Zanarini, M. C. (2004) The association between borderline personality disorder and chronic medical illnesses, poor health-related lifestyle choices, and costly forms of health care utilization. *Journal of Clinical Psychiatry*, **65**, 1660–1665.

Frost-Gaskin, M., O'Kelly, R., Henderson, C., *et al* (2003) A welfare benefits outreach project to users of community mental health services. *International Journal of Social Psychiatry*, **49**, 251–263.

Fryers, T., Melzer, D. & Jenkins, R. (2003) Social inequalities and the common mental disorders. *Social Psychiatry and Psychiatric Epidemiology*, **38**, 229–237.

Fryers, T., Melzer, D., Jenkins, R., *et al* (2005) The distribution of the common mental disorders: social inequalities in Europe. *Clinical Practice and Epidemiology in Mental Health*, **1**, 14–25.

Fryers, T. & Russell, O. (2003) Applied epidemiology. In *Seminars in the Psychiatry of Learning Disability* (2nd edn) (eds W. Fraser & M. Kerr), pp. 16–48. Gaskell.

Gordon, D., Levitas, R., Pantazis, C., *et al* (2000) *Poverty and Social Exclusion in Britain.* Joseph Rowntree Foundation.

Gossop, M., Marsden, J. & Stewart, D. (1998) *NTORS at One Year, The National Outcome Research Study: Changes in Substance Treatment Use, Health and Criminal Behaviour One Year after Intake.* Department of Health.

Green, H., McGinnity, A., Meltzer, H., *et al* (2005) *Mental Health of Children and Young People in Great Britain, 2004.* Office for National Statistics.

Grove, B. (2008) *Factors Influencing Recovery from Serious Mental Illness and Enhancing Participation in Family, Social and Working Life* (State-of-Science Review: SR-B9). Government Office for Science (http://www.foresight.gov.uk/Mental%20Capital/SR-B9_MCW.pdf).

Hansard (2008) Written Answers to Questions. Wednesday 14 May 2008 (http://www.publications.parliament.uk/pa/cm200708/cmhansrd/cm080514/text/80514w0001.htm#08051473000127).

Harrington, R. (2002) Affective disorders. In *Child and Adolescent Psychiatry* (4th edn) (eds M. Rutter & E. Taylor), pp. 463–485. Blackwell Science.

Harris, E. C. & Barraclough, B. (1998) Excess mortality of mental disorder. *British Journal of Psychiatry*, **173**, 11–53.

Hatcher, S. (1994) Debt and deliberate self-poisoning. *British Journal of Psychiatry*, **164**, 111–114.

Hayes, R. L. & Halford, W. K. (1996) Time use of unemployed and employed single male schizophrenic subjects. *Schizophrenia Bulletin*, **22**, 659–669.

Hayes, T. (2000) Stigmatizing indebtedness: implications for labelling theory. *Symbolic Interaction*, **23**, 29–46.

Help the Aged (2008) *Spotlight on Older People in the UK.* Help the Aged.

Hills, J. (2007) *Ends and Means: The Future Roles of Social Housing in England* (CASE Report 34). Economic and Social Research Council Research Centre for the Analysis of Social Exclusion.

Hintikka, J., Kontula, O., Saarinen, P., *et al* (1998) Debt and suicidal behaviour in the Finnish general population. *Acta Psychiatrica Scandinavica*, **98**, 493–496.

Hippisley-Cox, J., Vinogradova, Y., Coupland, C., *et al* (2006a) *A Comparison of Survival Rates for People with Mental Health Problems and the Remaining Population with Specific Conditions.* Disability Rights Commission.

Hippisley-Cox, C., Parker, C., Coupland, C., *et al* (2006b) *Use of Statins in Coronary Heart Disease Patients with and without Mental Health Problems.* Disability Rights Commission.

Home Office (2001) *British Crime Survey.* Home Office.

Hopton, J. L. & Hunt, S. M. (1996) Housing conditions and mental health in a disadvantaged area of Scotland. *Journal of Epidemiology and Community Health*, **50**, 1637–1649.

Hyndman, S. J. (1990) Housing dampness and health amongst British Bengalis living in East London. *Social Science and Medicine*, **30**, 131–141.

James, K. (2003) *Access to Adult Education for People with Mental Health Needs. Report of a National Postal Survey of Colleges of Further Education and Local Authority Adult Education Services.* NIACE and NIMHE.

Jenkins, R., Bhugra, D., Bebbington, P., *et al* (2008) Debt, income and mental disorder in the general population. *Psychological Medicine*, **38**, 1485–1493.

Johnson, J. G., Cohen, P., Dohrenwend, B. P., *et al* (1999) A longitudinal investigation of social causation and social selection processes involved in the association between socioeconomic status and psychiatric disorders. *Journal of Abnormal Psychology*, **108**, 490–499.

Johnstone, E. C., Crow, T. J., Johnson, A. L., *et al* (1986) The Northwick Park Study of first episodes of schizophrenia. I. Presentation of the illness and problems relating to admission. *British Journal of Psychiatry*, **148**, 115–120.

Kai, J., Crosland, A. & Drinkwater, C. (2000) Prevalence of enduring and disabling mental illness in the inner city. *British Journal of General Practice*, **50**, 992–994.

Kessler, R. C., Foster, C. L. Saunders, W. B., *et al* (1995) Social consequences of psychiatric disorders. I. Educational attainment. *American Journal of Psychiatry*, **152**, 1026–1032.

Kim-Cohen, J. (2003) Prior juvenile diagnosis in adults with mental disorder. *Archives of General Psychiatry*, **60**, 709–717.

Kim-Cohen, J., Caspi, A., Moffitt, T. E., *et al* (2003) Prior juvenile diagnoses in adults with mental disorder: developmental follow-back of a prospective longitudinal cohort. *Archives of General Psychiatry*, **60**, 709–717.

Lee, S., Tsang, A., Breslau, J., *et al* (2009) Mental disorders and termination of education in high-income and low- and middle-income countries: epidemiological study. *British Journal of Psychiatry*, **194**, 411–417.

Leff, J. & Warner, R. (2006) *Social Inclusion of People with Mental Illness*. Cambridge University Press.

Lewis, G., Bebbington, P., Brugha, T., *et al* (1998) Socioeconomic status, standard of living, and neurotic disorder. *Lancet*, **352**, 605–609.

Lupton, R., Wilson, A., May, T. H., *et al* (2002) *A Rock and a Hard Place: Drug Markets in Deprived Neighbourhoods* (Home Office Research Study No. 240). Home Office.

Mackin, P., Bishop, D., Watkinson, H., *et al* (2007) Metabolic disease and cardiovascular risk in people treated with antipsychotics in the community. *British Journal of Psychiatry*, **191**, 23–29.

Maher, J. & Green, H. (2000) *General Household Survey – Carers 2000*. Office for National Statistics.

Marwaha, S. & Johnson, S. (2004) Schizophrenia and employment. *Social Psychiatry and Psychiatric Epidemiology*, **39**, 337–349.

Marwaha, S., Johnson, S., Bebbington, P., *et al* (2007) Rates and correlates of employment in people with schizophrenia in the UK, France and Germany. *British Journal of Psychiatry*, **191**, 30–37.

Maughn, B., Brock, A. & Ladva, G. (2004) *The Health of Children and Young People*. Office for National Statistics.

Mayers, C. A. (2000) Quality of life: priorities for people with enduring mental health problems. *British Journal of Occupational Therapy*, **63**, 591–597.

McCrone, P. & Thornicroft, G. (1997) Credit where credit's due. *Community Care*, **September**, 18–24.

Meich, R. A., Caspi, A., Moffitt, T. E., *et al* (1999) Low socioeconomic status and mental disorders: a longitudinal study of selection and causation during young adulthood. *American Journal of Sociology*, **104**, 1096–1131.

Meltzer, H. (2003) *Further analysis of the Psychiatric Morbidity Survey 2000*. Data prepared for the Social Exclusion unit. Quoted in *Mental Health and Social Exclusion* (p. 72), Social Exclusion Unit (2004), Office of the Deputy Prime Minister.

Meltzer, H. (2008) *The Mental Ill-Health of Children in Local Authority Care (State-of-Science Review: SR-B7)*. Government Office for Science.

Meltzer, H., Gill, B., Petticrew, M., *et al* (1995a) *The Prevalence of Psychiatric Morbidity among Adults Living in Private Households (OPCS Surveys of Psychiatric Morbidity in Great Britain, Report No. 1)*. HMSO.

Meltzer, H., Gill, B., Petticrew, M., *et al* (1995b) *Economic Activity and Social Functioning of Adults with Psychiatric Disorders (OPCS Surveys of Psychiatric Morbidity in Great Britain. Report No. 3)*. HMSO.

Meltzer, H., Gatward, R., Goodman, R., *et al* (2000) *The Mental Health of Children and Adolescents in Great Britain*. TSO (The Stationery Office).

Meltzer, H., Singleton, N., Lee, A., *et al* (2002) *The Social and Economic Consequences of Adults with Mental Disorders*. TSO (The Stationery Office).

Meltzer, H., Gatward, R., Corbin, T., *et al* (2003) *The Mental Health of Young People looked after by Local Authorities in England*. (TSO) The Stationery Office.

Melzer, D., Fryers, T. & Jenkins, R. (2004) *Social Inequalities and the Distribution of the Common Mental Disorders* (Maudsley Monographs 44). Psychology Press.

Mencap (2004) *Treat Me Right! Better Healthcare for People with Learning Disability*. Mencap.

Mencap (2007) *Death by Indifference: Following up the Treat Me Right! Report*. Mencap.

Mental Health Foundation (2001) *An Uphill Struggle: Poverty and Mental Health*. Mental Health Foundation.

Michael, J. (2008) *Healthcare for All: Report of the Independent Inquiry into Access to Healthcare for People with Learning Disabilities*. Independent Inquiry into Access to Healthcare for People with Learning Disabilities.

Mind (2008) *In the Red: Debt and Mental Health*. Mind.

Moran, P., Stewart, R., Brugha, T., *et al* (2007) Personality disorder and cardiovascular disease: results from a national household survey. *Journal of Clinical Psychiatry*, **68**, 69–74.

Morgan, C., Kirkbride, J., Hutchinson, G., *et al* (2008) Cumulative social disadvantage, ethnicity and first episode psychosis: a case control study. *Psychological Medicine*, **38**, 1701–1715.

Murphy, E. (1991) *After the Asylums*. Faber and Faber.

Musselwhite, C. B. A. & Haddad, H. (2007) *Prolonging the Safe Driving of Older People through Technology (SPARC Project Final report)*. Centre for Transport and Society, University of the West of England.

Nash, M. (2002) Voting as a means of social inclusion for people with a mental illness. *Journal of Psychiatric Mental Health Nursing*, **9**, 697–703.

National Audit Office (2007) *Improving Services and Support for People with Dementia*. National Audit Office (http://www.nao.org.uk/publications/nao_reports/06-07/0607604.pdf).

National Social Inclusion Programme (2007) *At Home? A Study of Mental Health Issues arising in Social Housing*. NSIP (http://www.socialinclusion.org.uk/publications/GNHFullReport.doc).

Nelson, G., Aubry, T. & Lafrance, A. (2007) A review of the literature on the effectiveness of housing and support, assertive community treatment, and intensive case management for persons with mental illness who have been homeless. *American Journal of Orthopsychiatry*, **77**, 350–361.

Nettleton, S. & Burrows, R. (1998) Mortgage debt, insecure home ownership and health: an exploratory analysis. *Sociology of Health and Illness*, **20**, 731–753.

Neuburger, J. (2003) *Housekeeping: Preventing Homelessness through Tackling Rent Arrears in Social Housing*. Shelter.

NICE (2002) *Schizophrenia: Core Interventions in the Treatment and Management of Schizophrenia in Primary and Secondary Care*. NICE.

NICE (2006a) *Alzheimer's Disease – Donepezil, Galantamine, Rivastigmine (Review) and Memantine*. NICE (http://guidance.nice.org.uk/TA111).

NICE (2006b) *Bipolar Disorder: The Management of Bipolar Disorder in Adults, Children and Adolescents, in Primary and Secondary Care*. NICE.

NIMHE (2003) *Personality Disorder: No Longer a Diagnosis of Exclusion. Policy Implementation Guidance for the Development of Services for People with Personality Disorder*. Department of Health.

Office of the Deputy Prime Minister (2004) *Mental Health and Social Exclusion (Social Exclusion Unit Report)*. ODPM.

Office of the Deputy Prime Minister (2006) *Sure Start to Later Life: Ending Inequalities for Older People*. ODPM.

Office for National Statistics (2002) *The UK 2000 Time Use Survey*. ONS.

Office for National Statistics (2004) *Labour Force Survey: Employment status by occupation and sex, April–June 2004.* ONS (http://www.statistics.gov.uk/STATBASE/Product.asp?vlnk=14248).

Osborn, D. P., Levy, G., Nazareth, I., *et al* (2007) Relative risk of cardiovascular and cancer mortality in people with severe mental illness from the United Kingdom's general practice research database. *Archives of General Psychiatry*, **64**, 242–249.

Pantazis, P., Gordon, D. & Levitas, R. (2006) *Poverty and Social Exclusion in Britain.* Policy Press.

Partners in Care (2004) *The Princess Royal Trust for Carers, Carers Health Survey.* Partners in Care.

Payne, S. (2006) *Mental Health, Poverty and Social Exclusion.* In Poverty and Social Exclusion in Britain (eds P. Pantazis, D. Gordon & R. Levitas). Policy Press.

Perkins, R. & Rinaldi, M. (2002) Unemployment rates among patients with long-term mental health problems: A decade of rising unemployment. *Psychiatric Bulletin*, **26**, 295–298.

Phelan, M., Stradins, L. & Morrison, S. (2001) Physical health of people with severe mental illness. *BMJ*, **322**, 443–444.

Pickett, K. E., James, O. W. & Wilkinson, R. G. (2006) Income inequality and the prevalence of mental illness: a preliminary international analysis. *Journal of Epidemiology and Community Health*, **60**, 646–647.

Pinfold, V. (2004) Social participation (Report prepared for the Social Exclusion Unit by Rethink). In *Mental Health and Social Exclusion.* Social Exclusion Unit, Office of the Deputy Prime Minister.

Platt, J. (1995) Vocational rehabilitation of drug users. *Psychological Bulletin*, **117**, 416–433.

Platt, L. (2002) *Parallel Lives? Poverty among Ethnic Minority Groups in Britain.* Child Poverty Action Group.

Prime Minister's Strategy Unit (2003) *Alcohol Misuse, Interim Analysis Paper.* Prime Minister's Strategy Unit.

Read, J. & Baker, S. (1996) *Not Just Sticks and Stones: A Survey of Stigma, Taboos and Discrimination Experienced by People with Mental Health Problems.* Mind.

Reading, R. & Reynolds, S. (2001) Debt, social disadvantage and maternal depression. *Social Science and Medicine*, **53**, 442–454.

Richardson, J. & Joughin, C. (2000) *The Mental Health Needs of Looked after Children.* Gaskell.

Rinaldi, M., Perkins, R., Hardisty, J., *et al* (2006) Not just stacking shelves. *A Life in the Day*, **10**, 8–14.

Royal College of Psychiatrists (2007) *Healthcare Commission National Audit of Violence 2006–7. Final Report – Working Age Adult Services.* Royal College of Psychiatrists' Centre for Quality Improvement.

Sainsbury Centre for Mental Health (2002) *An Executive Briefing on Adult Acute Inpatient Care for People with Mental Health Problems.* Sainsbury Centre for Mental Health.

Sainsbury Centre for Mental Health (2003) *Getting a Move On* (Briefing 25). Sainsbury Centre for Mental Health.

Sainsbury Centre for Mental Health (2004) *The Supporting People Programme and Mental Health* (Briefing 26). Sainsbury Centre for Mental Health.

Samele, C., Seymour, L., Morris, B., *et al* (2006) *A Formal Investigation into Health Inequalities Experienced by People with Learning Difficulties and People with Mental Health Problems – Area Studies Report.* Disability Rights Commission.

Sayce, L. (2000) *From Psychiatric Patient to Citizen: Overcoming Discrimination and Social Exclusion.* Macmillan.

Sayer, S. (2010) Politicians must recognise that people with learning disabilities have a right to vote too. *The Guardian*, 20 January (http://www.guardian.co.uk/society/joepublic/2010/jan/20/learning-disabilities-rights-vote-election).

Schachar, R. & Tannock, R. (2002) Syndromes of hyperactivity and attention deficit. In *Child and Adolescent Psychiatry* (4th edn) (eds M. Rutter & E. Taylor), pp. 399–418. Blackwell Science.

Scharf, T., Phillipson, C., Smith, A.E., *et al* (2002) *Growing Older in Socially Deprived Areas*. Help the Aged (http://www.helptheaged.org.uk/NR/rdonlyres/924DF9BD-3489-434C-9769-6E0317453490/0/growing_older_in_socially_deprived_areas.pdf).

Schneider, J. (2007) *Better Outcomes for the Most Excluded. Report for Social Exclusion Task Force*. Institute of Mental Health.

Scottish Intercollegiate Guidelines Network (2001) *Attention Deficit and Hyperkinetic Disorders in Children and Young People* (SIGN Report No.52). SIGN.

Seebohn, P. & Scott, J. (2004) *Addressing Disincentives to Work Associated with the Welfare Benefits Systems in the UK and Abroad*. Social Enterprise Partnership.

Seebohm, P. & Secker J. (2005) What do service users want? In *New Thinking about Mental Health and Employment* (eds B. Grove, J. Secker & P. Seebohm). Radcliffe.

Shand, F. & Mattick, R. P. (2002) Results from the 4th National Clients of Treatment Service Agencies census: changes in clients' substance use and other characteristics. *Australian and New Zealand Journal of Public Health*, **26**, 352–357.

Shimitras, L., Fossey, E. & Harvey, C. (2003) Time use of people living with schizophrenia in a north London catchment area. *British Journal of Occupational Therapy*, **66**, 46–54.

Singleton, N., Maung, N. A. Cowie, A., *et al* (2002) *Mental Health of Carers*. TSO (The Stationery Office).

Skantze, K., Malm, U., Denker, S. J., *et al* (1992) Comparison of quality of life with standards of living in schizophrenic out-patients. *British Journal of Psychiatry*, **161**, 797–801.

Skodol, A. E., Gunderson, J. G., McGlashan, T. H., *et al* (2002) Functional impairment in schizotypal, borderline, avoidant, or obsessive-compulsive personality disorders. *American Journal of Psychiatry*, **159**, 276–283.

Slade, M., McCrone, P. & Thornicroft, G. (1995) Uptake of welfare benefits by psychiatric patients. *Psychiatric Bulletin*, **19**, 411–413.

Smith, M. (2010) *Jury Service – Rethink Briefing January 2010*. Rethink (http://www.rethink.org/how_we_can_help/campaigning_for_change/breaking_down_the_wall/jury_service.html).

Social Care Institute for Excellence (2003) *Alcohol, Drug and Mental Health Problems: Working with Families*. SCIE.

Strydom, A., Livingston, G., King, M., *et al* (2007) Prevalence of dementia in intellectual disability using different diagnostic criteria. *British Journal of Psychiatry*, **191**, 150–157.

Targosz, S., Bebbington, P., Lewis, G., *et al* (2003) Lone mothers, social exclusion and depression. *Psychological Medicine*, **33**, 715–722.

Taylor, M. P., Pevalin, D. J. & Todd, J. (2007) The psychological costs of unsustainable housing commitments. *Psychological Medicine*, **37**, 1027–1036.

Taylor, S. J. (1994) Debt and deliberate self-harm. *British Journal of Psychiatry*, **164**, 848–849.

Teplin, L., McClelland, G., Abram, K., *et al* (2005) Crime victimisation in adults with severe mental illness: comparison with the National Crime Victimization Survey. *Archives of General Psychiatry*, **62**, 911–921.

Thornicroft, G. (1991) Social deprivation and rates of treated mental disorder. Developing statistical models to predict psychiatric service utilisation. *British Journal of Psychiatry*, **158**, 475–484.

Thornicroft, G. (2006) *Shunned: Discrimination against People with Mental Illness*. Oxford University Press.

Trauer, T., Duckmanton, R. A. & Chiu, E. (1998) A study of the quality of life of the severely mentally ill. *International Journal of Social Psychiatry*, **44**, 79–91.

Tsemberis, S., Gulcur, L. & Nakae, M. (2004) Housing First, consumer choice and harm reduction for people with a dual diagnosis. *American Journal of Public Health*, **94**, 651–656.

van Schrojenstein Landman-de Valk, H. M. J. & Walsh, P. N. (2008) Managing health problems in people with intellectual disabilities. *BMJ*, **337**, 1408–1412.

Waddell, G. & Burton, K. (2006) *Is work good for your health and wellbeing?* TSO (The Stationery Office).

Waghorn, G. & Lloyd, C. (2005) The employment of people with mental illness. *Australian E-Journal for the Advancement of Mental Health*, **4** (suppl.), 1–43.

Walsh, E., Moran, P., Scott, C., *et al* (2003) Prevalence of violent victimisation in severe mental illness. *British Journal of Psychiatry*, **183**, 233–238.

Weeder, T. (1986) Comparison of temporal patterns and meaningfulness of the daily activities of schizophrenic and normal adults. *Occupational Therapy in Mental Health*, **6**, 27–48.

Weich, S. & Lewis, G. (1998*a*) Poverty, unemployment and common mental disorders: population based cohort study. *BMJ*, **317**, 115–119.

Weich, S. & Lewis, G. (1998*b*) Material standard of living, social class and the prevalence of the common mental disorders in Great Britain. *Journal of Epidemiology and Community Health*, **52**, 8–14.

Weich, S., Lewis, G. & Jenkins, S. P. (2001) Income inequality and the prevalence of common mental disorders in Britain. *British Journal of Psychiatry*, **178**, 222–227.

West, P. (1984) Social stigma and community recreational participation by the mentally and physically handicapped. *Therapeutic Recreation Journal*, **18**, 41–49.

Whitley, E., Gunnell, D., Dorking, D., *et al* (1999) Ecological study of social fragmentation, poverty and suicide. *BMJ*, **319**, 1034–1037.

WHO World Mental Health Survey Consortium (2004) Prevalence, severity, and unmet need for the treatment of mental disorders in the World Health Organization World Mental Health Surveys. *JAMA*, **291**, 2581–2590.

Wilkinson, R. & Pickett, K. (2009) *The Spirit Level: Why More Equal Societies Almost Always Do Better*. Penguin.

Woodward, L. J. & Fergusson, D. M. (2001) Life course outcomes of young people with anxiety disorders in adolescence. *Journal of the American Academy of Child and Adolescent Psychiatry*, **40**, 1086–1093.

World Health Organization Commission on Social Determinants of Health (2008) *Closing the Gap in a Generation: Health Equity through Action on the Social Determinants of Health (Final Report)*. World Health Organization.

CHAPTER 9

Social exclusion in specific social groups and individuals with mental health problems

Jed Boardman, Alan Currie, Helen Killaspy, Kwame McKenzie and Gillian Mezey

There seems no doubt that people with mental health problems are at risk of exclusion from many aspects of society, but it is also recognised that certain social identity groups are similarly at risk. In this chapter we examine the ways in which people with mental health problems who belong to these identity groups may be disadvantaged. In fact, they may be considered to be doubly disadvantaged, excluded by the nature of their ethnicity, culture or skin colour, their gender or sexual identity, or their faith and perhaps also by their mental health problems, or by the interaction of these characteristics. The idea of double disadvantage may be an oversimplification of the status of these groups – the disadvantage is unlikely to be straightforwardly additive – but it serves to illustrate the many ways in which disadvantage may operate. In addition, there are certain groups in society that are defined by their exclusion – prisoners, refugees and asylum seekers, the homeless – and the occurrence of mental health problems in these groups is higher than in the general population. They are excluded by their lack of liberty, lack of citizen status and lack of essential material needs.

Women with mental health problems

Women with mental health problems are especially vulnerable to exclusion in the areas of family activity and access to physical healthcare. Mental health problems are associated with the experience of domestic violence, which has an impact on social activity, income, leisure activities, and mental and physical health. Female mentally disordered offenders have particular problems.

Family activity

Women with mental health problems have as many children as those in the general population with the exception of women with schizophrenia and those with anorexia. The fertility rate for women with a diagnosis of schizophrenia is lower than that for other women (Howard *et al*, 2002).

This is not fully explained by prescribed medication, especially as fertility is likely to increase with increasing use of atypical antipsychotics (Howard *et al*, 2002). Two-thirds of women with long-term psychoses have children (McGrath *et al*, 1999; Howard *et al*, 2001) and the majority describe motherhood as rewarding and central to their lives (Diaz-Caneja & Johnson, 2004).

The exclusion of many women with mental health problems is influenced by their increased risk of problems during the perinatal period and beyond. Recent confidential enquiries into maternal deaths have highlighted the contribution of diagnosed mental health problems, which are one of the leading causes of death during pregnancy and 1 year postpartum (Confidential Enquiry into Maternal and Child Health (CEMACH), 2007). Women with a history of psychosis, particularly bipolar disorder, are at increased risk of relapse in the postnatal period (Harlow *et al*, 2007). Women with severe mental health problems are at increased risk of obstetric complications, including congenital malformations (Bennedsen *et al*, 2001), stillbirth and neonatal deaths (Webb *et al*, 2005). In addition, women with a range of mental health problems are less likely to attend antenatal appointments (Kelly *et al*, 1999). They are more likely to smoke and drink alcohol during pregnancy and are less likely to have their smoking and alcohol consumption addressed by antenatal care services than other women in obstetric services (Howard *et al*, 2003; Shah & Howard, 2006). After giving birth, women with mental health problems may experience difficulty looking after their child, although the majority of women with psychotic disorders admitted to psychiatric mother and baby units in the UK do not need Social Services' support on discharge (Howard *et al*, 2004). Nevertheless, a significant proportion of mothers with psychoses and severe personality disorders who have parenting difficulties may lose custody of their infant (Wang & Goldschmidt, 1994; Howard *et al*, 2003). Losing custody of a child can cause profound distress in these women (Apfel & Handel, 1993) but many do not know how to navigate legal and social services when custody issues arise (Sands *et al*, 2004). Women with mental illness are reluctant to seek help with childcare because they are frightened that their children will be taken away (Herle & McGrath, 2000; Krumm & Becker, 2006). Mental health services often leave childcare needs unmet, which makes many mothers with mental health problems reluctant to seek help for their problems (Chernomas *et al*, 2000; Edwards & Timmons, 2005).

The presence of a mental health problem may have an impact on family life in other ways. For example, women with mental illness are more likely to marry a person with a psychiatric disorder (Rutter & Quinton, 1984; Lancaster, 1999), have lower marriage rates and higher divorce rates than women without mental illness (Goldman, 1982), and describe the support or assistance received from fathers as being characteristically low (Mowbray *et al*, 1995). Women are more likely to be in single-parent households than men and single mothers are more likely to experience depression (Targosz *et al*, 2003). In addition to the spectre of loss of custody of their children, mental health problems in mothers can have an impact on the cognitive, emotional and behavioural development of their children (Murray *et al*, 1996; Pilowsky *et al*, 2006). However, effective treatment of maternal depression has a positive effect on both mothers and their children (Weissman *et al*, 2006). There are several mother and baby units in the UK for mothers who are ill in the perinatal period, though some areas have no in-patient mother and baby unit at all (Elkin *et al*, 2009). There are almost no such units for women with older children, though separate services for women have been developed where women in crisis can be admitted with their children (Killaspy *et al*, 2000).

Domestic violence and domestic abuse

Domestic violence affects family activity, social activity, finances, access to civic opportunities and leisure activities. Sexual violence against women is prevalent and represents a significant public health issue, alongside domestic abuse (Krug *et al*, 2002). Both domestic and sexual violence are associated with adverse health and social outcomes for women. Higher rates of domestic violence have been found in women with mental health problems who are in contact with mental health services compared with rates in the community (Post *et al*, 1980; Cascardi, *et al*, 1996; Dienemann *et al*, 2000). Domestic violence is associated with mental health problems, including depression, post-traumatic stress disorder, anxiety, insomnia, alcohol and drug abuse, suicide attempts and exacerbation of psychotic symptoms (Golding, 1999; Campbell, 2002; Neria *et al*, 2005).

There is a complex inter-relationship between mental health problems and abusive violence: mental health problems may be precipitated by abuse, but severe and chronic mental illness can also put women at risk of abuse. This may be as a result of their illness, medication, living conditions or co-occurring substance misuse which can contribute to increased vulnerability. In addition to the physical and psychological morbidity associated with domestic violence, its victims may have limited access to money, small social networks and fewer opportunities to participate in the wider community as a result of being controlled by the abuser (British Medical Association, 2007). Women from Black and minority ethnic groups, particularly immigrant groups, who experience domestic violence also find it harder to access services. Women may also be particularly vulnerable to violence within mental health services, for example sexual abuse and harassment by male patients on mixed-sex wards (Mezey *et al*, 2005).

Most domestic violence remains undetected by mental health services internationally (Rose *et al*, 1991; Wurr & Partridge, 1996; Young *et al*, 2001; Walby & Allen, 2004). Health professionals rarely enquire about domestic violence and service users are reluctant to disclose such experiences if not asked directly (Goodwin *et al*, 1988; Dill *et al*, 1991; Richardson *et al*, 2001; Walby & Allen, 2004; Read *et al*, 2005; Howard *et al*, 2008). There

175

appears to be a number of barriers to routine enquiry about domestic violence, including: a lack of training and confidence in staff, the severity of psychological disturbance and an associated fear of exacerbating it, the clinician's beliefs about the reliability of client's account, and the gender of the clinician (Little & Hamby, 1996; Mitchell *et al*, 1996; Read & Frazer, 1998; Agar & Read, 2002; Walby & Allen, 2004). When service users do disclose information about domestic violence, the response of mental health services is frequently inadequate (Little & Hamby, 1996; Agar & Read, 2002; Read *et al*, 2005). The Royal College of Psychiatrists' (2002) guidelines recommend that all patients be asked about partner violence as part of the clinical assessment and the key interventions cited are establishing safety, treating mental health problems, providing information about local resources and assessing current and future risk. In addition, the Department of Health began a pilot implementation project for women who have suffered violence and abuse, as part of the Victims of Violence and Abuse Prevention Programme (VVAPP) *Health and Mental Health Programme Implementation Guide*, in partnership with the Home Office VVAPP programme (Department of Health, 2005*b*, 2006).

Access to physical healthcare

Access to physical healthcare has been covered in Chapter 8, but women may face some specific difficulties. Women with mental health problems have difficulty accessing contraception (McLellan & Ganguli, 1999) and physical screening programmes such as those for cervical and breast cancer (Carney & Jones, 2006; Werneke *et al*, 2006). They also have specific difficulties in receiving optimal care during pregnancy.

Patients as parents

As we noted in Chapter 8, a substantial number of people who use mental health services and others with a diagnosis of mental health problems are parents. The children of these parents may be living with their birth parent/ parents, in stepfamilies, with relatives, in foster care or in other informal or formal care arrangements which may change frequently. Fathers are less likely than mothers to be actively caring for their children (Nicholson *et al*, 1999). Around 68% of women and 54.5% of men with any diagnosable mental health problems are parents (Nicholson *et al*, 2002); 59% of women and 25% of men with a diagnosis of psychosis are parents and 42% live with their children (Hearle *et al*, 1999). The prevalence of all personality disorders in the UK is about 4% (Coid *et al*, 2006) and a significant proportion of such individuals will be parents, especially those diagnosed with borderline personality disorder, who are more likely to be female. There are between 200 000 and 300 000 children in England and Wales and between 41 000 and 59 000 children in Scotland whose parents (one or both) have a serious drug problem (Advisory Council on the Misuse of Drugs, 2003). Many others live with a parent with alcohol misuse. Of those with drug misuse, only 37% of fathers and 64% of mothers are still living with their children and the more serious the drug problem, the less likely this is. Most children not living with their natural parents live with other relatives and about 5% of all children are in care (Advisory Council on the Misuse of Drugs, 2003).

The effects of the parents' mental health problems can be exerted from conception onwards and the impact is felt long beyond early childhood, into teenage years and adult life. Diagnosis alone conveys little about the risks and there are several ways in which parental mental ill health can influence not only child development, but also safety, adjustment, transition to adulthood and future parenthood. The transmission of this risk from parent to child could be genetic, the effect of drugs, alcohol or smoking in pregnancy, or caused by antenatal anxiety and stress and postpartum depression, all of which are known to impair the infant's cognitive and emotional development, and these effects are detectable up to and including adolescence (O'Connor et al 2002; Grace et al, 2003; Talge et al, 2007). Parental mental health problems may act directly (via symptoms or the side-effects of medication) or indirectly (through neglect, absence, the effects of third parties), and lead to: physical and emotional abuse or neglect; domestic violence; dangerously inadequate supervision; other inappropriate parenting practices; the presence of toxic substances in the home (prescribed and non-prescribed); exposure to criminal or other inappropriate adult behaviour; and social isolation. These risks will interact with, and exacerbate, the poverty and material deprivation and the social disadvantages such as joblessness and educational under-attainment experienced by people with mental health problems (Chapter 8). Mothers with mental health problems are more likely to report severe financial difficulty and physical health problems than other low-income urban populations and experience an excess of crises including loss of significant others, assaults and other negative life events (Mowbray et al, 2000). In addition to the stresses children living in poverty are exposed to, those whose parents are mentally ill may also experience prejudice and discrimination. Similarly, children with emotional or behavioural disorders can have an adverse influence on parental mental health.

Parents who have a personality disorder are likely to struggle because their capacity to manage and self-soothe their own arousal is limited and they may not be able to soothe their child's distress, but instead respond with hostility or fear. This can lead to a vicious cycle, in which the child gets more distressed and the parent becomes either more frightened or frightening, making it likely that the child will become insecurely attached. If the parent feels helpless and hostile, they are more likely to treat their child as an adult or peer, which may then lead to role reversal or attack behaviours.

Children may also experience: intermittent or permanent separation (resulting from admissions or receipt into care); inadequate accommodation and/or frequent changes in residence; interrupted or otherwise unsatisfactory education and socialisation. Losses may also arise in relation to the suicide or early death of a parent. The children of some mentally ill parents, particularly those of single parents, may be placed in the position of becoming a young carer. An estimated 25–30% of all young carers are looking after a parent with a mental illness. They may be taking on caring tasks and duties in addition to school or college work and these may fluctuate in response to changes in their parent's mental health. Such a role limits their social opportunities and may lead to stigma and discrimination from peers (Aldridge & Becker, 2003).

Black and minority ethnic individuals with mental health problems

In Chapter 7 we outlined the historical, cultural and social determinants that may lead to disparities and exclusion of Black and minority ethnic groups. Here we will concentrate on how such factors may interact with services for people with mental health problems leading to social exclusion. Not surprisingly, this is a complex phenomenon.

Put simply, people from Black and minority ethnic backgrounds in the UK are more likely to suffer social exclusion because of their economic and sociocultural position in society. Recent migrants and other linguistically and culturally isolated groups may be at most risk, but the cycle of disadvantage and despair seen in some inner city areas where such people tend to stay affects all who live there, not just the most recent immigrants. People with mental health problems are socially excluded because of stigma and disabilities associated with their illness; these often are not accommodated in the workplace and recovery-oriented work is not pursued to optimise individual recovery.

In those of Black and minority ethnic status, the two types of safety net that decrease exclusion and may promote recovery – mental health and social services, and family and community – may not be sufficient to balance the impact of the social determinants of inequity and mental health problems. This is in part because of differences in the accessibility, attractiveness and effectiveness of government mental health services for ethnically diverse populations but also because some hard-pressed families and communities have limited capacity to offer support and instrumental help to those who develop health problems.

Inequalities in rates of illness and service use

That ethnic minorities get unequal care in psychiatry is well documented. A snapshot of inequalities in the receipt of care is taken each spring in the Count Me In census by the Care Quality Commission. This has been running for 5 years and is a census of all people in mental health and learning disability in-patient units in England and Wales on one particular day. The 2009 census also included those on a community treatment order who were out-patients. The census records the ethnicity of all those individuals and in 2009 reports information for 31 786 individuals who were either in-patients on the mental health wards of 264 NHS and independent healthcare organisations or on a community treatment order on census day (1371 patients were on a community treatment order and of these, 118 were in-patients on census day). In 98% of cases ethnicity data are available (Care Quality Commission, 2010).

In the 2009 census, 6% of all patients reported that English was not their first language. Although the NHS still has inadequate interpreting services, the cost of providing high-quality interpretation has led some to suggest that future migrants should be expected to learn English rather than services being tailored to meet their unique linguistic needs. However, the most accurate accounts of a person's illness history are best given in the language that they are most used to speaking. Interpretation and translation services are needed if the NHS is going to offer equitable care.

Although 92% of the UK population is White British, only 76% of the Count Me In census sample were. The other groups were: 10% Black or White/Black mixed, 4% other White, 3% South Asian (Indian, Pakistani and Bangladeshi), 2% White Irish and 3% from other ethnic groups (including Chinese). At a population level, the Indian and Chinese groups had similar rates of admission to hospital as the White British (which was lower than average for the whole population), but all other ethnic groups had higher rates of admission than the White group. Rates were particularly high in the Black Caribbean, Black African, White/Black Caribbean mixed and White/Black African mixed groups – over three times higher than for White British. The 'other Black' group had rates nine times higher than the White British. It is of note that these figures were similar to those observed in previous Count Me In censuses. There was no evidence of a decline in admission rates over the 5 years of the census in Black and minority ethnic groups.

In hospital there are significant treatment differences. For instance, seclusion rates are higher than average among the other White and White/Black Caribbean mixed groups. Furthermore, the median duration of stay from the day of admission to the day of census were among the longest for patients from the Black Caribbean and White/Black Caribbean mixed groups, and among the shortest for patients from the Chinese, South Asian, Black African, White British and other groups.

Pathways to care are different for different groups. Rates of referral from GPs and community mental health teams were lower than average among Black and White/Black mixed groups, but rates of referral from the criminal justice system were increased. These findings echo those in first-episode groups, where Black of African origin groups have less GP and more prison justice system involvement (Morgan et al, 2005; Care Quality Commission, 2010).

Numerous studies have reported increased rates of involuntary admission to hospital for certain Black and minority ethnic groups (Bhui et al, 2003).

The Count Me In censuses are no different. Patients from the Black Caribbean, Black African, other Black and White/Black Caribbean mixed groups, and those in the other White group have been reported to be more likely to have been detained against their will or on a community treatment order in all 5 years of the census. Black Caribbean and other Black groups are also more likely to be detained in the community on forensic orders (Care Quality Commission, 2010).

The Count Me In census is hospital-based. Community-based surveys report a variety of differences in rates of mental health problems and access to, and use of, services in Black and minority ethnic groups. For instance, people from Black and ethnic minority groups are less likely to contact a mental health service or professional after a suicide attempt than White British (Crawford et al, 2005). Indeed, differential rates of suicide, with high rates in some South Asian groups and in people of African origin in hospital, have been documented, but these have not attracted a targeted service response (Bhui & McKenzie, 2008; McKenzie et al, 2008).

In the EMPIRIC study, a survey of a representative sample of 5000 people in Great Britain (Sproston & Nazroo, 2002), there were small but statistically significant variations in the prevalence of common mental disorders across ethnic groups. Compared with White population Irish men and Pakistani women had higher rates and Bangladeshi women lower rates of common mental disorders. Somatic symptom scores were elevated among Bangladeshi men and South Asian women (especially those of Indian and Pakistani origin). The researchers commented that the failure to give added weight to these symptoms may have resulted in underestimates of the prevalence of the common mental disorders among some South Asian groups.

In addition to differences in rates of illness, differences in service use were documented (Sproston & Nazroo, 2002). Black and minority ethnic groups were all more likely to have seen their GP recently than White British. Those with depression were more likely to have seen a GP recently irrespective of ethnicity. However, for Black and minority ethnic individuals their GP visits were less likely to be for an emotional or stress-related problem than for White British. In other words it would seem that Black and minority ethnic respondents with common mental disorders were at least as likely to see their GP as White British but less likely to see them and get treatment for depression. In addition, access to counsellors or psychologists was highest among the White, Irish and Black Caribbean individuals (Sproston & Nazroo, 2002).

Social support

In general those who are socioeconomically deprived have less capacity to support others. In addition there are reports of higher levels of stigma related to mental illness in some ethnic groups. This could lead to further exclusion and diminish the readiness of groups to offer support to those with mental health problems. However, it is difficult to find evidence to support the latter point. Levels of support in UK ethnic minority groups for people with mental illness tend to reflect levels of support for people who do not have mental illness.

Some of the best information on social support comes from the EMPIRIC study. This reported that in South Asian groups there were higher levels of family involvement and people were more likely to be married. However, in all Black and minority ethnic groups there were higher levels of negative aspects of close relationships. In terms of social networks, it was evident that, overall, Black and minority ethnic individuals had more contact with friends than relatives. Perhaps surprisingly, though, social support *per se* was not strongly related to a decreased rate of common mental disorders, but the negative aspects of close relationships were associated with an increased rate of those disorders.

On the other hand, although they reported large social circles and had relatively close contact with relatives and friends, Black Caribbean people received less confiding/emotional and practical support than others. Bangladeshi informants received high levels of emotional and practical support from their closest person, but also experienced very high levels of negative influence. Thus, close intimate relationships may have both advantages and disadvantages for mental health.

It is also interesting to note the relatively small friendship networks of Indian and Pakistani women in comparison with men. Some studies have suggested that smaller social networks precede the onset of common mental disorder and it is possible that the smaller networks contribute to the higher rates of common mental disorder, depressive episodes, anxiety disorders, and mixed anxiety and depressive disorder found in Pakistani women (Stansfield & Sproston, 2002).

Increasing social inclusion in mental health services for Black and minority ethnic individuals

Two concepts may be useful in considering how to improve mental health services and decrease social exclusion for Black and minority ethnic individuals. One is the concept of differential treatment because of the way the mental health system works. The other is the concept of fundamental social causes.

Systematic institutionalised differential treatment

The concept of systematic institutional differential treatment (sometimes referred to as institutional racism) often makes people uncomfortable. This is because people usually take offence at the perceived slur of racism in their ranks. The discussion usually descends into questions about whether the profession or service is racist instead of what can be done to improve services for specific groups.

Institutionalised differential treatment is supposed to:

1 Focus on the actions of institutions rather than individuals.

People may act in good faith and not harbour racist attitudes but perpetuate discriminatory practices because of systems set up by the institution.

2 Target the results of practice rather than the intent.

Proved disparities in health, the reasons for them and the ways that services can change to reduce disparities between groups should be the focus for action rather than looking for intent or racist ideology.

3 Acknowledge that the connection and interaction between medicine and a discriminatory social world may be important in producing the disparities.

Poor educational provision for some minority groups means that many will not meet the criteria for entry to medical school.

4 Take into account how the history of the NHS affects patients' perceptions.

For example, knowledge of high rates of more coercive treatment of African–Caribbeans by psychiatrists may lead to a delay in presentation with mental illness.

5 Acknowledge other forms of social stratification and their effects.

As we see in this chapter, gender, social class or sexual orientation may interact with ethnic background to increase disparities.

6 Acknowledge the fact that discrimination may change with time and with the type of institution.

Overt racism may be replaced by more subtle racism but the disparities between ethnic groups may remain the same.

7 Identify the problem as ideological.

Health disparities are brought about and perpetuated not only by culture, class and sociopolitical forces external to medicine but also by the ideology of the medical profession that leads to ineffective or no action in the face of disparities and to a lack of concerted effort to teach or discuss racism in medicine in undergraduate and postgraduate curriculums. Moreover, the emphasis on the biomedical model undermines the anthropological research that is needed to properly document the perceptions, needs and aspirations of minority ethnic groups (McKenzie, 1999).

Taking up the last point, it is of interest that in the EMPIRIC study the qualitative interviews demonstrated what the respondents saw as important. Much of this highlighted factors that get relatively scant attention in medicine, such as the fact that experiences of racism are pervasive and powerful and at times are considered to 'strike right at the heart of people's ability to live tolerable lives' (O'Connor & Nazroo, 2002). Another study underlined this reporting that previous experiences of racism were associated with adherence to treatment and length of hospital stay (unpublished; further details available from K.M. on request).

Fundamental social causes

Link's concept of fundamental social causation is a useful way of thinking about how social exclusion occurs both in wider society and within psychiatry (Link & Phelan, 1995). The idea of fundamental social causes will not be new to most. It posits that the driver of health disparities are factors such as access to new information, education, influence, money and the ability to use health messages. Decreasing the disparity requires action targeted at these fundamental social causes rather than specific illnesses as these are epiphenomena. Moreover, even if the particular illness disparity is dealt with over time, new disparities will emerge as society changes. The issue here is that social exclusion makes one group a repository of particular social ills even if those ills change over time.

This concept is important for those considering service improvement. Generic policies aimed at improving mental health services may actually lead to increased disparities. This is because they interact with the fundamental social causes. A simple example would be an information website on local mental health services. Because of their social situation, English language proficiency, money and education, Black and minority ethnic individuals in general will have limited access to the website, limited access to information, and the gap between their care and that of the White population may increase. Unless interventions are targeted at the fundamental causes or have remedial plans to make up for their impact, health innovation may increase ethnic disparities (Link & Phelan, 1995).

Service development for Black and minority ethnic groups

Institutionalised differential treatment and the fundamental social causes offer significant challenges to those wanting to improve mental health services for Black and minority ethnic groups. The first highlights the breadth of change that is needed to deliver improved services across a number of different parts of the social world and the second highlights the depth of change that is required.

The social exclusion of ethnic minorities plays out in different ways for different ethnic groups but is a reflection of fundamental social causes. In the UK, disparities in rates of illness, access to care, outcome and satisfaction with services have been reported. However, more often than not such disparities are not measured and ethnic minorities suffer in silence. When disparities are reported the focus of discussions gets side-tracked into questions about whether the data are correct and whose fault the problems are (McKenzie & Bhui, 2007). In response policy improvements such as Delivering Race Equality (Department of Health, 2005a) are set up, with little funding or leverage on providers, a remit significantly to change the access, outcome and satisfaction with services for Black and minority ethnic groups and with 5 years to do it. Indeed, Delivering Race Equality was only allowed to focus on two of the seven aspects of systematic differential treatment that should be considered and not surprisingly has had modest impact.

If the aim is to improve social inclusion in mental health services for individuals from ethnic minorities, then some fundamental work on the power structures in psychiatry and the way that it engages with the community will have to be undertaken. It is difficult to envisage how this can be achieved unless psychiatry is more community-based, diagnoses are emic (based on intrinsic cultural distinctions) as opposed to etic (based on universal models) and we offer care from a truly multicultural perspective. Mental health services are developed to cater for the dominant economic or cultural group. Ethnic minorities will not receive equitable care unless this changes.

The problems faced will be different for different ethnic groups. This reflects differences in culture, socioeconomic status and the group's fit within the dominant society. However, there are some similarities caused by the generally lower socioeconomic status of ethnic minority groups, varying degrees of social isolation, acculturation, the impact of migration, and differences in illness models between minority ethnic groups and the services. The need is for a service model that properly engages such populations and takes note of what they say and want. Rather than an add-on to specific forms of work, the community voice needs to be a fundamental hard-wired part of a learning and listening service (McKenzie, 2008). Bolt-on policies that are motivated only by the equity and legal agendas, devoid of realistic appraisals of the challenge for timescales required for change, are unlikely to deliver the sustainable shifts towards effective services. The fundamental cause in the wider world is access to power. The fundamental social cause in psychiatry is no different.

In order to develop equitable services we need to consider a multi-level approach. Working from the patient outwards a non-exhaustive list would include the levels shown in Box 9.1. Any policy to increase social inclusion would need to be multi-level. There would need to be policy work, community development work and specific work on health and linked services. Increasing inclusion in hard-pressed services and multiply-disadvantaged urban areas is challenging enough. However, added to this there will be a need to understand the aspirations and desires of different cultural groups and generations so that inclusion offers real and relevant opportunities.

Asylum seekers and refugees

Refugees and asylum seekers are among the most marginalised groups in the UK, excluded by the very nature of their status – they do not have the same rights as British citizens. They suffer high rates of psychological problems and there is no national strategy to meet their mental health needs.

The terms asylum seeker and refugee mean different things – the terms are legal classifications that vary from country to country. In the UK an asylum seeker is a person who has made a formal application to the Home

Box 9.1   A multi-level approach to developing equitable services for Black and minority ethnic groups

Level 1. Development of clinical skills, attitudes and knowledge

Level 2. Development of better support for clinicians, for example interpreting services or advocacy

Level 3. Development of service delivery models and training that are culturally acceptable

Level 4. Improvements in access to services – pathways into care and out of care

Level 5. Improvements in community influence of commissioning of secondary care

Level 6. Cross-cultural improvements in primary care

Level 7. Support and development of non-statutory/voluntary sector alternatives

Level 8. Culturally acceptable and valid health promotion strategies in public health

Level 9. A legislative framework that supports service development

Level 10. Wider social policy aimed at the social determinants of health and fundamental social causes of disparities and an acknowledgement of the role of racial discrimination in the rates and outcomes of ill health

Level 11. Mixed-methods community-informed research to develop expertise, evidence and innovation, to monitor change and outcomes

Level 12. Health impact assessment and remedial plans to ensure that all service improvements decrease rather than increase disparities.

Office for asylum status and is waiting for a decision. A refugee is a person whose asylum application has been successful. They are granted permission to stay in the country under the terms of the 1951 United Nations' Convention on the Status of Refugees, which states that a refugee must be outside their country; have a well-founded fear of persecution because of his or her race, religion, nationality, membership of a social group or political opinion; and be unable or unwilling to return to the country for fear of persecution. If the person does not meet refugee criteria they still may qualify for humanitarian protection or discretionary leave.

The process of seeking asylum can be long and drawn out. If an initial application is turned down this may lead to an appeal. A person's application can only be considered failed when the legal process, including all appeals, has been exhausted. Even then there may be clear reasons why the Home Office cannot remove them from the country, such as ill health or if their country is deemed too dangerous.

There are approximately 10 million asylum seekers and refugees worldwide (UNHCR, 2006a), most of whom are in low-income countries, sometimes in refugee camps; 23% of asylum seekers and refugees are in Europe and only 3% in the UK. The number of applicants who receive refugee status reflects the policies and practices and ease of entry rather than the numbers of people legitimately seeking asylum. If the size of the domestic populations is taken into account, the UK ranks 14th in the EU for the numbers of applications. Less than 0.5% of the UK population is an asylum seeker or refugee. There has been a fall in applications for asylum in the UK over the past decade, from 91 600 in 2001 to 30 840 applications in 2005. In 2005, the main nationalities applying to the UK were Iranian, Eritrean, Chinese, Somali and Afghan. The majority of the principal (head of family) applicants in 2005 were under 35 years old and male, but there were a significant number (approximately 3000) of unaccompanied asylum-seeking children (Heath *et al*, 2006). Although the number of asylum seekers and refugees in the UK is low, they are concentrated in certain parts of certain cities. In London they make up 5% of the population and form 11% of the caseloads of some community mental health teams (McColl & Johnson, 2006).

Asylum seekers and refugees can present with complex medical needs, including infectious diseases, mental health problems and complications from injuries due to trauma, including torture and violence. Asylum seeker and refugee groups are often considered as one, but they have different social risk factors, not least because asylum seekers are still dealing with uncertainty due to unresolved status and because UK laws and social policy change. There is also much diversity within groups. The vast majority of asylum seekers and refugees have no mental illness, but there are increased levels of psychopathology and mental illness in refugee and asylum seeker groups, in particular anxiety and depression. Refugees resettled in Western countries are about 10 times more likely to have post-traumatic stress disorder than age-matched general populations in those countries (Fazel *et al*, 2005). Other studies suggest that there may be more somatic presentation of psychological problems (Tribe, 2002; Van Ommeren *et al*, 2002).

Post-migration problems

There is also evidence that post-migration problems have a significant impact on psychological well-being. In a survey on in-patients, Iverson & Morken (2004) found the asylum seekers had much higher rates of post-traumatic stress disorder than refugees (45% *v.* 11%), possibly because of the high level of stress associated with the pathways into asylum. In male Iraqi refugees in the UK, Gorst-Unsworth & Goldenberg (1998) found that psychological morbidity was associated with poor social support, separation from children, lack of contact with political organisations in exile, low confidant support and a low number of social activities. A meta-analysis of studies comparing the mental health of refugees with that of control groups from the host countries found that refugees (including asylum seekers and internally displaced people) had an overall increase in psychopathology (Porter & Haslam, 2005). However, the analysis found that increase in psychopathology was not an inevitable consequence of acute wartime stress. Refugees who were older, more educated, female, had a higher pre-displacement socioeconomic status and rural residence had worse mental health outcomes. Morbidity was significantly associated with post-migration factors such as a lack of permanent accommodation and restricted opportunity to work.

Social exclusion

Asylum seekers are excluded by the very nature of their status and the exclusion of both asylum seekers and refugees is also determined by factors that may increase their risk of mental ill health. Many asylum seekers and refugees have experienced pre-migration adversities such as war, imprisonment, genocide, physical and sexual violence, witnessing violence to others, traumatic bereavement, starvation, homelessness, lack of healthcare. Their journey to the UK may be hazardous and associated with separation from families and communities.

The adversities faced after migration, including aspects of the asylum system, can compound the impact that social isolation, poverty and cultural alienation have. These adversities may be summarised as 'seven Ds'.

1   *Discrimination.* Asylum seekers and refugees are often stigmatised in host countries: the UNHCR (2006*b*) condemned the attitudes of politicians and the press who have turned asylum seekers and refugees into 'victims of intolerance' and 'faceless bogymen'. Negative attitudes and public hostility to asylum seekers increase social exclusion and risk of psychological distress.

    Cultural differences and religious beliefs of asylum seekers may be different from the majority population in the UK and this may exacerbate social exclusion, particularly if the person is isolated from a similar cultural or religious group. It may also cause considerable difference in the ways in which mental health needs are expressed and in the requirements for treatment. For example, a Western model of trauma may not be the most helpful means of addressing complex issues the asylum seekers face. Many asylum seekers either do not speak English or speak English as a second language. Access to interpreters remains variable within the health services, as does their quality.

2   *Detention.* Detention removes asylum seekers from taking part in the ordinary life of the population and worsens their health, yet health service provision to detainees is unsatisfactory (Silove *et al*, 2001; Fazel & Silove, 2006). Approximately 25000 people were held in ten removal centres in the UK in 2004–2005, including increasing numbers of children (Amnesty International UK, 2005; Save the Children, 2005).

3   *Dispersal.* A Home Office department, the National Asylum Support Service (NASS) is responsible for support arrangements for destitute asylum seekers. The package of support can involve enforced dispersal across the country, often to locations with few resources for asylum seekers. They may be given no choice in where they are sent, be moved many times, and the arrangement of transfer can be chaotic. Social isolation, often exacerbated by few family ties in the host country, limitations of language, cultural differences and frequent changes in sites of accommodation through dispersal all lead to social exclusion as well as disrupting the continuity of any care.

4   *Destitution.* Asylum seekers are not entitled to mainstream welfare benefits nor access to employment. There are no central statistics on destitution in asylum seekers in the UK, but local reports (Patel & Kerrigan, 2004: Save the Children, 2005; Lewis, 2007) and pressure has led to some changes to government policies which could make asylum seekers more destitute, such as the Section 55 of the National Immigration and Asylum Act 2002.

5   *Denial of healthcare.* All asylum seekers and refugees are entitled to free primary healthcare services. However, in April 2004 UK law changed so that failed asylum seekers are now no longer eligible for free secondary healthcare, except in cases that are deemed immediately necessary or life-threatening.

6   *Delayed decisions.* Asylum seekers live with instability and uncertainty in many aspects of their lives, including temporary housing, dispersal, and possible deportation linked with increasing government requirements to limit this form of migration. In addition, the length of the asylum process adversely affects health (Steel *et al*, 2006) and may double the risk of diagnosable mental health problems after 2 years of delay (Laban *et al*, 2004). Under the New Asylum Model introduced in March 2007, the Home Office is trying to speed up decisions and to improve their quality, but the balance may not be right. There is concern that the timescale between applying, submitting evidence and receiving a decision is now too short (in some cases only 11 days). This may be insufficient for a newly arrived asylum seeker to access the help required to make a proper application.

7   *Denial of the right to work.* Asylum seekers are denied the basic right of work to which UK citizens are entitled. They are initially prevented from undertaking paid work, but if they do not have an initial decision on their asylum status after 12 months they can then apply for permission to work. Lack of work can inhibit social integration and increase poverty.

The importance of post-migration factors is that many of them can be modified in the host country. Sensitive social policy can minimise risk factors for illnesses in asylum seeker and refugee groups and is vital for a preventative health strategy. The worst outcomes were found for those displaced internally in their own country, living in temporary or institutional accommodation and experiencing restricted economic opportunity.

Addressing environmental needs such as housing, opportunities for employment, and access to English language classes will aid integration and social cohesion for asylum seekers. Government committees such as the Joint Committee on Human Rights emphasise the need to address these issues. The draft strategy for refugee integration in London (Mayor of London, 2007) recommends that for healthcare it is vital that the evidence base is increased, confusion around the rights to access to care is reduced, appropriate training for all healthcare professionals is offered and there is better linking with voluntary sector agencies and the NHS.

Access to mental health services for asylum seekers is variable and service provision may take many different forms. The response of services must be considered in the light of the complex social and health needs of asylum seekers and will often require a sensitive, multidisciplinary approach from specialists in the field. Whether asylum seekers should be initially assessed and treated within generic mental health services or be offered specialist care remains unclear and will likely be influenced by other factors that also affect inclusion issues, for example the needs of women, children and those of the family as a whole, the supportive interventions required, and particular needs such as writing court reports or supporting applications for housing.

Social inclusion policies and practices for these groups need to address matters in the political, social, cultural and medical fields. Addressing areas of social exclusion has been shown to bear upon mental health outcomes and reduce post-migration adversity, although it is recognised that further work is needed to provide a broader evidence base for assessing the mental health needs of asylum seekers than is currently feasible. The five areas of integration – civic, economic, social, interpersonal and healthcare – all highlight where asylum seekers do not have rights or equality of access. Asylum seekers should have greater access to services that would meet many basic human rights and refugees should have access to community life – integrated and socially cohesive. This would enable participation through appropriate choices, safety, respect, housing, relationships and employment. In addition, the serious consequences of community fragmentation and inter-racial, cultural and religious divides may all be better addressed.

The Royal College of Psychiatrists' (2007) position statement on improving services for refugees and asylum seekers emphasises that three main areas of action are required to promote health and to prevent the development of mental and physical illness in those groups in the UK. First, a public policy that minimises the impact of social risk factors for physical and mental illness; second, equitable access to a full range of health, social care and legal services that are capable of delivering appropriate and high-quality care; and finally, public bodies should be organised to fulfil their duties under national and international law.

Sexual orientation and mental health problems

At least 5% of people in the UK are gay, lesbian or bisexual (Johnson et al, 2001). Homosexual people are at higher risk of mental disorder, suicidal ideation, substance misuse and deliberate self-harm than heterosexual people – in a systematic review King et al (2007a) found a two- to fourfold excess in suicide attempts, whereas the risk of depression, anxiety or alcohol/drug dependence was at least 1.5 times higher relative to heterosexuals. Lesbian and bisexual women were found to be particularly at risk of suicidal ideation, drug and alcohol dependence (four times higher than heterosexual women), whereas the lifetime risk of suicide attempts in gay men was four times that of heterosexual men.

Despite these high levels of psychological morbidity, psychiatry has a regrettable history with regard to its attitudes to homosexuality, which was until recently considered a mental disorder. In 1973, the American Psychiatric Association declassified homosexuality as a mental disorder but retained a diagnosis of 'egodystonic homosexuality' for people who were distressed about being homosexual. This latter diagnosis was removed in 1987 from the revised third edition of the *Diagnostic and Statistical Manual of Mental Disorders* (DSM–III) and rephrased as 'sexual disorder, not otherwise specified: marked and persistent distress about one's sexual orientation' and it remains in this form in DSM–IV. Similarly, the WHO dropped the diagnosis 'homosexuality' from its *International Classification of Diseases* (ICD) in 1992, but retained 'egodystonic sexual orientation' in ICD–10, under 'disorders of adult personality and behaviour', described as 'when an individual wishes their sexual orientation were different and may seek treatment to change it'. Clearly this is intended for gay and bisexual people. Heterosexual people who wish to be homosexual are rarely described. This history of pathologisation of homosexuality was reflected in the attitudes of professionals. Negative views of homosexuality persisted until recently among healthcare professionals including GPs (Bhugra & King, 1989), medical students and psychiatric trainees (Chaimowitz, 1991; Evans et al, 1993), psychoanalysts and psychotherapists (Bartlett et al, 2001).

Over the past few years there has been a great deal of legislation reflecting British society's increasing tolerance of homosexuality. For example: in 2001, an equal age of consent was introduced; in 2002, same-sex spouses were recognised as nearest relatives under the Mental Health Act; in 2003, homophobic assault was recognised as a hate crime; in 2003, Section 28 of the Local Government Act 1988 (the law banning councils and schools in England and Wales from intentionally promoting homosexuality) was repealed; in 2003, the Victorian laws on Gross Indecency and Buggery were repealed; and in 2005, the Civil Partnership Act was introduced in the UK. Although the visibility and rights of lesbian, gay, bisexual and transgender people have increased, prejudice, homophobic attacks and minimal or stereotypical media representation still pervade. Furthermore, homosexual service users continue to report pathologisation of their sexual orientation (McFarlane, 1998; King & McKeown, 2003; King *et al*, 2007*b*), prejudice, harassment and even violence from mental health staff (Golding, 1997). This marginalisation is not only unacceptable, it also makes services unattractive to this group of people.

Sexual orientation may not be a constant 'state' and not everyone who identifies themselves as lesbian, gay, bisexual or transgender necessarily wants to be 'out' in any or every situation. This presents a particular challenge for mental health staff in knowing how and when to ask about sexual orientation. Staff may be silenced by their own lack of knowledge about issues relating to sexual orientation or uncomfortable with asking about it and wary of saying the wrong thing. Diversity training in mental health has never focused routinely on issues of sexual orientation and staff necessarily fall back on anecdotal knowledge, and sometimes prejudice, and are left ill equipped to deal with issues related to sexual orientation among their service users and colleagues.

All mental health staff should be adequately skilled to provide appropriate mental health services accessible to lesbian, gay, bisexual and transgender clients. Specialist services provided by the non-statutory sector may also appeal to some service users and reduce burden on the NHS, especially for individuals with less severe mental health problems.

The Royal College of Psychiatrists' Gay, Lesbian and Bisexual Special Interest Group has developed a training pack for mental health professionals which has been endorsed by the College and is being taken up through diversity programmes within individual trusts. The aim is to give staff skills to enquire sensitively about sexual orientation rather than assuming service users are heterosexual, and to aid staff's understanding of how an individual's sexual orientation may or may not be related to their current mental health problems. Psychiatrists and other mental health professionals need to recognise the reparatory work required to gain the confidence of homosexual people as a first step in providing them with a socially inclusive service. As clinical leaders, psychiatrists have a key role in facilitating their social inclusion through equipping themselves with the appropriate skills to enquire and take into account service users' sexual orientation in their assessment. In addition, discriminatory practices secondary to staff or service users' sexual orientation should be addressed in the same way as discrimination on the grounds of any other aspect of diversity.

Faith groups and mental health problems

There are few epidemiological data specifically looking at rates of mental illness and social exclusion in the UK among different faith groups. There is, however, some evidence concerning the use of mental health services among two particular faith groups. This is derived from evidence based on qualitative interviews showing that both Orthodox Jews and Muslims are reluctant to use mainstream psychiatric services.

Orthodox Jews

For the Orthodox Jewry, Lowenthal (2006) discusses barriers in the strictly Orthodox Jewish community in the UK to seeking help for mental health problems. These barriers chiefly include stigma, concerns about violating Jewish religious law and other concerns about conflicts between the values inherent in psychotherapy and Jewish values. Psychotherapy, psychology, psychiatry and psychoanalysis tend to be identified as a nebulous group associated with strong concerns about how 'kosher' (religiously acceptable) it is to use these services. For Jews, having a psychiatric history may negatively affect future marriage prospects and is thus stigmatising. In relation to the violation of religious laws, particularly in psychotherapy, there are concerns that prohibitions about unrelated men and women being together in public places will be broken. Furthermore, because of the Jewish emphasis on being respectful to parents, not speaking disrespectfully about them, it may be difficult, if not impossible, to fully engage in psychoanalytic therapy. There are also prohibitions about speaking badly about others, which again may impinge on the psychoanalytic process. There is frequently a conflict between traditional religious values and secular knowledge. Psychiatry and psychology are held to be atheistic and godless and thus Orthodox Jews are wary of any interaction with these disciplines. There often is a conflict within the Jewish diaspora between tradition and secularisation, with some Jewish groups encouraging self-imposed ghettoisation and restricted contact with the outside world.

There is evidence that Orthodox Jews (Charedim) need mental health services and psychological help as much as the general population. Although there have been suggestions of distinctive patterns for specific disorders in Jews (Fallin *et al*, 2004; Frosh *et al*, 2005; Shifman *et al*, 2004), it appears that the general prevalence of mental health problems is roughly similar to that of other groups. Lowenthal (2006) points out that rabbis are overwhelmed with pastoral and counselling work and that they would welcome more professional support, although they do refer for professional help. There is limited evidence that Orthodox Jews resort to prayer, frequently approach rabbis for help with mental health issues and only go to statutory services in which the patient can remain anonymous. They often travel a long distance from home in order to keep their identities anonymous. They also use culturally sensitive services specially organised by the Jewish population (Lowenthal & Rogers 2004).

Muslims

Similarly, there is little population-level data about rates of illness among Muslims in Britain and their use of psychiatric and psychological services. Much of the research on attitudes towards psychiatry is based upon anthropological work. Dein *et al* (2008) conducted an anthropological study looking at understanding attitudes towards psychiatry among Bangladeshi

Muslims in London. The study showed that members of the community expressed distrust of mainstream psychiatry. They saw psychiatric services as custodial and stigmatising. Few would readily admit to having attended psychiatric consultations. They felt that mainstream psychiatrists did not understand their culture or their needs (their mental health problems may be expressed in the idiom of spirit possession by Jinn spirits). Rather than accessing mental health services, members of the community frequently consult imams and traditional healers, who often charge exorbitant sums of money. This research emphasised the need for British psychiatry to incorporate a cultural perspective when working with Muslim patients.

There is emerging evidence that Islamophobia may have significant negative effects on the mental health and healthcare of Muslim families and children. Despite substantive differences in healthcare systems in the UK and the USA, social structure and political forces play similar roles in the health of Muslim children in both countries (Leard *et al*, 2007). In the UK, service users in the local Muslim communities have pleaded for mental health professionals to take into account their religious and spiritual needs, yet literature suggests that services fail to meet such needs (Greasley *et al*, 2001). This is hardly surprising since mental health professionals receive scant training on the role of religion in an individual's experience of suffering. Global events such as the World Trade Center bombings and the consequent perceived persecution of Muslims worldwide may worsen attitudes towards Muslims in Britain.

Prisoners with mental health problems

Like asylum seekers and refugees, people in prison are excluded by the very nature of their status – they have been deprived of their liberty. In addition, prisoners have extremely high rates of mental health problems and typically come from backgrounds characterised by multiple forms of disadvantage. The number of people in prison has doubled over the past 20 years, with half the increase happening in the past decade, and now exceeds 82 000 in England and Wales. This is the highest rate of imprisonment relative to population size of any country in Western Europe. The UK government has forecast that the prison population could be as high as 101 900 by 2014 (Ministry of Justice, 2007).

Mental health problems are common in prisoners (Meltzer, 2008*a*). The most comprehensive source of data on prevalence is a survey of psychiatric morbidity among prisoners in England and Wales carried out in 1997 for the Office for National Statistics (Singleton *et al*, 1998). The survey showed that over 90% of all prisoners have some kind of mental health problem (this includes psychosis, common mental health problems, personality disorder, alcohol misuse and drug dependence). The overall prevalence of mental disorder among prisoners is about four times as high as in the general population of working age (Singleton *et al*, 1998) and 8% of prisoners have a psychotic disorder, compared with 0.5% in the wider population. Multiple

193

diagnoses are extremely common: over 70% of prisoners have more than one mental health problem (compared with less than 5% in the general population) and those with a psychosis are likely to have three or four other problems. Over the past 10 years there have been around 750 deaths by suicide in prison, equivalent to an annual suicide rate of 1 per 1000, about 10 times as high as the rate in the wider community. Almost a third of suicides occur within the first week of someone arriving in prison and one in seven within 2 days of admission (Prison Reform Trust, 2007).

Prisoners often come from excluded families and maintain these early disadvantages into adult life. Factors that indicate exclusion are shown in Box 9.2 and it is clear that they are much more common in prisoners than the general population (Social Exclusion Unit, 2002). Many of the problems persist, sometimes in aggravated form, after release from prison. For example, 42% of released prisoners have no fixed abode (Niven & Stewart, 2005) and 70% have no employment or placement in training or education on release (Williamson, 2006).

Mental healthcare in prison

Recent years have seen significant changes in prison mental healthcare, including a transfer of responsibility for the funding and provision of services from the prison service to the NHS. Particularly important has been the establishment of a network of multidisciplinary mental health in-reach teams, intended to provide specialist services throughout the prison estate, equivalent to those provided by community-based mental health teams for the population at large. In 2007, there were over 350 in-reach workers providing services in 102 hospitals (Brooker *et al*, 2008). Notwithstanding this extra provision, prison mental healthcare remains underdeveloped and in-reach teams have been hindered by limited resourcing, constraints

---

Box 9.2   The social exclusion of prisoners

Prisoners are more likely than the general population to:

- have been taken into care as a child: 27% (*v.* 2% in the general population)
- have regularly truanted from school: 30% (*v.* 3%)
- have no qualifications: 52% men and 71% women (*v.* 15%)
- have numeracy at or below Level 1 (unlikely to get any basic qualification): 65% (*v.* 23%)
- be unemployed: 67% in the 4 weeks before imprisonment (*v.* 5%)
- be receiving welfare benefits: 72% immediately before imprisonment (*v.* 14%)
- be in debt: 48% with a history of debt (*v.* 10%)
- be homeless: 32% before imprisonment (*v.* 0.9%).

Source: Social Exclusion Unit (2002)

imposed by the prison environment and wide variations in local practice. The resources currently available for mental healthcare in prisons are only about a third of the amount required to deliver standards of service equivalent to those in the wider population (Sainsbury Centre for Mental Health, 2008).

Continuity of care between prison and the community is a major challenge and work done in prisons is often undone when a prisoner is released. Many released prisoners have nowhere to live and only about half of those leaving prison are registered with a GP (Social Exclusion Unit, 2002). Because of frequent movements within the prison estate, many prisoners end up in establishments that are distant from their normal place of residence and this hampers liaison between in-reach teams and local services. Finally, community mental health services are sometimes reluctant to take on responsibility for people released from prison, even if they were involved with them before.

Women in prison

Women account for only about 5% of the prison population, but their numbers have increased particularly rapidly, from around 2000 in 1995 to more than 4500 today. Within magistrates' courts the chance of a woman receiving a custodial sentence has increased sevenfold (Carter, 2003). A large proportion are in custody for short stays, either on remand (a fifth of the female prison population) or with short sentences (over 60% of sentences are for 6 months or less). Women are most commonly held for theft and handling (42%) and 37% are held for drug offences.

Because of the relatively small numbers of women in prison, they are more likely than men to be imprisoned far from home: in 2006, the average distance was 58 miles from home and 60% were held in prisons outside their home region (Prison Reform Trust, 2007). These findings indicate a rapid turnover of women prisoners, with the concomitant difficulty of offering treatment and support, and result in remand prisons such as Holloway (women-only) in London, where 90% of the prisoner population changes within 1 month.

The Prisons and Probation Ombudsman's (2004) independent report comments on the vulnerability of women in remand, noting the effect of external factors such as fractured relationships and unstable living arrangements as well as most women being affected by multiple drug dependence or mental health problems, often in combination. The report further comments that 'It is difficult to see that repeatedly imprisoning them, without support in the community upon discharge, serves either their interests or those of society' (p. 16).

As with male prisoners, over 90% of women in prison have a diagnosable mental health problem (Singleton *et al*, 1998). The prevalence of psychosis is particularly high, affecting an estimated 13% of female prisoners, compared with 0.5% in the general population (Singleton *et al*, 1998). Unlike in the community, proportionately more women than men die by suicide in prison, and five times more self-harm, with over half of all recorded incidents of self-harm occuring in the female estate (Corston, 2007). Many female prisoners, whatever their indicative crime, have a drug/multiple drug and/ or alcohol addiction/problem that requires detoxification as they enter. Over half of female remand prisoners (54%) and 41% of female sentenced prisoners are drug-dependent (of these, 43% and 21% respectively are dependent on opiates) (Kesteven, 2002). A substantial proportion of the women's prison population have an identified learning disability – 11 % of remanded women have an IQ of 65 (IQ below 70 classifies a person with special needs) (Butler & Kousoulou, 2006).

Children and young people in prison

Nearly 15% of people in prison are under 21 years old. Young people in prison have an even greater prevalence of poor mental health than adults, with 95% having at least one mental health problem and 80% having more than one (Lader *et al*, 2000). Few have any qualifications or had worked before entering prison and most had traumatic experiences in earlier life. They are 18 times more likely to die by suicide in prison than young people in the community.

In addition to those directly experiencing imprisonment, much larger numbers of children and young people are affected because their mothers or fathers are in custody (Prison Reform Trust, 2007) – almost 60% of men and two-thirds of women in prison have dependent children under 18. More children are affected by imprisonment than by divorce. Each year nearly 18 000 children are separated from their mothers by imprisonment, over 150 000 have a parent in prison at any one time, and during their time at school 7% of all children experience their fathers' imprisonment (Prison Reform Trust, 2007). Only 5% of the children of women prisoners remain in their own homes once their mother has been sentenced, in part because as many as a third of female prisoners lose their homes while in custody. In most cases the children are looked after by other relatives, but 12% are in care, with foster parents or have been adopted. About 30% of the children of prisoners suffer significant mental health problems, compared with 10% of children in the general population (Social Exclusion Unit, 2002).

Black and minority ethnic prisoners

People from Black and minority ethnic groups account for around one in ten of the general population but in prison this rises to about one in four. This can partly be explained by the presence of foreign nationals in British prisons, who account for 35% of minority ethnic prisoners (Prison Reform Trust, 2007). The rate of diagnosed mental health problems is lower among prisoners from minority ethnic groups than among the White prison population. This may be due to a number of reasons, including lower rates of referral and recognition (Durcan & Knowles, 2006).

Homelessness, social exclusion and mental health problems

Homelessness may be seen as the extreme end of social exclusion, the place where the most alienated and excluded in society end up (Timms & Balazs, 1997). The evidence suggests that, historically, there have always been significant numbers of people with mental health problems in homeless populations. Even in the heyday of the asylums, the institutions for the poor continued to accommodate large numbers of so-called 'pauper lunatics'. The descendants of these institutions were the large direct-access hostels for homeless people (the 'spikes'), Salvation Army hostels and Rowton Houses that were to be found in the working class areas of every UK city.

However, in the 1980s the landscape changed. With the escalation of inner-city property values, these institutions were sold off to voluntary sector organisations, downsized and often converted into high-income housing. Different solutions to 'warehousing' had to be found if the persistence of large numbers of street homeless people – not just the mentally ill – was to be avoided. From the early 1990s, central government funding was deployed in a number of initiatives, including the Homeless Mentally Ill Initiative (Craig *et al*, 1995), which funded several specialist teams in London as well as a number of projects outside the capital. In London, homeless funding was centralised under the umbrella of the Rough Sleepers Initiative, but more recently the centralised funding has been re-deployed to individual boroughs. In Scotland, the Homelessness etc. (Scotland) Act 2003 aims to give every homeless person a right to a home by 2012. The significance of this is that it will get rid of the idea of 'priority need' and the notion of 'intentional' homelessness, both significant barriers to housing for those with mental health problems, substance dependence or personality disorders.

The voluntary sector continues to be in the forefront of service provision for homeless people.

Homelessness in the UK

Obtaining accurate figures for the numbers of homeless people is difficult in almost any country. This is not just because governments may be reluctant to reveal the true size of the problem, as there are considerable problems with estimating the size of homeless populations. The number of homeless people tends to be hidden (National Coalition for the Homeless, 2007) and changes relatively quickly in response to changes in the law or local policing practices. Individuals who become homeless may only be so for a short period and this temporal dimension is rarely recorded. People recorded as homeless by housing and benefits agencies are a selected sample, omitting those who are most alienated and excluded from the benefit and other systems.

Many governments do not collect national data on homelessness and those that do tend to use different definitions of housing type. For instance, in many countries it is impossible to disaggregate supported housing from homeless hostels. This makes international comparisons extremely difficult. A survey by the European Federation of National Organisations Working with the Homeless (FEANTSA) (Edgar *et al*, 2004) noted that 7 out of 15 European countries surveyed collected no official data at all on homelessness. Moreover, on those countries that did collect statistics, the report commented that 'these all take a different approach to data collection, have not covered all agencies and most do not include municipal or statutory services' (p. 8). Surveys tend to be local, irregular and not collated on a regional or national basis.

Current figures on the number of homeless in Great Britain are difficult to gather, not least because the routine data sources have significant limitations. The charity for homeless people, Crisis, and the Public Health Resource Unit (Rees, 2009) estimated the numbers of single homeless people in Great Britain using information on: 'rough sleepers'; people staying in hostels and shelters; people staying in bed and breakfast and other boarded accommodation; squatters; and concealed households (those living with friends or family, but without any explicit right to do so and in accommodation that is in some way unsatisfactory). They estimated there to be between 310 000 and 380 000 single homeless people, of which around a quarter are in hostels, bed and breakfast accommodation or facing imminent threat of eviction on the grounds of debt. The remaining three-quarters are from concealed households.

In the UK, responsibility for homelessness has passed through several government departments but now rests with the Department of Communities and Local Government. One official measure of homelessness is that of the number of households accepted as being owed the main homelessness duty by local authorities under the homeless legislation ('homelessness acceptances'). The long-term trend for local authority homelessness acceptances – mainly of families with children – was slowly upward for many years but has declined since 2003. The number of households living in temporary accommodation has been falling since the end of 2005, reaching 77 510 by April 2009 (Fig. 9.1). The reasons for this decline are not yet clear. Although it gives cause for cautious optimism, it does not represent the homeless populations in which serious mental illness has been historically found – hostel dwellers and rough sleepers.

Even in the UK, which has one of the more sophisticated systems for collecting homelessness data, the reasons for homelessness are couched in broad housing categories (such as the end of a short-term tenancy, loss of rented housing, mortgage arrears and rent arrears) which give no hint as to the nature of the problems underlying these housing crises.

Refugees and asylum seekers are also at risk of homelessness and many have mental health problems (Pernice & Brook, 1994; Palmer, 2006). Although these groups do not fall into the conceptual category of

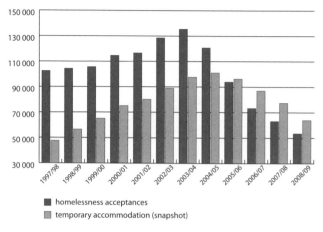

Fig. 9.1 Homelessness acceptances. Source: Communities and Local Government (http://www.communities.gov.uk/housing/homelessness/homelessnesstrends/).

homelessness under UK legislation, their predicament often produces many of the same problems and, albeit in unknown numbers, they contribute to the numbers of street homeless. At the end of December 2003, 80 125 asylum seekers (including dependants) were being supported by the National Asylum Support Service (NASS), 13% lower than the end of December 2002: 49 760 asylum seekers were being supported in NASS accommodation and 30 360 were receiving subsistence only support.

Street homeless

The UK government is the only European government to have constructed a long-term strategy to reduce street homelessness. This is a potent political issue, as although this group may be the tip of the iceberg of a range of homeless situations, they represent the milieu where one is likely to find the most disadvantaged and alienated people, with a constant two-way flow from the street to hostels or night shelters and back again. Using figures from counts of rough sleepers carried out from January 2007 to June 2008, 483 people were sleeping rough on the streets of England on any single night, with half of them in London (Rees, 2009). Figures gathered by homeless agencies suggest that in London alone over 3000 people slept rough at some point during 2008 (Rees, 2009). Most street homeless are men and about 20% are women. The figures for rough sleeping in England since 1998 are shown in Fig. 9.2. These are based on regular surveys of street hostel populations.

For the reasons outlined above, these figures are a significant underestimate of street homelessness. However, their value lies in the trends they suggest, for example that the government's 1999 target of reducing street homelessness by two-thirds by 2002 (Rough Sleepers Unit,

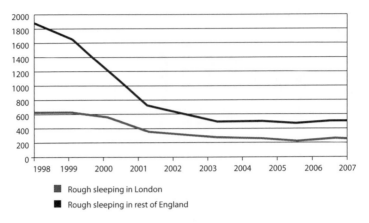

Fig. 9.2 Rough sleepers in England 1998–2007. Source: Communities and Local Government (2007).

1999) was almost achieved. However, it also appears that the numbers of street sleepers in both London and the rest of the UK have remained at their 2003 levels. It is likely that this obstinate residuum is made up of long-term street sleepers, usually with drug, alcohol or mental health problems, those relapsing back into street sleeping for the same reasons, new arrivals on the street from 'traditional' sources, and refugees, asylum seekers and economic migrants from Eastern Europe.

Homelessness and mental health problems

Recent data on the number of homeless people who have mental health problems are also hard to ascertain, not least because most of the published figures are from the 1980s and 1990s, but also because of the variety of survey methods used to assess the type and extent of mental health problems among the homeless (Meltzer, 2008*b*). This picture is often incomplete as most of the research covers the homeless population that are street homeless or in direct access hostels and does not cover those in second-stage accommodation, temporary housing or in unstable accommodation. Figures from the 1996 Office of Population, Censuses and Surveys studies of psychiatric morbidity in Great Britain showed that 38% of residents of homeless hostels had a common mental health problem, 8% had a psychosis and 16% were alcohol dependent (Gill *et al*, 1996). Scott (1993) found rates of mental health problems at 30% to 50% among the homeless, mostly psychoses and personality dysfunction; 20% of these people also had substance abuse, and many had physical health problems. Among the middle-aged group in hostels the prevalence of psychoses is particularly high, but in younger people (under 25 years old) depression, anxiety and impulsive self-harm are common (Dean & Craig, 1999). Over a third of homeless day centre users and 40% of those using soup runs had mental health problems, and 15–20% of these had been in a psychiatric in-patient unit (Bines, 1994). Rates of deliberate self-harm and attempted suicide are high in homeless people (Cullum *et al*, 1995; Haw *et al*, 2006).

In spite of point prevalence rates for schizophrenia of up to 30% in homeless hostels (Scott, 1993), over 60% of those diagnosed were receiving no specialist mental health service (Bines, 1994). The UK studies do not suggest that those with serious mental illness who become homeless are ex-patients from the large institutions that closed, but are a younger group of service users (Craig & Timms, 1992; Leff, 1993). This may reflect the failure of community-based mental health services to provide for their needs as many had past contact with services (Bines, 1994; Langdon *et al*, 2001; O'Neill *et al*, 2007).

Less is known about homeless women but their risk of street homelessness is less than it is for men (Marpasat, 1999). In inner London hostels 50–60% of women had been previously admitted to psychiatric hospital and a similar proportion had a diagnosis of schizophrenia (Marshal & Jeered, 1992; Tacchi & Scott, 1996). Data from the Office for National Statistics shows that a third of women living in temporary accommodation had depression and anxiety, particularly the younger women, and many of these women had children and were from South Asian backgrounds (Sims & Victor, 1999). In Birmingham, between 45% and 50% of homeless mothers experience depression and substance misuse and about one-third of children admitted to hostels have significant mental health problems (Vostanis *et al*, 1997).

Recent changes in the homeless population

Although there are no readily available and reliable published figures, the experience of all inner London homeless mental health teams has been that over the past 10 years there has been: a gradual growth in the number of refugees and failed asylum seekers presenting to homelessness services with post-traumatic stress disorder and adjustment disorders; a decline in the number of older men with schizophrenia; continuing presentations of those with unrecognised first-episode psychosis and dropping out from other psychiatric services; and the emergence of personality disorder as a major issue for homelessness services. Many people who are homeless fall into the category of adults described in Chapter 8 as having 'chaotic lives and multiple needs' or 'facing chronic exclusion' (Bloor *et al*, 2007; Schneider, 2007). The factors promoting the pathway into homelessness are typical of this group and reinforce the nature of their exclusion (Box 9.3). Notably, of the people described as 'of no fixed abode' in the Oxford area, not only did many of them have a history of deliberate self-harm, recent contact with mental health services, current alcohol or drug abuse and/or were described as having personality disorders, but they were likely to be male, jobless, socially isolated, have financial problems, a criminal record, have been a recent victim of violence or have been violent towards others (Haw *et al*, 2006).

Box 9.3   Pathways to homelessness

- Unemployment
- Problem drinking among middle aged men
- Drug misuse among teenagers
- Lack of low-rent housing
- Marital break-up
- Clashes with family or friends
- Leaving local authority care
- Leaving the armed forces
- Leaving prison
- Episode of mental illness
- Children of homeless families
- Very few people choose to have no home

Source: Timms & Balazs (1997)

Conclusion

The evidence presented in this chapter reinforces that people with mental health problems are often excluded. In this case this may relate both to the mental health problems and to other aspects of the person's identity. For others with mental health problems their increased presence in certain excluded groups, such as prisoners, gives them a particular disadvantage. As we have already seen in several chapters in this book, the direction of causality is often not clear – is the increased presence of mental health problems a result of the person's identity or situation or is the opposite the case? Do people with mental health problems face a greater likelihood of homelessness or do the conditions of having no accommodation compound the risk of mental health problems? What does seem likely is that the experience of mental health problems, combined with the conditions of exclusion and the social and legal forces that produce these conditions, reduces the likelihood of escaping from the predicament in which the individual finds him- or herself. As a result, such people present particular challenges for governments and for mental health and social care services.

Summary

The identity groups of people with mental illness that we have examined in this chapter are excluded to differing degrees and in different ways. Many of these groups are doubly (or more) excluded as a result of their mental health problems and their social identity.

Prisoners, the homeless, and refugees and asylum seekers are by the nature of their situation excluded; this creates particular problems for those with mental ill health.

References

Advisory Council on the Misuse of Drugs (2003) *Hidden Harm – Responding to the Needs of Children of Problem Drug Users*. Advisory Council on the Misuse of Drugs.

Agar, K. & Read, J. (2002) What happens when people disclose sexual or physical abuse to staff at a community mental health centre? *International Journal of Mental Health Nursing*, **11**, 70–79.

Aldridge, J. & Becker, S. (2003) *Children Caring for Parents with Mental Illness: Perspectives of Young Carers, Parents and Professionals*. Policy Press.

Amnesty International UK (2005) *Seeking Asylum is not a Crime: Detention of People Who Have Sought Asylum*. Amnesty International.

Apfel, R. J. & Handel, M. H. (1993) *Madness and Loss of Motherhood: Sexuality, Reproduction and Long-term Mental Illness*. American Psychiatric Publishing.

Bartlett, A., King, M. & Phillips, P. (2001) Straight talking: an investigation of the attitudes and practice of psychoanalysts and psychotherapists in relation to gays and lesbians. *British Journal of Psychiatry*, **179**, 545–549.

Bennedsen, B. E., Mortensen, P. B., Olesen, A. V., *et al* (2001) Congenital malformations, stillbirths and infant deaths among children of women with schizophrenia. *Archives of General Psychiatry*, **58**, 674–679.

Bhugra, D. & King, M. B. (1989) Controlled comparison of attitudes of psychiatrists, general practitioners, homosexual doctors and homosexual men to male homosexuality. *Journal of the Royal Society of Medicine*, **82**, 603–605.

Bhui, K. & McKenzie, K. (2008) Rates and risk factors by ethnic group for suicides within a year of contact with mental health services. *Psychiatric Services*, **59**, 414–420.

Bhui, K., Stansfeld, S., Hull, S., *et al* (2003) Ethnic variations in pathways to and use of specialist mental health services in the UK: systematic review. *British Journal of Psychiatry*, **182**, 105–116.

Bines, W. (1994) *Health of Single Homeless People*. Centre for Housing Policy, University of York.

Bloor, R., Crome, I., Astari, A., *et al* (2007) *Service Responses and Outcomes for Adults Described as Having Chaotic Lives and Multiple Needs*. A Scoping Exercise. Clinical Effectiveness Support Unit and Keele University.

British Medical Association (2007) *Domestic Abuse*. A Report from the BMA Board of Science. British Medical Association.

Brooker, C., Gojkovic, D. & Shaw, J. (2008) *The 2nd National Survey of Prison In-Reach*. Report to the Department of Health. Department of Health.

Butler, P. & Kousoulou, D. (2006) *Women at Risk: The Mental Health of Women in Contact with the Judicial System*. Care Services Improvement Partnership.

Campbell, J. (2002) Health consequences of intimate partner violence. *Lancet*, **359**, 1331–1336.

Care Quality Commission, National Mental Health Development Unit (2010) *Count Me in 2009. Results of the 2009 National Census of Inpatients and Patients on Supervised Community Treatment in Mental Health and Learning Disability Services in England and Wales*. Care Quality Commission.

Carney, C. P. & Jones, L. E. (2006) The influence of type and severity of mental illness on receipt of screening mammography. *Journal of General Internal Medicine*, **21**, 1097–1104.

Carter, P. (2003) *Managing Offenders, Reducing Crime – A New Approach*. Research, Development & Statistics Directorate, Home Office.

Cascardi, M., Mueser, K. T., DeGiralomo, J., *et al* (1996) Physical aggression against psychiatric inpatients by family members and partners. *Psychiatric Services*, **47**, 531–533.

CEMACH (2007) *Saving Mothers' Lives: Reviewing Maternal Deaths to Make Motherhood Safer, 2003–2005*. The Seventh Report of the Confidential Enquiries into Maternal Deaths in the United Kingdom. CEMACH.

Chaimowitz, G. A. (1991) Homophobia among psychiatric residents, family practice residents and psychiatric faculty. *Canadian Journal of Psychiatry*, **36**, 206–209.

Chernomas, W. M., Clarke, D. E. & Chisholm, F. A. (2000) Perspectives of women living with schizophrenia. *Psychiatric Services*, **51**, 1517–1521.

Coid, J., Yang, M., Tyrer, P., *et al* (2006) Prevalence and correlates of personality disorder in Great Britain. *British Journal of Psychiatry*, **188**, 423–431.

Communities and Local Government (2007) *Homelessness Statistics and Rough Sleeping – 10 Years from the Target. Policy Briefing 20*. Department of Communities and Local Government.

Corston, Baroness Jean (2007) *The Corston Report: A Review of Women with Particular Vulnerabilities in the Criminal Justice System*. Home Office.

Craig, T. & Timms, P. W. (1992) Out of the wards and onto the streets? Deinstitutionalization and homelessness in Britain. *Journal of Mental Health*, **1**, 265–275.

Craig, T., Bayliss, E., Klein, O., *et al* (1995) *The Homeless Mentally Ill Initiative*. Department of Health.

Crawford, M. J., Nur, U., McKenzie, K., *et al* (2005) Suicidal ideation and suicide attempts among ethnic minority groups in England: results of a national household survey. *Psychological Medicine*, **35**, 69–77.

Cullum., S., O'Brien, S., Burgess, A., *et al* (1995) Deliberate self-harm: the hidden population. *Health Trends*, **27**, 130–132.

Dean, R. & Craig, T. (1999) *Pressure Points: Why People with Mental Health Problems become Homeless*. Crisis.

Dein, S., Alexandra, M. & Napier, D. (2008) Folk psychiatry and contested notions of misfortune among East London Bangladeshis. *Transcultural Psychiatry*, **45**, 31–55.

Department of Health (2005a) *Delivering Race Equality in Mental Health Care: An Action Plan for Reform Inside and Outside Services and the Government's Response to the Independent Inquiry into the death of David Bennett*. Department of Health.

Department of Health (2005b) *Responding to Domestic Abuse: A Handbook for Health Professionals*. Department of Health.

Department of Health (2006) *Tackling the Health and Mental Health Effects of Domestic and Sexual Violence and Abuse*. Department of Health.

Diaz-Caneja, A. & Johnson, S. (2004) The views and experiences of severely mentally ill mothers – a qualitative study. *Social Psychiatry and Psychiatric Epidemiology*, **39**, 472–482.

Dienemann, J., Boyle, E., Baker, D., *et al* (2000) Intimate partner abuse among women diagnosed with depression. *Issues Mental Health Nursing*, **21**, 499–513.

Dill, D. L., Chu, J. A., Grob, M. C., *et al* (1991) The reliability of abuse history reports: a comparison of two inquiry formats. *Comprehensive Psychiatry*, **32**, 166–169.

Durcan, G. & Knowles, K. (2006) *London Prison Mental Health Services: A Review* (Policy Paper 5). Sainsbury Centre for Mental Health.

Edgar, B., Meert, H. & Doherty, J. (2004) *Third Review of Statistics on Homelessness in Europe: Developing an International Definition of Homelessness*. FEANTSA (http://www.feantsa.org/files/transnational_reports/EN_StatisticsReview_2004.pdf).

Edwards, E. & Timmons, S. (2005) A qualitative study of stigma among women suffering postnatal illness. *Journal of Mental Health*, **14**, 471–481.

Elkin, A., Gilburt, H., Slade, M., *et al* (2009) A National Survey of Psychiatric Mother and Baby Units in England. *Psychiatric Services*, **60**, 629–633.

Evans, J. K., Bingham, J. S., Pratt, K., *et al* (1993) Attitudes of medical students to HIV and AIDS. *Genitourinary Medicine*, **69**, 377–380.

Fallin, M., Lassiter, V., Wolynic, P., *et al* (2004) Genome Y Linkage scan for bipolar disorders susceptibility, Loci, Ashkinizi Jewish families. *American Journal of Human Genetics*, **75**, 204–219.

Fazel, M. & Silove, D. (2006) Detention of refugees. *BMJ*, **332**, 251–252.

Fazel, M., Wheeler, J. & Danesh, J. (2005) Prevalence of serious mental disorder in 7000 refugees resettled in western countries: a systematic review. *Lancet*, **365**, 1309–1314.

Frosh, S., Lowenthal, C., Lindsey, C., *et al* (2005) Preference of emotional behaviour disorders amongst strictly orthodox Jewish children in London. *Clinical Child Psychology and Psychiatry*, **10**, 351–368.

Gill, B., Meltzer, H., Hinds, K., *et al* (1996) *OPCS Surveys of Psychiatric Morbidity in Great Britain: Report 7: Psychiatric Morbidity among Homeless People*. HMSO.

Golding, J. (1997) *Without Prejudice: The Mind Lesbian, Gay and Bisexual Health Awareness Research*. Mind.

Golding, J. M. (1999) Intimate partner violence as a risk factor for mental disorders: a meta-analysis. *Journal of Family Violence*, **14**, 99–132.

Goldman, H. H. (1982) Mental illness and family burden: a public health perspective. *Hospital Community Psychiatry*, **33**, 557–560.

Goodwin, J., Attias, R., McCarthy, T., *et al* (1988) Reporting by adult psychiatric patients of childhood sexual abuse. *American Journal of Psychiatry*, **145**, 1183–1184.

Gorst-Unsworth, C. & Goldenberg, E. (1998) Psychological sequelae of torture and organised violence suffered by refugees from Iraq. Trauma-related factors compared with social factors in exile. *British Journal of Psychiatry*, **172**, 90–94.

Grace, S. L., Evindar, A. & Stewart, D. E. (2003) The effect of postpartum depression on child cognitive development and behaviour: a review and critical analysis of the literature. *Archives of Women's Mental Health*, **6**, 263–274.

Greasley, P., Chiu, L. & Gartland, M. (2001) The concept of spiritual care in mental health nursing. *Journal for Advanced Nursing*, **33**, 629–637.

Harlow, B. L., Vitonis, A. F., Sparen, P., *et al* (2007) Incidence of hospitalization for postpartum psychotic and bipolar episodes in women with and without prior pre-pregnancy or prenatal psychiatric hospitalizations. *Archives of General Psychiatry*, **64**, 42–48.

Haw, C., Hawton, K. & Casey, D. (2006) Deliberate self-harm patients of no fixed abode: a study of characteristics and subsequent deaths in patients presenting to general hospital. *Social Psychiatry and Psychiatric Epidemiology*, **41**, 918–925.

Hearle, J. & McGrath, J. (2000) Motherhood and schizophrenia. In *Women and Schizophrenia* (eds D. J. Castle, J. McGrath & J. Kulkarni). Cambridge University Press.

Hearle, J., Plant, K., Jenner, L., *et al* (1999) A survey of contact with offspring and assistance with child care among parents with psychotic disorders. *Psychiatric Services*, **50**, 1354–1356.

Heath, T., Jeffries, R. & Pearce, S. (2006) *Asylum Statistics United Kingdom 2005*. Home Office Statistical Bulletin (http://rds.homeoffice.gov.uk/rds/pdfs06/hosb1406.pdf). Home Office.

Howard, L. M., Kumar, R. & Thornicroft, G. (2001) Psychosocial characteristics and needs of mothers with psychiatric disorders. *British Journal of Psychiatry*, **178**, 427–432.

Howard, L. M., Leese, M., Kumar, C., *et al* (2002) The general fertility rate in women with psychotic disorders. *American Journal of Psychiatry*, **159**, 991–997.

Howard, L. M., Goss, C., Leese, M., *et al* (2003) Medical outcome of pregnancy in women with psychotic disorders and their infants in the first year after birth. *British Journal of Psychiatry*, **182**, 63–67.

Howard, L. M., Thornicroft, G., Salmon, M., *et al* (2004) Predictors of parenting outcome in women with psychotic disorders discharged from mother and baby units. *Acta Psychiatrica Scandinavica*, **110**, 347–355.

Howard, L. M., Hunt, K., Seneviratne, T., *et al* (2008) *CAN-M: Camberwell Assessment of Need for Mothers*. RCPsych Publications.

Iverson, V. C. & Morken, G. (2004) Differences in acute psychiatric admission between asylum seekers and refugees. *Nordic Journal of Psychiatry*, **58**, 465–470.

Johnson, A., Mercer, C., Erens, B., *et al* (2001) Sexual behavior in Britain: partnerships, practices and HIV risk behaviors. *Lancet*, **358**, 1835–1842.

Kelly, R. H., Danielsen, B. H., Golding, J. M., *et al* (1999) Adequacy of prenatal care among women with psychiatric diagnoses giving birth in California in 1994 and 1995. *Psychiatric Services*, **50**, 1584–1590.

Kesteven, S. (2002) *Women who Challenge: Women Offenders and Mental Health Issues*. A Nacro Policy report. Nacro.

Killaspy, H., Dalton, J., McNicholas, S., *et al* (2000) Drayton Park, an alternative to hospital admission for women in acute mental health crisis. *Psychiatric Bulletin*, **24**, 101–104.

King, M. & McKeown, E. (2003) *Mental Health and Social Well-being of Gay Men, Lesbians and Bisexuals in England and Wales*. Mind.

King, M., Semlyen, J., See Tai, S., *et al* (2007a) *Mental Disorders, Suicide, and Deliberate Self Harm in Lesbian, Gay and Bisexual People: A Systematic Review*. National Institute for Mental Health in England.

King, M., Semlyen, J., Killaspy, H., *et al* (2007b) *A Systematic Review of Research on Counselling and Psychotherapy for Lesbian, Gay, Bisexual and Transgender People*. Report for British Association for Counselling.

Krug, E. G., Dahlberg, L. L., Mercy, J. A., *et al* (2002) *World Report on Violence and Health*. WHO.

Krumm, S. & Becker, T. (2006) Subjective views of motherhood in women with mental illness: a sociological perspective. *Journal of Mental Health*, **15**, 449–460.

Laban, C. J. Gernaat. H. B. P. E., Komproe, I. H. (2004) Impact of a long term asylum procedure on the prevalence of psychiatric disorders in Iraqi asylum seekers in the Netherlands. *Journal of Nervous and Mental Diseases*, **192**, 843–851.

Lader, D., Singleton, N. & Meltzer, H. (2000) *Psychiatric Morbidity among Young Offenders in England and Wales*. Office for National Statistics.

Lancaster, S. (1999) Being there: How parental mental illness can affect children. In *Children of Parents with Mental Illness* (ed. V. Cowling). Australian Council for Educational Research.

Langdon, P. E., Yaguez, L., Brown, J., *et al* (2001) Who walks through the 'revolving door' of a British psychiatric hospital? *Journal of Mental Health*, **10**, 525–533.

Leard, L., Amer, M., Barnett, E, *et al* (2007) Muslim patients and health disparities in the UK and US. *Archive of Diseases in Childhood*, **92**, 922–926.

Leff, J. (1993) All the homeless people – where do they all come from? *BMJ*, **306**, 669–670.

Lewis, H. (2007) *Destitution in Leeds*. Joseph Rowntree Trust.

Link, B. & Phelan, J. (1995) Social conditions as fundamental causes of disease. *Journal of Health and Social Behavior*, **35**, 80–94.

Little, L. & Hamby, S. L. (1996) Impact of a clinician's sexual abuse history, gender and theoretical orientation on treatment issues related to childhood sexual abuse. *Professional Psychology: Research and Practice*, **27**, 617–625.

Lowenthal, K. (2006) Strictly orthodox Jews and the relations with psychotherapy and psychiatry. *World Cultural Psychiatry Research Review*, **1**, 128–132.

Lowenthal, K. & Rogers, M. B. (2004) Culture-sensitive counselling, psychotherapy and support groups in the Orthodox-Jewish community: how they work and how they are experienced. *International Journal of Social Psychiatry*, **50**, 227–240.

Marpasat, M. (1999) An advantage with limits: the lower risk for women of becoming homeless. *Population*, **54**, 885–932.

Marshal, C. & Jeered, J. L. (1992) Psychiatric morbidity in homeless British women. *British Journal of Psychology*, **160**, 761–768.

Mayor of London (2007) *London Enriched: The Mayor's Draft Strategy for Refugee Integration in London*. Greater London Authority.

McColl, H. & Johnson, S. (2006) Characteristics and needs of asylum seekers and refugees in contact with London community mental health teams: a descriptive investigation. *Social Psychiatry and Psychiatric Epidemiology*, **41**, 789–795.

McFarlane, L. (1998) *Diagnosis: Homophobic. The Experiences of Lesbians, Gay Men and Bisexuals in Mental Health Services*. PACE.

McGrath, J. J., Hearle, J., Jenner, L., *et al* (1999) The fertility and fecundity of patients with psychoses. *Acta Psychiatrica Scandinavica*, **99**, 441–446.

McKenzie, K. (1999) Something borrowed from the blues? *BMJ*, **318**, 616–617.

McKenzie, K. (2008) Improving mental healthcare for ethnic minorities. *Advances in Psychiatric Treatment*, **14**, 285–291.

McKenzie, K. & Bhui, K. (2007) Better mental healthcare for minority ethnic groups – moving away from the blame game and putting patients first. *Psychiatric Bulletin*, **31**, 368–369.

McKenzie, K., Bhui, K., Nanchahal, K., *et al* (2008) Suicide rates in people of South Asian origin in England and Wales: 1993–2003. *British Journal of Psychiatry*, **193**, 406–409.

McLellan, J. D. & Ganguli, R. (1999) Family planning and parenthood needs of women with severe mental illness: clinicians' perspective. *Community Mental Health Journal*, **35**, 369–380.

Meltzer, H. (2008a) *The Mental Ill-Health of Prisoners. Report for Foresight Review Mental Capital and Wellbeing: Making the Most of Ourselves in the 21st Century. State-of-Science Review: SR-B5.* Government Office for Science.

Meltzer, H. (2008b) *The Mental Ill-Health of Homeless People. Report for Foresight Review Mental Capital and Wellbeing: Making the Most of Ourselves in the 21st Century. State-of-Science Review: SR-B6.* Government Office for Science.

Mezey, G., Hassell, Y. & Bartlett, A. (2005) Safety of women in mixed-sex and single-sex medium secure units: staff and patient perceptions. *British Journal of Psychiatry*, **187**, 579–582.

Ministry of Justice (2007) *Prison Population Projections 2007–2014, England and Wales.* Ministry of Justice.

Mitchell, D., Grindel, C. G. & Laurenzano, C. (1996) Sexual abuse assessment on admission by nursing staff in general hospital psychiatric settings. *Psychiatric Services*, **47**, 159–164.

Morgan, C., Mallett, R., Hutchinson, G., *et al* (2005) Pathways to care and ethnicity. 2: Source of referral and help-seeking: report from the ÆSOP study. *British Journal of Psychiatry*, **186**, 290–296.

Mowbray, C. T., Oyserman, D., Zemencuk, J. K., *et al* (1995) Motherhood for women with serious mental illness: pregnancy, childbirth and the postpartum period. *American Journal of Orthopsychiatry*, **65**, 21–38.

Mowbray, C., Schwartz, S. & Bybee, D. (2000) Mothers with a mental illness: stressors and resources for parenting and living. *Families in Society*, **81**, 118.

Murray, L., Hipwell, A., Hooper, R., *et al* (1996) The cognitive development of 5-year-old children of postnatally depressed mothers. *Journal of Child Psychology and Psychiatry*, **37**, 927–935.

National Coalition for the Homeless (2007) *How Many People Experience Homelessness?* National Coalition for the Homeless.

Neria Y., Bromet, E., Carlson, G., *et al* (2005) Assaultive trauma and illness course in psychotic bipolar disorder: findings from the Suffolk county mental health project. *Acta Psychiatrica Scandinavica*, **111**, 380–383.

Nicholson, J., Nason, M. W. & Calabresi, A. O. (1999) Fathers with severe mental illness: characteristics and comparisons. *American Journal of Orthopsychiatry*, **69**, 134–141.

Nicholson, J., Biebel, K. & Katz-Levy, J. (2002) The prevalence of parenthood in adults with mental illness: implications for state and federal policymakers, programs, and providers. In *Mental Health, United States, 2002* (eds R. W. Manderscheid & M. J. Henderson), pp. 120–137. United States Department of Health and Human Services.

Niven, S. & Stewart, D. (2005) *Resettlement Outcomes on Release from Prison in 2003.* Home Office.

O'Connor, W. & Nazroo, J. (eds) (2002) *Ethnic Differences in the Context and Experience of Psychiatric Illness: A Qualitative Study.* TSO (The Stationery Office).

O'Connor, T. G., Heron, J., Golding, J., *et al* (2002) Maternal antenatal anxiety and children's behavioural/emotional problems at 4 years: report from the Avon Longitudinal Study of Parents and Children. *British Journal of Psychiatry*, **180**, 502–508.

O'Neill, A., Casey, P. & Minton, R. (2007) The homeless mentally ill: an audit from an inner city hospital. *Irish Journal of Psychological Medicine*, **24**, 62–66.

Palmer, D. (2006) Imperfect prescription: mental health perceptions, experiences and challenges faced by the Somali community in the London Borough of Camden and service responses to them. *Primary Care Mental Health*, **4**, 45–56.

Patel, B. & Kerrigan, S. (2004) *Hungry and Homeless.* The Refugee Council.

Pernice, R. & Brook, J. (1994) Relationship of migrant status (refugee or immigrant) to mental health. *International Journal of Social Psychiatry*, **40**, 177–188.

Pilowsky, D. J., Wickramaratne, P. J., Rush, A. J., *et al* (2006) Children of currently depressed mothers: a STAR*D ancillary study. *Journal of Clinical Psychiatry*, **67**, 126–136.

Porter, M. & Haslam, N. (2005) Pre-displacement and post-displacement factors associated with the mental health of refugees and internally displaced persons: a meta-analysis. *JAMA*, **294**, 602–612.

Post, R. D., Willett, A. B., Franks, R. D., *et al* (1980) A preliminary report on the prevalence of domestic violence among psychiatric inpatients. *American Journal of Psychiatry*, **137**, 974–975.

Prison Reform Trust (2007) *Bromley Briefings: Prison Factfile*. Prison Reform Trust (http://www.prisonreformtrust.org.uk/uploads/documents/factfile5dec.pdf).

Prisons and Probation Ombudsman for England and Wales (2004) *Annual Report 2003–2004* (Cm 6256). Home Office (http://www.ppo.gov.uk/docs/annual-report-03041.pdf/).

Read, J. & Fraser, A. (1998) Staff response to abuse histories of psychiatric inpatients. *Australian and New Zealand Journal of Psychiatry*, **32**, 206–213.

Read, J., van Os, J., Morrison, A. P., *et al* (2005) Childhood trauma, psychosis and schizophrenia: a literature review with theoretical and clinical implications. *Acta Psychiatrica Scandinavica*, **112**, 330–350.

Rees, S. (2009) *Mental Ill Health in the Adult Single Homeless Population: A Review of the Literature*. Crisis.

Richardson, J., Feder, G., Eldridge, S., *et al* (2001) Women who experience domestic violence and women survivors of sexual abuse: a survey of health professionals' attitudes and clinical practice. *British Journal of General Practice*, **51**, 468–470.

Rose, S. M., Peabody, C. G. & Stratigeas, B. (1991) Undetected abuse among intensive case management clients. *Hospital and Community Psychiatry*, **42**, 499–503.

Rough Sleepers Unit (1999) *Coming in from the Cold: The Government's Strategy on Rough Sleeping*. Department of the Environment, Transport and the Regions.

Royal College of Psychiatrists (2002) *Domestic Violence* (CR102). Royal College of Psychiatrists.

Royal College of Psychiatrists (2007) *Improving Services for Refugees and Asylum Seekers: Position Statement*. Royal College of Psychiatrists (www.rcpsych.ac.uk/docs/Refugee%20asylum%20seeker%20consensus%20final.doc).

Rutter, M. & Quinton, D. (1984) Parental psychiatric disorder: effects on children. *Psychological Medicine*, **14**, 853–880.

Sainsbury Centre for Mental Health (2008) *Short-Changed: Spending on Prison Mental Health Care*. Sainsbury Centre for Mental Health.

Sands, R. G., Koppelman, N. & Solomon, P. (2004) Maternal custody status and living arrangements of children of women with severe mental illness. *Health Social Work*, **29**, 317–325.

Save the Children (2005) *No Place for a Child*. Save the Children.

Schneider, J. (2007) *Better Outcomes for the Most Excluded*. Report for Social Exclusion Task Force, February 2007. Institute of Mental Health.

Scott, J. (1993) Homelessness and mental illness. *British Journal of Psychiatry*, **162**, 314–324.

Shah, N. & Howard, L. (2006) Screening for smoking and substance misuse in pregnant women with mental illness. *Psychiatric Bulletin*, **30**, 294–297.

Shifman, S., Bronstein, M., Sternfeld, M., *et al* (2004) COMT: A common susceptibility gene in bipolar disorder and schizophrenia. *American Journal of Medical Genetics Part B: Neuropsychiatric Genetics*, **128B**, 61–64.

Silove, D., Steel, Z. & Mollica, R. (2001) Refugees – detention of asylum seekers: assault on health, human rights, and social development. *Lancet*, **357**, 1436–1437.

Sims, J. & Victor, C. R. (1999) Mental health of the statutorily homeless population: secondary analysis of the psychiatric morbidity surveys. *Journal of Mental Health*, **8**, 523–532.

Singleton, N., Meltzer, H. & Gatward, R. (1998) *Psychiatric Morbidity among Prisoners in England and Wales*. Office for National Statistics.

Social Exclusion Unit (2002) *Reducing Re-Offending by Ex-Prisoners*. Office of the Deputy Prime Minister.

Sproston, K. & Nazroo, J. (eds) (2002) *Ethnic Minority Psychiatric Illness Rates in the Community (EMPIRIC) Quantitative Report*. TSO (The Stationery Office).

Stansfield, S. & Sproston, K. (2002) Social support and networks. In *Ethnic Minority Psychiatric Illness Rates in the Community (EMPIRIC) Quantitative Report* (eds K. Sproston & J. Nazroo), pp: 117–136. TSO (The Stationery Office).

Steel, Z., Silove, D., Brooks, R., *et al* (2006) Impact of immigration detention and temporary protection on the mental health of refugees. *British Journal of Psychiatry*, **188**, 58–64.

Tacchi, M. J. & Scott, J. (1996) Characteristics of homeless women living in London hostels. *Psychiatric Services*, **47**, 196–198.

Talge, N. M., Neal, C. & Glover, V. (2007) Antenatal maternal stress and long-term effects on child neurodevelopment: how and why? *Journal of Child Psychology and Psychiatry and Allied Disciplines*, **48**, 245–261.

Targosz, S., Bebbington, P., Lewis, G., *et al* (2003) Lone mothers, social exclusion and depression. *Psychological Medicine*, **33**, 715–722.

Timms, P. & Balazs, J. (1997) ABC of mental health: mental health on the margins. *BMJ*, **315**, 536–539.

Tribe, R. (2002) Mental health of refugees and asylum-seekers. *Advances in Psychiatric Treatment*, **8**, 240–247.

UNHCR (2006a) *State of the Refugees: Human Displacement in the New Millenium*. Oxford University Press.

UNHCR (2006b) Refugees: Victims of Intolerance. *Refugees Magazine*, **142**, UNHCR (http://www.unhcr.org/publ/PUBL/44508c182.pdf).

Van Ommeren, M., Sharma, B., Sharma, G. K., *et al* (2002) The relationship between somatic and PTSD symptoms among Bhutanese refugee torture survivors: examination of comorbidity with anxiety and depression. *Journal of Traumatic Stress*, **15**, 415–421.

Vostanis, P., Grattan, E., Cumella, S., *et al* (1997) Psychosocial functioning of homeless children. *Journal of the American Academy of Child and Adolescent Psychiatry*, **36**, 881–889.

Walby, S. & Allen, J. (2004) *Domestic Violence, Sexual Assault and Stalking: Findings from the British Crime Survey. Home Office Research Study 276*. Home Office.

Wang, A. R. & Goldschmidt, V. V. (1994) Interviews of psychiatric inpatients about their family situation and young children. *Acta Psychiatrica Scandinavica*, **90**, 459–465.

Webb, R., Abel, K., Pickles, A., *et al* (2005) Mortality in offspring of parents with psychotic disorders: a critical review and meta-analysis. *American Journal of Psychiatry*, **162**, 1045–1056.

Weissman, M. M., Pilowsky, D. J., Wickramaratne, P. J., *et al* (2006) Remissions in maternal depression and child psychopathology. *JAMA*, **295**, 1389–1398.

Werneke, U., Horn, O., Maryon-Davis, A., *et al* (2006) Uptake of screening for breast cancer in patients with mental health problems. *Journal of Epidemiology and Community Health*, **60**, 600–605.

Williamson, M. (2006) *Improving the Health and Social Outcomes of People Recently Released from Prisons in the UK: A Perspective from Primary Care*. Sainsbury Centre for Mental Health.

Wurr, J. C. & Partridge, I. M. (1996) The prevalence of a history of childhood sexual abuse in an acute adult inpatient population. *Child Abuse and Neglect*, **20**, 867–872.

Young, M., Read, J., Barker-Collo, S., *et al* (2001) Evaluating and overcoming barriers to taking abuse histories. *Professional Psychology: Research and Practice*, **32**, 407–414.

CHAPTER 10

Social exclusion and people with mental health problems: developing a clearer picture

Jed Boardman

In the previous chapters, we have seen that there is an association between mental health problems and social exclusion across all the domains that have been examined (material, productivity, social, political and health). This differs across the range of disorders and is influenced by the person's socioeconomic and social identity group. It is clear that mental health problems are a significant risk factor for poor economic, health and social outcomes, however the direction of causality is often difficult to establish. Nevertheless, it would appear that the causal pathways can operate in both directions and that mental health problems can be both a cause and consequence of exclusion. This emerging complexity of the causal relationships requires further exploration and in this chapter we shall try to build a descriptive model of exclusion and mental health problems. We will explore further the relationship between mental health problems and exclusion and examine some of the main drivers, but first it is necessary to introduce the related topic of mental health and well-being.

Mental health and well-being

There is a growing literature on mental health and well-being (psychological well-being or positive mental health) which focuses on people's strengths in contrast to their deficits. This echoes the long-standing literature on health, as opposed to ill health or disease, which in the 20th century was encapsulated by the World Health Organization's (WHO) definition of health as:

> a state of complete physical, mental and social well-being and not merely the absence of disease or infirmity (WHO, 1948).

This perspective is now reflected in their definition of positive mental health as:

> a state of well-being in which the individual realizes his or her own abilities, can cope with the normal stresses of life, can work productively and fruitfully, and is able to make a contribution to his or her community (WHO, 2005).

Essentially, mental well-being is about people's lives going well (Huppert, 2008) and is concerned not only with a positive subjective state (emotion and cognition), but also with social functioning and interaction and the ability to deal with adversity and painful emotions. It combines two elements (Huppert, 2005; Lyubomirsky *et al*, 2005; Friedli, 2009):

1   hedonic, or feeling good, which covers positive feelings of subjective well-being, satisfaction with life, happiness or contentment with other emotions such as interest, engagement, confidence, affection
2   eudemonic, or functioning effectively psychologically, which involves engagement, fulfilment, developing one's potential, a sense of meaning, having control over one's life, a sense of purpose, working towards valued goals, and having positive relationships.

The indicators of well-being include resilience, self-esteem, self-efficacy, optimism, life satisfaction, hopefulness, a sense of coherence and meaning in life, and social integration.

Mental health and mental ill health are not necessarily separate concepts and their measures have been seen as existing on two psychometrically distinct, but correlated, continua in populations (Keyes, 2002a; Huppert & Whittington, 2003; Keyes, 2005). Thus an absence of mental illness does not necessarily mean the presence of mental health, and people with mental health problems can still experience many aspects of positive mental health (Friedli, 2009). This is a key to understanding the ideas of recovery.

Evidence for the importance of mental well-being comes from a range of sources including neuroscience, experimental psychology, developmental studies, and cross-sectional and longitudinal survey data (Huppert, 2008). These studies suggest that an individual's mental health reflects the influence of inherent factors (genes and early biological programming), as well as factors present during the life course such as maternal attachment, parental behaviour and education. In general terms, positive emotions lead to positive cognitions, positive behaviours and an increased cognitive capacity; and in turn these cognitions, behaviours and capabilities influence positive emotions in a virtuous cycle (Huppert, 2008). The notion of well-being is neither shared across all communities across the world, nor identical at all periods of history, and is a relatively recent concept in the Western world. Nevertheless, three near-universal themes do seem apparent: material security, health status and the nature of stresses and adversity, all of which are reflected in the current literature (Littlewood, 2008).

Linked to this idea of positive mental health is that of resilience. Resilience can be seen as an ability to react and adapt positively when things go wrong (Bartley, 2006). The concept emerges from the commonly observed phenomena that not all people exposed to risk factors have poor outcomes and that known risk factors do not fully explain variations in mortality, morbidity or other outcomes. Thus other factors must be present that protect individuals against the noxious effects of risk factors, or modulate or buffer against their impact. These 'health assets' may reflect a person's genetic inheritance or the effects of their early life, or may be cultural or social and thus may operate at an individual or collective level. This has led to an extension of the concept of individual resilience to apply to places or communities (Friedli, 2009).

The literature on well-being broadens the individual perspective to one that can focus on populations. In classical epidemiology the focus is on the distribution and causes of disease in populations, and the equivalent of this in well-being literature is salutogenesis, which focuses on the distribution and causes of health and well-being (Antonovsky, 1979; Morgan *et al*, 2004). The application of the population perspective is based on a familiar public health model (Rose, 1992) that makes the observation that the variation of personal characteristics in a population, for example blood pressure, cholesterol levels or mental health, tends to form continuous distributions (Fig. 10.1). This suggests that a shift in the distribution of health characteristics, or moving the average towards the healthy end of the scale, will result in benefit to the entire population. Figure 10.1 shows how this might apply to mental well-being. This type of distribution is familiar and can be seen when questionnaire measures, for example the General Health Questionnaire, are used in community surveys (Cox *et al*, 1987; Rose, 1992). People with diagnosable mental health problems form the left-hand tail of the distribution, whereas people at the other end of the scale are 'flourishing'. These flourishing individuals 'have enthusiasm for life and are actively and proactively engaged with others and social institutions' (Keyes, 2002*b*: p. 262). The largest group of people have moderate mental health, but a significant number are 'languishing'. Population surveys indicate that people with mental health problems represent about 20% of the adult population, depending on the range of problems included and how the cut-off or threshold to measure mental ill health is defined. The 'languishing'

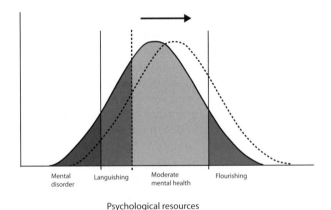

Mental disorder | Languishing | Moderate mental health | Flourishing

Psychological resources

Fig. 10.1 The mental health spectrum. The bold arrow reflects the effect of shifting the mean of the mental health spectrum. Source: Huppert (2008).

group is of particular interest as they may be represented by individuals who have 'subclinical' or 'borderline' mental health problems such as 'minor depression'. These individuals may not reach the threshold for a diagnosis of a mental health problem but they do experience symptoms and may have poor functioning, their lives may be empty and they may 'live a life of quiet desperation' (Thoreau, 1854; Keyes, 2002b). They may be at increased risk of depression, especially when faced with life stressors (Brown et al, 1986, 1990) or physical disorders (Keyes, 2004). This group may also contain significant numbers of young people highlighted in a UNICEF report (2007) who it is thought may be seeking to fill a void in their lives (Keyes, 2004; Huppert, 2008). There are no current UK data on the languishing or flourishing groups, but data from the USA suggest that 17% of adults are flourishing and 11% are languishing (Keyes, 2002b).

The population approach to prevention would suggest that a shift in mental health to the right side of the distribution in Fig. 10.1 would produce an increase in those flourishing and a decrease in those with mental health problems and those at risk of such problems. Thus a public health approach to increasing flourishing provides an alternative to an approach that focuses exclusively on the treatment and prevention of disorder. However, although there is evidence in favour of this approach from observational studies, evidence from intervention studies that enhance mental well-being is lacking (Huppert, 2008).

One hypothetical reason for promoting positive mental health is that even if mental health problems remain, other outcomes may be modified. These include healthier lifestyles, better physical health, higher education attainment, greater productivity, improved relationships and quality of life, and greater social cohesion and engagement (WHO, 2004; Jané-Llopis et al, 2005; Barry & Jenkins, 2007; Friedli, 2009) (Box 10.1).

Influences on positive mental health

The potential effectiveness of the population approach to mental well-being depends on the risk and vulnerability factors being the same for mental health problems (or what some refer to as 'mental ill-being', Huppert, 2008) and mental well-being. Indeed, many of the drivers are the same for both these phenomena, but some are not (Huppert, 2008). This applies to factors operating at the individual level (genes, mother–infant attachment, parenting style, adverse life events) or at the social level (poverty, unemployment, sigma and discrimination). Personality variables such as neuroticism are associated with common mental health problems, whereas extraversion is associated with mental well-being (van Os et al, 2001; Kendler et al, 2005; Huppert, 2008). Positive styles of thinking and intrinsic motivation link to well-being rather than ill health (Huppert, 2008) but intentional activities, those over which we have control, are also important drivers of well-being (Lyubomirsky et al, 2005; Huppert, 2008).

Box 10.1   Outcomes associated with positive mental health

Physical health:

- mortality
  - living longer (Danner *et al*, 2001; Levy *et al*, 2002)
- morbidity
  - overall health (Benyamini *et al* 2000)
  - lower stroke incidence and better chances of survival (Ostir *et al* 2000, 2001)
  - protection from heart disease (Kubzansky & Kawachi, 2000; Bunker *et al*, 2003; Keyes, 2004)

Health behaviour:

- improved sleep, exercise, diet (Pressman & Cohen, 2005; Mental Health Foundation, 2006*a*)
- reduction of alcohol intake and smoking (Mental Health Foundation, 2006*b*)
- reduction of delinquent activity (Windle, 2000)

Productivity:

- improved well-being or positive affect reduces sickness absence and increases performance/productivity (Cropanzano & Wright, 1999; Pelled & Xin, 1999; Wright & Staw, 1999; Harter *et al*, 2003; Keyes, 2005; Lyubomirsky *et al*, 2005)

Crime:

- Small improvements in emotional adjustment in children may have a significant impact on subsequent crime rates (Scott *et al*, 2001; Fergusson *et al*, 2005; Keyes, 2006)

Educational outcomes:

- in a longitudinal study, effects associated with a high-quality home learning environment on children's development were stronger than for other traditional measures of disadvantage such as parental social class, education or income (Sylva *et al*, 2007)

Pro-social behaviour:

- cross-sectional studies show correlation between well-being, social ties and pro-social behaviour such as participation, civic engagement and volunteering (Diener & Seligman, 2002; Lyubomirsky *et al*, 2005; Pressman & Cohen, 2005)
- in a longitudinal study, positive affect predicted participation in volunteering but volunteering also increased positive affect (Thoits & Hewitt, 2001).

Gender links with common mental health problems but not well-being, whereas age and marital status show complex and variable associations to both (Huppert, 2008). The main socioeconomic factors tend to show similar influences on both well-being and mental ill health (Huppert, 2008). For example, the social gradient seen for mental health problems (Chapter 8) is also seen in all levels of well-being (Ryff & Singer, 1998; Dolan *et al*, 2008). Income inequality is also associated with well-being and with mental health problems (Alesina *et al*, 2004; Pickett *et al*, 2006). Employment is associated with both, but the effects of unemployment appear to operate predominantly on well-being rather than on the symptoms of mental ill health (Huppert & Whittington, 2003).

One proviso that must be borne in mind is the overall contribution of these drivers to mental well-being. Socioeconomic and demographic factors account for about 10% of the variation in well-being between individuals, compared with personality factors (neuroticism and extraversion), which account for about 20% (Huppert, 2008).

Causes and consequences of social exclusion

The causes of social exclusion are difficult to pin down. Traditionally, the conditions of exclusion may be seen as a cause of mental health problems (Faris & Dunham, 1939; Hollingshead & Redlich, 1958; Castle *et al*, 1993) or their consequence (Goldberg & Morrison, 1963; Hare *et al*, 1972). Multiple pathways lead to the same outcomes. Some factors are clearly bi-directional: deficits in close personal relationships may be a cause *and* a consequence of mental health problems. In addition, there is a surplus of 'third variables' which confound causal pathways: poverty may be seen to contribute to *both* a lack of social participation *and* mental illness. Notwithstanding these problems, a number of major social variables can be considered to have some causal influence in driving social exclusion (Office of the Deputy Prime Minister, 2004). We will consider three: poverty, lack of social capital, and stigma.

Poverty

As we have seen in previous chapters, poverty has played a central role in the development of the concept of social exclusion and is a major risk factor in almost all the domains of exclusion that have been proposed. Concepts of poverty and social exclusion are not identical, but nevertheless the relationship between the two is such that it would make little sense not to think of poverty as having a major influence on exclusion.

The precise relationship between poverty and mental health problems is difficult to analyse and interpret. A clear association between economic disadvantage and a raised prevalence of mental ill health is well established (see Chapter 8), but the strength of this association varies greatly both by type of mental health condition and by age group. For example, the Office for National Statistics' (ONS) survey of psychiatric morbidity among adults in private households showed that the prevalence of any type of mental disorder among people living in households with an income of less than £200 a week (the poorest 14% of the population at the time of the survey) was 28.5%. In comparison, prevalence among individuals living in the top income group (household income over £500 a week) was 22.4% (Meltzer *et al*, 2002). Mental health problems, defined broadly, are therefore more common among the poor than among the rich by about a quarter. But, again according to the ONS survey, the prevalence of severe mental health problems (psychosis) is about nine times higher among the poor than the rich. A separate ONS survey (Green at al, 2005) showed that income-related differences in the general prevalence of mental ill health appear to be more pronounced among children than they are among adults. Thus, the prevalence of any mental disorder is about three times as high among children living in the poorest 15% of households, compared with those in the top income range. This is clearly much greater than the difference found among adults.

So, what can we make of these associations between a raised prevalence of mental health problems and poverty? Poverty itself is not a simple or well-defined concept and may be standing as a proxy for a range of other variables that have a more direct causal association with mental ill health. For example, unemployment is a major cause of low income among adults of working age and it is now well established that unemployment is bad for mental health (Waddell & Burton, 2006). However, the statistics may show an association between low income and mental health problems, but does this reflect the causal influence of low income *per se*, or rather, does it reflect the negative psychological impact of being involuntarily out of work? If it is the latter, then a policy aimed at raising the incomes of the unemployed through higher benefits may have limited effects on mental health compared with the alternative of helping people back into work.

The dynamic of poverty and social exclusion is important here and adds another layer of complication to the analysis (see also Chapter 7). In general, it is a mistake to think of the poor as a fixed or static group whose composition remains unchanged year after year. Longitudinal studies show that 'people can experience different types of poverty, that the majority of people who experience poverty move out of poverty, and that many more people experience poverty over a period of time than they do at any one moment in time' (Smith & Middleton, 2007: p. 1). To illustrate, between 1991 and 1997 almost half of those living in poverty in any one year had left the following year and as many as a third of the population experienced poverty in at least one year at that time, but less than 2% did so in every year. People may therefore variously experience transient, intermittent or persistent poverty. Virtually nothing is known about how these differences in the nature of economic disadvantage relate to the prevalence of mental illness.

Finally, there remain unresolved questions about the direction of causation between poverty and mental ill health. Does poverty cause mental illness, or does mental illness cause poverty (perhaps operating through the negative effects of mental illness, particularly severe mental illness, on the capacity to earn)? These negative effects include not only the immediate incapacitating consequences of mental illness on occupational functioning, but also stigma among employers and a lack of effective or appropriate support from the statutory services in helping people into work. The most sensible conclusion is that the causation does, indeed, run in both directions. However, in the absence of a firm understanding of the relative magnitudes (and the precise underlying causal mechanisms in each case) it is difficult to think how effective interventions or policy initiatives can be most appropriately designed.

Social capital

Since Putnam's pioneering work on social capital (see Chapter 3), two complementary strands have developed within the literature (Falzer, 2007). The first is the 'classic' view, based primarily on Putnam's ideas, which conceptualises social capital as part of the political processes of macro-social entities. In this view, social capital is a characteristic of communities. It is a 'community stock' which strengthens the fabric of society and promotes values such as citizenship, reciprocity and diversity. These benefits then cascade downwards through the community, improving its collective health and thereby the health of its individual members. The other strand takes a micro-level analysis, more located in individual social networks. It defines social capital as the aggregate of potential resources that are available to individuals through their networks of interpersonal relationships. In particular, these networks facilitate access to economic, cultural and information resources which then benefit the individual directly. These two overlapping conceptions of social capital are important in our understanding of the relationship between social capital and social inclusion and the research evidence regarding the possible contribution of social capital to the prevention of mental health problems.

The research on social capital and mental health problems has been summarised by De Silva et al (2005), who undertook a meta-analysis of more than 50 studies and concluded that there was, indeed, evidence for an association at an individual level between measures of social capital and mental disorders. This applied regardless of whether the measures of social capital were objective (e.g. participation in networks, social roles) or subjective (e.g. trust, confidence, feeling supported). The nature of this association suggested an inverse relationship, with lower levels of objective and subjective social capital being associated with higher levels of symptoms. This association applied to both adults and children. However, there was clearly some confounding in that some aspects of mental disorders (e.g. social withdrawal) were also measures of objective deficits in social capital. The associational nature of this relationship also made causal interpretation difficult. On the other hand, there was much less evidence for any association between macro-level social capital measures and mental disorders, with the possible exception of suicide and schizophrenia, although in the latter case there were again problems with confounding.

These data suggest there is a stronger evidence for the association between micro-level measures of social inclusion and mental disorders than between macro-level measures. But does this mean that we should discount the importance of a broader social viewpoint? Falzer (2007) argues that we should not, and suggests that we need to continue to consider both aspects. Thus, it is clearly insufficient to think in terms of simply enhancing social inclusion (employment rates, access to stable housing, etc.) without thinking of the wider social context in which such interventions will operate (friends, families, the wider public). Falzer refers to these wider social benefits as a 'strategic surplus' and goes on to explain the important, practical implications:

> A service user who joins the employment market by working at an entry level job may achieve the short-term goal of becoming employed, but the opportunity to turn this achievement into a resource for recovery can quickly reach a dead end ... On the other hand, if the service provider assists the consumer to use the pursuit of employment as an opportunity to become acquainted with the neighbourhood and the local economy, meet prospective employers, and develop vocational and social interests, then the therapeutic strategy is not merely targeting a short-term goal, but potentiating a long-term gain. Development and use of social capital is a product of the strategic surplus that transcends the achievement of therapeutic goals (p. 40).

There is one variable that may have a particularly important influence on the accumulation of this strategic surplus and that is stigma.

Stigma

The notion that one of the major obstacles to social inclusion for people with mental health problems arises from stigma is hardly an unexpected or new idea (Goffman, 1963). Thornicroft's (2006) helpful framework of ignorance, prejudice and discrimination, summarised in Chapter 3, gives us a clear way of seeing how stigma can directly exclude people with mental health problems from the areas of participation outlined in Chapter 8, including access to jobs, education, travel, decent living conditions, and social and civic participation, through the attitudes and actions of individuals and institutions. There is also an indirect pathway through which stigma may operate, through the internalisation by people with mental health problems of these wider societal attitudes.

From the accounts of service users we know that they often experience loss of hope, lack of control and powerlessness, particularly when dealing with social institutions. They may also expect to be discriminated against. Personal experiences of ignorance, prejudice and discrimination along with reactions to failure and rejection and the expected discriminatory attitudes of others can lead to an internalisation of these experiences, sometimes known as 'self-stigmatisation' (Corrigan & Watson, 2002). Self-stigmatisation is a 'complex set of expectations, actions, reactions, inhibitions, avoidance, loss of confidence, and social withdrawal' (Thornicroft, 2006: p. 152), all of which can contribute to further exclusion in the form of a vicious cycle. In addition, these emotions, cognitions, attitudes and behaviours all reflect the poor mental well-being of people with mental health problems and are contrary to the core aspects of hope, agency and opportunity that are associated with recovery.

But stigma is not just confined to the person's mental health problems. As we saw in Chapter 9, people with mental health problems have other social identities and they also experience stigma and discrimination in relation to these, which further contributes to their exclusion and to the development of their internalised negative beliefs about self. In addition, for many people who are socially excluded there is the stigma of poverty. The damaging effects of poverty go beyond the lack of material resources that are required to live a just, valued and healthy life; they are reinforced by the effects of prejudice, discrimination and humiliation that further undermine people's sense of pride, dignity and shame and in turn influence their health and well-being. Wealth may be a marker for social status, success and respectability, but poverty is stigmatising (Marmot & Wilkinson, 2007). Indeed, we have seen a hardening of the attitudes of the public towards the poor in recent decades and a greater tolerance of excessive wealth (Sefton, 2009). Recipients of benefits are often seen as 'scroungers' and the public's attitudes towards people on low incomes are more negative and condemning than those they hold towards the rich, believing that people on benefits will not make a contribution to society and that certain levels of inequality are fair (Bamfield & Horton, 2009). The views marginalised people hold often contrast with these general public views. Mowlam & Creegan (2008) and Creegan et al (2009) looked at the views of people with learning disabilities, ex-offenders, ex-homeless, carers, unemployed people, care leavers and other vulnerable young people, all of whom had experienced challenging social problems and loss of opportunities, to collect their views on modern social problems. Responders identified a range of problems including the decline of family, community and values, increasing individualism and selfishness, poverty, crime and violence, and drugs. Although they attributed these problems to external factors, they also recognised the role of personal responsibility and choice. Importantly, they recognised that they were often unable to fulfil their own potential because of the limited nature of choices and opportunities put to them.

For people with mental health problems and learning disabilities, the humiliation of poverty and public attitudes reinforce the already real experience of stigma and discrimination because of mental ill health, their experience of poor treatment by some parts of the health services and the possible effects of low expectations of many health professionals. To this may be added the prejudice and discrimination associated with their gender, ethnicity or sexual orientation, their homelessness, their offender or refugee status. The effect is that of undermining their mental well-being.

Risk factors for social exclusion

These three social factors – poverty, social capital, stigma – may have a major causal role in driving social exclusion for people with mental health problems. We now need to build on this and consider possible risk factors and triggers.

Levitas *et al* (2007) discuss a number of possible risk factors for social exclusion, which are mainly historical and structural variables, including age, gender, ethnicity, educational disadvantage, lone parenting, a history of worklessness, an adverse family background, history of drug abuse and/ or contact with the criminal justice system, chronic physical ill health, long-standing deficits in social capital and living in a disadvantaged urban or rural community. These factors convey an increased risk of exclusion, but are not necessarily indicators in themselves. They are better regarded as variables that may precede the occurrence of social exclusion (and mental health problems) and contribute to its causality (vulnerability factors).

These variables therefore need to be assessed independently of the indicators of social exclusion, but require well-conducted longitudinal studies or experimental interventions to clarify their causal significance (see Chapter 3). At this point we should return to consider the role of mental health and well-being. We have already seen that many of the risk factors for mental ill health are the same for mental health and well-being, but ill health and health may also be linked in other ways, through the types of outcome that may be influenced by these health states.

Physical health, mental health problems and mental health and well-being

We have already seen that there is a clear association between mental health problems and physical morbidity and mortality (Chapter 8). However, there is also a burgeoning literature from naturalistic and longitudinal studies, experimental and intervention studies linking positive mental health to improved physical health and survival outcomes (Pressman & Cohen, 2006; Huppert, 2008; Friedli, 2009). Importantly, it appears that positive emotions may have an effect on these outcomes independently of negative emotions (Huppert, 2008). The pathways through which these effects are exerted may be physiological, hormonal or immunological, behavioural (healthier lifestyles and health behaviours – e.g. diet, smoking, alcohol intake) or social (through social support and pro-social behaviour). These pathways are likely to have identical influences on the well-being of people with mental health problems, but the effects will be moderated by the person's mental ill health and by their material and social circumstances.

Income inequality, mental health problems, and mental health and well-being

Income inequality is associated with mental ill health and positive mental health, but in opposing directions (Alesina *et al*, 2004; Pickett *et al*, 2006). The possible links between poverty, exclusion and psychological ill health may be mediated by an absence of key components of well-being. There are inevitably a range of possible emotional and cognitive responses to relative deprivation, for example the effect of low status on identity and social relationships or on damaging behaviours (Rogers & Pilgrim, 2003; Wilkinson, 2005; Friedli, 2009) or the lack of a sense of control (Wilkinson, 1996, 2005). Lacking the basic necessities and the possibility of changing these matters reduces an individual's sense of control over their lives. The experience of a lack of control over one's material and social life may act as a mediating factor between the experience of poverty and exclusion and the experience of poor mental health.

Recovery and well-being

In earlier chapters, recovery concepts, although not traditionally part of the social exclusion literature, were given a central place and seen to play an important part in promoting inclusion and participation for people with mental health problems and learning disabilities. The central elements of recovery are hope, agency and opportunity, concepts that all represent aspects of positive mental health, for example resilience, self-esteem, self-efficacy, life satisfaction, hopefulness, a sense of coherence and meaning in life, and social integration. On the other hand, these central elements of recovery are all impeded in situations of disadvantage. In this way concepts of recovery may be seen as a means of pulling together social inclusion and mental well-being. Giving recovery ideas a central place in health and Social Services, and by default promoting positive mental health, contributes to improved outcomes for people with mental health problems, particularly those with long-term problems or younger people (Keyes, 2006).

Triggers of social exclusion

In addition to indicators and risk factors, we must also consider the role of triggers in social exclusion. Thus, individuals who are vulnerable by virtue of historical and structural disadvantages (high risk) may nevertheless require a triggering event before their trajectory into social exclusion becomes evident. Trigger factors may be such events as: loss of employment (including redundancy and retirement); development or relapse of mental health problems or physical illness; discharge from hospital; release from prison. Identification of trigger factors may have important implications for the provision of appropriate services which can intervene as appropriate points in the pathways to exclusion or can divert people away from social systems which may add to, rather than decrease, their social exclusion.

Contextual factors

There are several broader or contextual factors that influence the experience of social exclusion. These include the striking inequalities that exist within countries (Wilkinson, 1996, 2005; Wilkinson & Pickett, 2009) or the nature of the communities and physical and ecological environments that people live in. However, a particular context influencing people in the UK is the nature of social welfare policies and their associated attitudes that impinge on disadvantaged and excluded people, and which form the basis for the stigma associated with poverty.

Britain's welfare policies emanate from the past with the harsh treatment of the poor, the sequelae of the Poor Laws and means testing, the implied blame of the poor for their state, and the divisive effects of the attitudes to the deserving and undeserving poor (Ashford, 1987; Timmins, 1995; Jones & Novak, 1999). Although these policies and attitudes may have changed over the 20th century, their echoes often remain in our treatment and attitudes towards the poor. The modern context in which welfare policies are delivered is well illustrated in the comparative study of the welfare states in Sweden and Britain by Jones *et al* (2006). The British social security system has never received the same form of collective public support as the National Health Service, often being characterised as providing a fund for scroungers and cheats. Jones *et al* (2006) point out that the poor often feel abused and disrespected by welfare provision, and receive inadequate payments in an unpleasant and dehumanising context. The way in which politicians frame and portray economic inequality provides some of the context within which public attitudes are formed, and the public attitudes influence how governments act to address poverty (Joseph Rowntree Foundation, 2009; Sheldon *et al*, 2009). The press, while glorifying the members of *The Sunday Times*'s 'rich list', stigmatise the poor (Seymour, 2008). The exclusion of the poor is explicit:

> Most striking has been the distancing of those who receive social assistance from the rest of society – with welfare recipients always seen as a separate stratum in society, often with deviant behaviours and different living conditions – and an individualisation of the causes and consequences of social assistance (Jones *et al*, 2006: p. 438).

Jones *et al* go on to point out the effects of this on well-being:

> it is evident that the consequences of an individualised view of poverty can often be devastating, or at least make the struggle to survive more difficult. The sheer lack of respect and understanding given to the disadvantaged in Britain is highly corrosive of wellbeing, and all the more so because it is constant and overwhelming. We have had welfare recipients tell us how every interaction they have with the official welfare world is negative: no one has a good word to say to them; they spend hours shuttling between agencies in grimy offices that reinforce their powerlessness. Their time is of no account because they are considered to be of no account (p. 439).

To return to a point made in Chapter 3, the issue of social exclusion and mental health problems is concerned with substantive freedoms, in this case the 'ability to go about without shame' (Sen, 1999). Sen quotes Adam Smith's *An Enquiry into the Nature and Causes of the Wealth of Nations* (1776):

> By necessaries, I understand not only the commodities which are indispensably necessary for the support of life, but whatever the custom of the country renders it indecent for creditable people, even the lowest order to be without … a creditable day labourer would be ashamed to appear in public without a linen shirt.

Here again we see that material conditions are important for more than their value in providing for the basics of our day-to-day existence and, as Friedli (2009) points out, the absence of the shirt is an indicator of not only poverty, but shame 'that erodes the self-esteem, self worth, agency and confidence that are essential to flourishing wellbeing' (p. 37).

Developing a descriptive model

We are now at a point where it is possible to construct a descriptive model based on the factors that we have identified in Chapters 7, 8 and 9 and the constructs described above. In this we need to include the causal factors, triggers and risk factors involved in social inclusion/exclusion of people with mental health conditions, as well as the contextual factors that were described earlier. However, it would be helpful to identify a structure in which to include these factors and this can be borrowed from Phillipson & Scharf (2004), who identified four groups of conditions that might cause exclusion.

1   Condition-related characteristics: ways in which people with particular types of mental health condition might be disproportionately affected by certain kinds of losses or restrictions relating to income, health or reduced social ties. In this respect, some conditions might be more likely to make employment difficult, whereas others might reduce the quality of individual's social ties.

2   Cumulative disadvantage: way in which individuals and groups may acquire cumulative disadvantages across the life course. Reduced educational and work opportunities at early points in the life course may have long-term consequences in terms of reduced income in old age or limited awareness about how to access the full range of social and health services. Similarly, disrupted family and social relationships at earlier points in the life course may mean that individuals lack emotional and instrumental support in mid- and later life.

3   Community characteristics: highlight the way in which people with mental health conditions may experience disadvantage arising from the places in which they reside and provide a place for the concepts of social capital. For example, residence in some urban communities with high population turnover, declining socioeconomic status, and rising levels of crime and insecurity may undermine the ability of individuals to maintain stable social relationships. Residence in urban or rural communities characterised by a loss of public and commercial services may make it difficult for vulnerable people to access the local help and support that they need.

4   Forms of discrimination: impact of discriminatory behaviours and policies in generating exclusion of people with mental health conditions. This encompasses traditional debates about the stigmatisation of people with certain conditions, but is likely to be more deep-seated.

A descriptive model using these four groups of characteristics and incorporating causal and risk factors identified in Chapters 8 and 9 along with trigger factors is shown in Fig. 10.2.

Cycles of exclusion and cumulative risk factors

In addition to the four conditions above, the model must also acknowledge the dynamic nature of exclusion (Room, 2001). In the proposed model this is partly dealt with by the condition of cumulative disadvantage, which allows us to include life cycle effects and the interaction between risk and trigger factors over time. The Government's action plan on social exclusion (HM Government, 2006) presents consistent evidence for historical cycles of social disadvantage, whereby historical factors (e.g. family disruption, educational disadvantage, poverty) contribute to poor social outcomes (exclusion, mental ill health) and these then contribute to further disadvantage in the future (Rutter & Madge, 1997). This is also reflected in the notion of 'truncated opportunities', those opportunities that over the lifespan may be lost, limited or wasted through circumstances that have arisen or through people's own actions (Creegan, 2008). Opportunities thus may be limited early in life owing to, for example, being born into poverty or with a learning disability, or may arise later. A further dynamic is described by the cycles of exclusion which illustrate how risk factors and trigger factors interact. These have been described in the social exclusion report (Office of the Deputy Prime Minister, 2004: p. 20) and are illustrated in Fig. 10.3. Finally, our analysis also suggests that there may be a 'multiplier effect' for social disadvantage. Thus, having three risk factors together carries more than three times the risk of each added together. In other words, there is an amplification of social disadvantage – perhaps through the negative effects of stigma on well-being and resilience – which means that the most disadvantaged are cumulatively disadvantaged.

Poverty, exclusion and mental health – links

This approach allows us to develop some scenarios that illustrate how this model may operate for individuals with mental health problems. There may be many ways in which income, poverty, lack of necessities, poor neighbourhoods, isolation, low participation, etc. may influence a person's mental health. For example:

- being jobless gives a lack of structure and meaning, whereas fear of giving up benefits decreases the likelihood of seeking a new job, especially in the face of prejudice or the difficulty in accessing jobs owing to poor skills or poor literacy/numeracy
- being unable to afford insurance or savings increases financial worries and the fear of burglary or unanticipated needs such as replacing an essential item or having to travel unexpectedly
- being unable to afford basic repairs around the home and unable to create a pleasant or healthy home environment

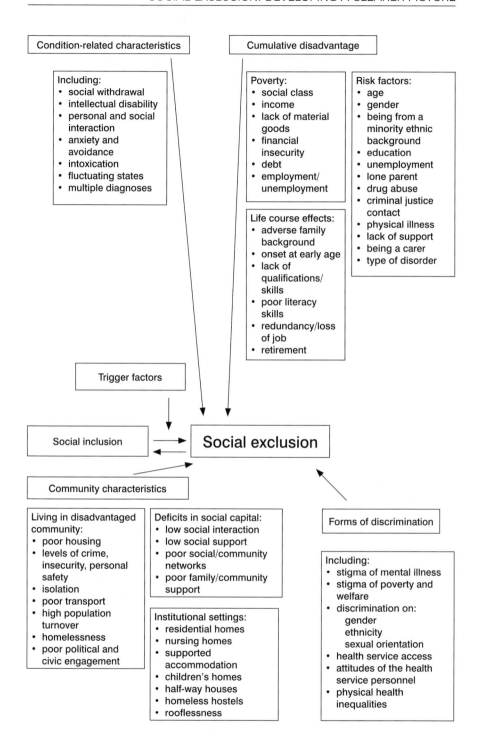

Fig. 10.2   Mental health problems and social exclusion – a descriptive model

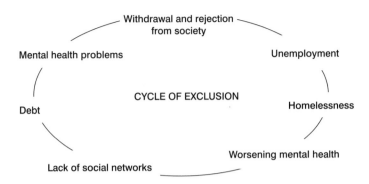

Fig. 10.3 A cycle of exclusion

- lack of clothes or difficulty getting around may decrease self-esteem and self-belief
- low mood, poor self-esteem, low drive, anxiety decrease the desire to engage with others, with low support increasing the likelihood of mood disorders in the presence of adverse events and difficulties
- having poor social skills and awkwardness with others increases the likelihood of prejudice and chances of being picked on or rejected by others or being a victim of crime or violence, especially when living in a deprived or high-crime neighbourhood (and a lack of opportunity to move away from the area owing to low income, debt and lack of savings).

These scenarios take many forms often involving multiple vicious cycles and are readily recognised among many of the people who use mental health services. In addition to these examples we may add the effects of the social environment. The environment (transport, pavements, public buildings) can be disabling and excluding for people with mobility difficulties (Oliver, 1990), but can also be so for people with mental health problems, owing to stigma and discrimination (Thornicroft, 2006). People with mental health problems commonly experience an inability to take part in social and civic activities, like going to the cinema, libraries, shops, cafés, football matches. Lack of the ability to take part in certain public events and activities is in itself excluding for the individual, as well as representing an indicator of wider social exclusion and cumulative effects on mental health.

Conclusion

In the previous few chapters we have accumulated a wealth of evidence to support the contention that people with mental health problems and those with learning disabilities are excluded from participation in many areas of society. Mental health problems are not equally spread across social groups – there are social inequalities in mental ill health. Although it is clear that this is the case across all forms of mental health problems, some groups are more at risk of exclusion than others. The size of this problem is huge, not least because mental health problems have a high prevalence and a high profile, larger than most other groups of physical disorders, but also because of their high personal, social and economic cost (Sainsbury Centre for Mental Health, 2003, 2008; McCrone *et al*, 2008).

We have tried to build up a picture of the relationship between mental health problems and social exclusion and have seen that in order to do this we need to take into consideration the nature of the mental health problems, material disadvantages, stigma and discrimination, and the effects of the wider community and society. However, this picture is rendered more complex due to the dynamic nature of exclusion – its effects across the life course and across generations and the interaction of the factors affecting exclusion. Added to this are the strong contextual effects of material factors, summarised by the association of poor health with income inequality and suggesting that above a certain level economic growth does not produce an increase in population health and may in fact be damaging (Layard, 2005; Pickett *et al*, 2006; Wilkinson & Pickett, 2009).

In this chapter we have introduced the notion of mental health and well-being and have seen that this overlaps with mental health problems – mental ill health and mental health have many shared drivers. Mental health problems predict a range of negative outcomes, whereas mental health and well-being predict positive outcomes across a range of domains. This suggests that the health of those with mental health problems be improved not only by direct treatment, but also through schemes designed to improve the health of populations or, where there are separate drivers for well-being, through interventions at, for example, the workplace and school level. This may play a part in facilitating recovery for people with mental health problems. However, the prominence of structural factors in driving exclusion implies that without attention being given to such matters as poverty, employment, education, housing, communities, rights and social justice there may be little chance of improving the status and outcomes of those with mental health problems. In Part 3 we will turn to the role of psychiatry and mental health services in addressing some of these matters.

Summary

Mental health and well-being offer another way of viewing the outcomes and concepts of recovery. Many of the risk and vulnerability factors for mental health problems are the same as those for mental health and well-being, with some exceptions.

Poverty, lack of social capital and stigma are key drivers of social exclusion in people with mental health problems. In creating a descriptive model for social exclusion and mental health problems risk factors, triggers and contextual factors all need to be considered in addition to condition-related characteristics, cumulative disadvantage, community characteristics and forms of discrimination; as well as cycles of exclusion and cumulative risk factors.

References

Alesina, A., Di Tella, R. & MacCulloch, R. (2004) Inequality and happiness: are Europeans and Americans different? *Journal of Public Economics*, **88**, 2009–2042.

Antonovsky, A. (1979) *Health, Stress and Coping*. Jossey-Bass.

Ashford, D. E. (1987) *The Emergence of Welfare States*. Blackwell.

Bamfield, L. & Horton, T. (2009) *Understanding Attitudes to Tackling Economic Inequality*. Joseph Rowntree Foundation.

Barry, M. M. & Jenkins, R. (2007) *Implementing Mental Health Promotion*. Churchill Livingstone.

Bartley, M. (ed.) (2006) *Capability and Resilience: Beating the Odds*. ESRC Human Capability and Resilience Research Network, UCL Department of Epidemiology and Public Health (http://www.ucl.ac.uk/capabilityandresilience/beatingtheoddsbook.pdf).

Benyamini, Y., Idler, E. L., Leventhal, H., *et al* (2000) Positive affect and function as influences on self-assessments of health: Expanding our view beyond illness and disability. *Journal of Gerontology: Psychological Sciences*, **55B**, P107–P116.

Brown, G. W., Bifulco, A., Harris, T., *et al* (1986) Life stress, chronic subclinical symptoms and vulnerability to clinical depression. *Journal of Affective Disorders*, **11**, 1–19.

Brown, G. W., Bifulco, A. & Andrews, B. (1990). Self-esteem and depression: 3. Aetiological issues. *Social Psychiatry and Psychiatric Epidemiology*, **25**, 235–243.

Bunker, S. J., Colquhoun, D. M., Esler, M. D., *et al* (2003) 'Stress' and coronary heart disease: psychosocial risk factors. National Heart Foundation of Australia position statement update. *The Medical Journal of Australia*, **178**, 272–276.

Castle, D. J., Scott, K., Wessely, S., *et al* (1993) Does social deprivation during gestation and early life predispose to later schizophrenia? *Social Psychiatry and Psychiatric Epidemiology*, **28**, 1–4.

Corrigan, P. W. & Watson, A. C. (2002) The paradox of self-stigma and mental illness. *Clinical Psychology: Science and Practice*, **9**, 35–53.

Cox, B. D., Blaxter, M., Buckle, A. C., *et al* (1987) *The Health and Lifestyle Survey*. Health Promotion Research Trust.

Creegan, C. (2008) *Opportunity and Aspiration: Two Sides of the Same Coin? Joseph Rowntree Foundation*.

Creegan, C., Warrener, M. & Kinsella, R. (2009) *Living with Social Evils – The Voices of Unheard Groups*. Joseph Rowntree Foundation.

Cropanzano, R. & Wright, T. A. (1999) A 5-year study of change in the relationship between well-being and job performance. *Consulting Psychology Journal: Practice and Research*, **51**, 252–265.

Danner, D. D., Snowdon, D. A. & Friesen, W. V. (2001) Positive emotions in early life and longevity: Findings from the nun study. *Journal of Personality and Social Psychology*, **80**, 804–813.

De Silva, M. J., McKenzie, K., Harpham, T., *et al* (2005) Social capital and mental illness: a systematic review. *Journal Epidemiology and Community Health*, **59**, 619–627.

Diener, E. & Seligman, M. E. (2002) Very happy people. *Psychological Science*, **13**, 81–84.

Dolan, P., Peasgood, T. & White, M. (2008) Do we really know what makes us happy? A review of the economic literature on the factors associated with subjective well-being. *Journal of Economic Psychology*, **29**, 94–122.

Falzer, P. R. (2007) Developing and using social capital in public mental health. *Mental Health Review Journal*, **12**, 34–42.

Faris, R. E. L. & Dunham, H. W. (1939) *Mental Disorders in Urban Areas*. Hafner.

Fergusson, D., Horwood, J. & Ridder, E. (2005) Show me the child at seven: the consequences of conduct problems in childhood for psychosocial functioning in adulthood. *Journal of Child Psychology and Psychiatry*, **46**, 837–849.

Friedli, L. (2009) *Mental Health, Resilience and Inequalities*. WHO Regional Office for Europe.

Goffman, I. (1963) *Stigma: Notes on the Management of Spoiled Identity*. Penguin Books.

Goldberg, E. M. & Morrison, S. L. (1963) Schizophrenia and social class. *British Journal of Psychiatry*, **109**, 785–802.

Green, H., McGinnity, A., Meltzer, H., *et al* (2005) *Mental Health of Children and Young People in Great Britain, 2004*. Palgrave MacMillan.

Hare, E. H., Price, J. S. & Slater, E. (1972) Parental social class in psychiatric patients. *British Journal of Psychiatry*, **121**, 515–524.

Harter, J. K., Schmidt, F. L. & Keyes, C. L. M. (2003) Well-being in the workplace and its relationship to business outcomes: A review of the Gallup studies. In *Flourishing: Positive Psychology and the Life Well-Lived* (eds C. L. M. Keyes & J. Haidt), pp. 205–224. American Psychological Association.

HM Government (2007) *Reaching Out: An Action Plan on Social Exclusion*. Cabinet Office.

Hollingshead, A. B. & Redlich, F. C. (1958) *Social Class and Mental Illness: A Community Study*. Wiley.

Huppert, F. A. (2005) Positive mental health in individuals and populations. In *The Science of Well-Being* (eds F. A. Huppert, B. Keverne & N. Baylis), pp. 307–340. Oxford University Press.

Huppert, F. A. (2008) *Psychological Wellbeing: Evidence Regarding Its Causes and Consequences* (State-of-Science Review: SR-X2). Government Office for Science.

Huppert, F. A. & Whittington, J. E. (2003) Evidence for the independence of positive and negative wellbeing: implications for quality of life assessment. *British Journal of Health Psychology*, **8**,107–122.

Jané-Llopis, E., Barry, M., Horsman, C., *et al* (2005) What works in mental helath promotion. *Promotion and Education*, **2** (suppl.), 9–25.

Jones, C. & Novak, T. (1999) *Poverty, Welfare and the Disciplinary State*. Routledge.

Jones, C., Burstrom, B., Marttila, A., *et al* (2006) Studying social policy and resilience in families facing adversity in different welfare state contexts – the case of Britain and Sweden. *International Journal of Health Services*, **36**, 425–442.

Joseph Rowntree Foundation (2009) *What are the Implications of Attitudes to Economic Inequality?* Joseph Rowntree Foundation.

Kendler, K. S., Kuhn, J. W., Vittum, J., *et al* (2005) The interaction of stressful life events and a serotonin transporter polymorphism in the prediction of episodes of major depression: A replication. *Archives of General Psychiatry*, **62**, 529–535.

Keyes, C. L. M. (2002a) The mental health continuum: from languishing to flourishing in life. *Journal of Health and Social Research*, **43**, 207–222.

Keyes, C. L. M. (2002b) Promoting a life worth living: Human development from the vantage points of mental illness and mental health. In *Promoting Positive Child, Adolescent and Family Development: A Handbook of Program and Policy Innovations* (eds R. M. Lerner, F. Jacobs & D. Wertlieb), pp. 257–274. Sage.

Keyes, C. L. M. (2004) The nexus of cardiovascular disease and depression revisited: the complete mental health perspective and the moderating role of age and gender. *Aging and Mental Health*, **8**, 266–274.

Keyes, C. L. M. (2005) Mental illness and/or mental health? Investigating axioms of the complete state model of health. *Journal of Consulting and Clinical Psychology*, **73**, 539–548.

Keyes, C. L. M. (2006) Mental health in youth: is America's youth flourishing? *American Journal of Orthopsychiatry*, **76**, 395–402.

Kubzansky, L. D. & Kawachi, I. (2000) Going to the heart of the matter: Do negative emotions cause coronary heart disease? *Journal of Psychosomatic Research*, **48**, 323–337.

Layard, R. (2005) *Happiness: Lessons from a New Science*. Allen Lane.

Levitas, R., Pantazis, C., Fahmy, E., *et al* (2007) *The Multidimensional Analysis of Social Exclusion: A Research Report for the Social Exclusion Task Force.*: The Cabinet Office.

Levy, B. R., Slade, M. D., Kunkel, S. R., *et al* (2002) Longevity increased by positive self-perceptions of aging. *Journal of Personality and Social Psychology*, **83**, 261–270.

Littlewood, R. (2008) *Comparative Cultural Perspectives on Wellbeing. Report for Foresight Review Mental Capital and Wellbeing: Making the Most of Ourselves in the 21st Century* (State-of-Science Review: SR-X5). Government Office for Science.

Lyubomirsky, S., King, L. & Diener, E. (2005) The benefits of frequent positive affect: does happiness lead to success? *Psychological Bulletin*, **131**, 803–855.

Marmot, M. & Wilkinson, G. (2007) Psychosocial and material pathways in relation to income and health: a response to Lynch *et al. BMJ*, **322**, 1233–1236.

McCrone, P., Dhanasiri, S., Patel, A., *et al* (2008) *Paying the Price: The Cost of Mental Health in England to 2026*. King's Fund.

Meltzer, H., Singleton, N., Lee, A., *et al* (2002) *The Social and Economic Consequences of Adults with Mental Disorders*. TSO (The Stationery Office).

Mental Health Foundation (2006a) *Feeding Minds: The Impact of Food on Mental Health*. Mental Health Foundation.

Mental Health Foundation (2006b) *Cheers? Understanding the Relationship between Alcohol and Mental Health*. Mental Health Foundation.

Morgan, A., Ziglio, E., Harrison, D., *et al* (2004) *Assets for Health and Development Programme Overview (AHDP): Making the Case*. WHO Regional Office for Europe.

Mowlam, A. & Creegan, C. (2008) *Modern-Day Social Evils: The Voices of Unheard Groups*. Joseph Rowntree Foundation.

Office of the Deputy Prime Minister (2004) *Mental Health and Social Exclusion*. Office of the Deputy Prime Minister.

Oliver, M. (1990) *The Politics of Disablement*. Macmillan.

Ostir, G. V., Markides, K. S., Black, S. A., *et al* (2000) Emotional wellbeing predicts subsequent functional independence and survival. *Journal of the American Geriatrics Society*, **48**, 473–478.

Ostir, G. V., Markides, K. S., Peek, M. K., *et al* (2001) The association between emotional wellbeing and the incidence of stroke in older adults. *Psychosomatic Medicine*, **63**, 210–215.

Pelled, L. H. & Xin, K. R. (1999) Down and out: An investigation of the relationship between mood and employee withdrawal behaviour. *Journal of Management*, **25**, 875–895.

Phillipson, C. & Scharf, T. (2004) *The Impact of Government Policy on Social Exclusion of Older People: A Review of the Literature*. Social Exclusion Unit, Office of the Deputy Prime Minister.

Pickett, K. E., James, O. W. & Wilkinson, R. G. (2006) Income inequality and the prevalence of mental illness: a preliminary international analysis. *Journal of Epidemiology and Community Health*, **60**, 646–647.

Pressman, S. & Cohen, S. (2005) Does positive affect influence health? *Psychological Bulletin*, **131**, 925–971.

Pressman, S. D. & Cohen, S. (2006) Does positive affect influence health? *Brain, Behavior and Immunity*, **20**,175–181.

Rogers, A. & Pilgrim, D. (2003) *Inequalities and Mental Health*. Palgrave Macmillan.

Room, G. (2001) Trajectories of social exclusion: The wider context. In *Breadline Europe: The Measurement of Poverty* (eds D. Gordon & P. Townsend), pp. 407–439. Policy Press.

Rose, G. (1992) *The Strategy of Preventative Medicine*. Oxford: Oxford University Press.

Rutter, M. & Madge, N. (1997) *Cycles of Disadvantage: A Review of Research*. Heinemann.

Ryff, C. D. & Singer, B. (1998) Middle age and well-being. *Encyclopaedia of Mental Health*, **2**, 707–719. Academic Press.

Sainsbury Centre for Mental Health (2003) *The Economic and Social Costs of Mental Illness* (Policy paper 3). Sainsbury Centre for Mental Health.

Sainsbury Centre for Mental Health (2008) *Mental Health at Work: Developing the Business Case* (Policy paper 8). Sainsbury Centre for Mental Health.

Scott, S., Spender, Q., Doolan, M., *et al* (2001) Multicentre controlled trail of parenting groups for child antisocial behaviour in clinical practice. *BMJ*, **323**, 194–197.

Sefton, T. (2009) Moving in the right direction? Public attitudes to poverty, inequality and redistribution. In *Towards a More Equal Society? Poverty, Inequality and Policy since 1997* (eds J. Hills, T. Sefton & K. Stewart). Policy Press.

Sen, A. (1999) *Development as Freedom*. Knopf.

Seymour, D. (2008) *Reporting Poverty in the UK: A Practical Guide for Journalists*. Joseph Rowntree Foundation.

Sheldon, R., Platt, R. & Jones, N. (2009) *Political Debate about Economic Inequality: An Information Resource*. Joseph Rowntree Foundation.

Smith, N. & Middleton, S. (2007) *A Review of Poverty Dynamics Research in the UK*. Joseph Rowntree Foundation.

Sylva, K., Melhuish, E., Sammons, P., et al (2007) *Effective Pre-School and Primary Education 3–11 Project (EPPE 3–11). A Longitudinal Study Funded by the DfES (2003–2008): Promoting Equality in the Early Years. Report to the Equalities Review*. Institute of Education (http://archive.cabinetoffice.gov.uk/equalitiesreview/upload/assets/www.theequalitiesreview.org.uk/promoting_equality_in_the_early_years.pdf).

Thoits, P. A. & Hewitt, L. N. (2001) Volunteer work and wellbeing. *Journal of Health and Social Behavior*, **42**,115–131.

Thoreau, H. D. (1854) *Walden; or, Life in the Woods*. (2004 edn: Princeton University Press: p. 8).

Thornicroft, G. (2006) *Shunned: Discrimination against People with Mental Illness*. Oxford University Press.

Timmins, N. (1995) *The Five Giants: A Biography of the Welfare State*. HarperCollins.

UNICEF (2007) *Child Poverty in Perspective: An Overview of Child Well-Being in Rich Countries, Innocenti Report Card 7*. UNICEF Innocenti Research Centre.

van Os, J., Park, S. B. G. & Jones, P. B. (2001) Neuroticism, life events and mental health: evidence for person–environment correlation. *British Journal of Psychiatry*, **178** (suppl. 40), s72–s77.

Waddell, G. & Burton, K. (2006) *Is Work Good for Your Health and Wellbeing?* TSO (The Stationery Office).

Wilkinson, R. G. (1996) *Unhealthy Societies: The Afflictions of Inequality*. Routledge.

Wilkinson, R. (2005) *The Impact of Inequality: How to Make Sick Societies Healthier*. The New Press.

Wilkinson, R. & Pickett, K. (2009) *The Spirit Level: Why More Equal Societies Almost Always Do Better*. Penguin.

Windle, M. (2000) A latent growth curve model of delinquent activity among adolescents. *Applied Developmental Science*, **4**, 193–207.

World Health Organization (1948) *Preamble to the Constitution of the World Health Organization as adopted by the International Health Conference, New York, 19–22 June, 1946; signed on 22 July 1946 by the representatives of 61 States (Official Records of the World Health Organization, no. 2, p. 100) and entered into force on 7 April 1948*. WHO (http://www.who.int/about/definition/en/print.html).

World Health Organization (2004) *Promoting Mental Health: Concepts, Emerging Evidence, Practice (Summary Report)*. WHO (http://www.who.int/mental_health/evidence/en/promoting_mhh.pdf).

World Health Organization (2005) *WHO European Ministerial Conference on Mental Health Briefing*. WHO (http://www.euro.who.int/document/mnh/ebrief08.pdf).

Wright, T. A. & Staw, B. M. (1999) Affect and favourable work outcomes: two longitudinal tests of the happy-productive worker thesis. *Journal of Organisational Behaviour*, **20**, 1–23.

CHAPTER 11

Finding acceptance: the experiences of people who use mental health services

Rosemary Wilson, Michael Osborne and Susan Brook

This chapter was co-written by three members of the National Social Inclusion Programme's (NSIP's) Reference Group. Although we all have considerable experience of mental distress, which has been, or is being, treated by mental health professionals, and of discussing and promoting socially inclusive practice, it can be seen that we all have different approaches to the topic of social inclusion. For one of us employment plays an important role, for another working as a volunteer alongside mental health professionals has been the key to inclusion, whereas the third argues strongly for the right to take time out, to stand back and reflect. This variation of perspectives should come as no surprise. Social inclusion – participating and being part of a community – is multi-faceted and personal, charged with different meanings and experiences. In this chapter we shall be looking at some of these facets and experiences.

We are aware that solving the problem of exclusion will require political and social changes. Discrimination remains a significant barrier. We cannot, for example, serve on a jury and we may be excluded from the workplace. We may be disadvantaged in financial matters, in foreign travel and in the job market. Public attitudes are still prejudicial and as common parlance bears out, people with mental health issues have been excluded throughout recorded history; we are 'round the bend', 'out of our mind', 'off our rocker'. But in this chapter we shall be focusing on how mental health practitioners can help us to achieve the more everyday forms of social inclusion by the way they interact with us and the treatment they offer. We will contribute examples of good and bad practice, which we have been given by other people using services to use anonymously and by referring to our own experiences.

It is important to recognise that we are not 'representative service users'. There is no such person, as each experience of life and distress is unique. We are, however, privileged to have access to a wide community of people who use services who perhaps feel more able to talk about their experiences to us rather than to professionals, because there is no perceived imbalance of power. Traditionally it was called the views of the smoke-room; more accurately now it is the outcome of peer support, the use of storytelling to gain understanding which has been practised since time immemorial. Of course, in the consulting room we tell our stories; however, the clinicians tend to guide us in the time available to them to reveal what they feel they need to hear about, whereas we may hold back details out of politeness, fear, embarrassment or a simple need for privacy.

Our original intent was to combine our views into one coherent entity, but we have chosen to present three individual accounts, believing that the reader will learn by recognising our different approaches and use of language, our different experiences and aspirations to reflect that each person is unique, that there can be no one-size-fits-all outcome and that clinicians must be prepared to stand alongside each person they see professionally and learn where they have come from, where they are at present and where they would like to be in the future. Quite probably that will not be the place the professional or society at large would choose for us; different people choose very different life paths. But are we to be made 'normal'? Do we have any real sense of what 'normal' is? What is normal for one individual or community may be unbelievably strange to another. Certainly the path that professionals may consider the best for the people who use their services today is not the path mental health professionals even 20 years ago would have considered appropriate and it may again be radically different in another 20 years' time. Similarly, the goals of the people who use mental health services will change, but much more quickly; as they move forward or even simply look up from the ground, different perspectives and horizons will present themselves and they may choose to pursue a new path. The success of social inclusion can be measured by the number of new opportunities the person feels empowered to embrace.

Michael: Living with depression

It goes without saying that it is very important that service users are socially included in all activities that are beneficial for a satisfactory role in society. Social inclusion means the service user getting back into the main stream of life. It means having employment, going out for enjoyment, having friends and being on closer terms with any family that they have. Being excluded from all this for long periods makes most people very unhappy and discontented. Furthermore, it is very likely that their mental condition will deteriorate.

When a person is working and is subsequently off ill with, for example, depression they may quickly lose contact with their workplace (Case study 11.1). Workmates do not contact them and I heard of one case where a person was never contacted when off ill for 9 months. They were thus excluded from all personal news and work news. After a long time off work they lose their work image and so lose their sense of belonging anywhere. No contact with employer, workmates or other staff exacerbates this condition until the prospect of returning to work becomes an insurmountable problem.

When a person is off from work with depression, psychiatrists and GPs often tell them that they should go out and do things. Of course this is right, they should, but if workmates see them out at the pub or at a football match, the word goes round that they are malingering and not really ill. They may also feel that they have to stay in, in case personnel come to call. Owing to other people's ignorance and misleading perceptions about depression, the doctor's perfectly reasonable suggestions for improvement are not followed. Other attitudes that are met at work may also stand in the way. An office manager once told a service user that 'depression is not a real illness'. This denies the reality of their experiences and excludes them from daring to be off ill, so when they do take time off because they cannot go on any longer, they face a burden of guilt and the fear that they may be sacked (Case study 11.2). If, because of this, they continue working when ill, the illness can get to unbearable and dangerous proportions.

It is helpful if psychiatrists have close involvement with line managers to explain to them about mental illness. They could explain that an ill person may be told to get out more and that it should not be condemned as malingering. They could also explain the nature and effects of stigma, the need for involvement of an ill person in facilitating their return to work and the importance of making adjustments at work.

Stigma remains when the person returns to work. One of the really excluding items is when they are not given a piece of work 'because it might upset you' or because 'we don't want to make you ill again'. This puts them apart from their workmates; it turns them into a 'special case'. It excludes them while in work.

Case study 11.1

After 10 years' involvement with mental health services, Jack was asked to identify the significant others in his life. Whereas he had previously been a family man with a wide circle of work colleagues and other friends, he could now only identify his psychiatrist and his care coordinator.

Case study 11.2

During the first year of mental health difficulties, the assessment described 'nervous breakdowns'. The carer was advised to find the service user non-stressful work as a cleaner, despite their education, skills and qualifications. After failing to turn up for work because of deteriorating mental health, they were sacked – another family member said not to argue, as this would mean having to send in the medical certificate, showing reason for absence as psychosis, and 'as everyone knows, this means schizophrenia'.

In some cases friends, relatives and work colleagues may observe aspects of the behaviour of a depressed person that may lead to them avoiding that person. This, in turn, may deepen the person's sense of isolation and rejection. It also gives the impression that depression invites exclusion. When depressed, people are very often quiet and withdrawn and this may provoke the belief that they are a miserable so and so, stand-offish or just plain stupid, whereas they can quietly enjoy company without talking, and gain from just being part of a group. However, most people do not allow them to take their place in society at their desired pace and so often they are pressed to take part, which can be very unsettling to them. Friends also think when the person is depressed that they have not enjoyed themselves because they have not spoken or laughed much. After a while they do not invite them out or visit them anymore.

Attending a day centre for those with an enduring history of mental health problems can be beneficial. This can give a real sense of inclusion because the person becomes part of a community of people with similar experiences. Some structure is given to the day and the person can discuss their problems freely, without fear of stigma or lack of understanding. This is like belonging to a club that is free of stigma. However, it is not 'real' life. It is also not real inclusion, but it is nevertheless a great step forward and an improvement from the difficult experience of isolation. The need for activity, structure and a meaningful day can be thus fulfilled and contribute towards improvement, and a good day centre can provide this. A sense of involvement is also important. Encouragement to become involved in the centre's business meetings and taking part in training, self-help groups and activities is beneficial, as a person finds that they have something to offer. This can make them feel worthwhile and helps in developing self-confidence and a feeling of being useful. Another great confidence booster is learning – going to a further education college is a valuable form of inclusion, as the class often becomes a social group (Case study 11.3).

Going with someone to the theatre, cinema and sports events gives not only a sense of doing something but also a sense of purpose and brings

Case study 11.3

In response to service user demand a voluntary service offered literacy and numeracy classes in partnership with a local college. Uptake far exceeded expectations.

Case study 11.4

A user-delivered voluntary service set up a football afternoon for people using its services. As a result the usual trend for accessing counselling was reversed. There were more people from a socially deprived area and more men than women.

people together. These activities can be organised by the day centre. Some of the best forms of inclusion are achieved through music, sports activities and education (Case study 11.4). They are most beneficial especially in reducing stigma – if you play a musical instrument, do sport or have knowledge, people will respect you no matter what condition you may have. Encouraging people with mental health issues to arrange activities by themselves can be particularly rewarding. Forming a sports team, perhaps a seven a side football team that play in local leagues, or a snooker team that competes against other clubs, are good examples. It also gets people out in the evening, which is often a barrier to be overcome by those with mental health problems.

There are many other examples of initiatives that can promote inclusion. Some colleges of further education hold classes in day centres, which brings the public into the centres and makes it easier for the service users to attend. This means that the public can recognise that the service users are not violent and are 'just like themselves'. Such openness may also result in the exposure of prejudice, as happened in the case of two members of the public refusing to enter a day centre 'in case they were stabbed'.

Treatment of the service user in the NHS varies and, like the curate's egg, is good in parts. What the patient mostly craves is to be listened to – how can you understand their condition if you do not listen to them? To be treated with dignity and respect is also an understandable and common wish – a caring and understanding manner by a psychiatrist is really desired. Too often service users report that 'he never looked at me', 'she kept looking at her watch', and 'they treated me as though I was dirt'. These statements are a sad indictment of some practitioners in the hospital service. General practitioners may also get the same bad reports and reports of poor treatment in accident and emergency departments are legion. Nevertheless, there are many reports of excellent treatment by good and caring psychiatrists and other staff. I have personal experience of first-class treatment throughout my 40 years in secondary care, and only a few weeks ago a service user gave me a letter to pass on to the psychiatrist and ward staff in praise of the fine treatment and service given while he was confined to a hospital ward.

Lack of information is frequently reported as a problem. Often the person does not get a diagnosis of their condition or information on their medication. For many people a diagnosis is important, as it gives a label to their illness and something to tell to family, friends and employers (Case study 11.5). It can feel very stigmatising when someone asks you what is wrong and you say that you do not know. Too often people unfamiliar with mental ill health say 'There's nothing wrong with you, you just want to pull yourself together'. On the other hand, some people do not like to have a diagnosis, as they believe it gives them a label, and feel that they are then treated as 'an illness' rather than as a whole person. On its own a diagnosis gives a narrow view of a person's condition. You are not just a 'depression' to be cured. You are a person with other needs than just your illness – needs for better housing, social contact, relaxing activities and often financial support. Being looked at holistically makes one feel a whole person with more to you than just an illness – this is most helpful.

Unfortunately, it is only when the service user is well that they are capable of complaining of bad treatment. It is also at this stage that they can give compliments for their treatment.

Those suffering from mental ill health often have bothers when they have physical ailments. General practitioners, when approached about a physical illness by someone who uses mental health services, may take the attitude that 'it is all in the mind' and discount the physical illness. I have heard of a case where a GP would not accept that the patient had a stomach ulcer and persistently claimed that their frequent vomiting and bad indigestion were caused by 'nerves'. In such cases the person is excluded from treatment (Case study 11.6).

The ideas associated with recovery are a great help towards moving you on. Small wins in facing the day – getting up an hour earlier, often getting up at all, going out when there is no need to, or trying to read a book when you have trouble concentrating – are all steps forward (Case study 11.7). Having hope of getting better, of meeting someone special, a job opportunity – all these bring you towards wellness. People have recovered, do recover, and will still recover from mental illness.

Otherwise the service user can still live with their illness. The label does not have to define you, even if the effects of the problem can still give you setbacks. You can be depressed without being a 'depressive'. You can have

---

Case study 11.5

Judith reported that her GP repeatedly asked her what condition she would like to be identified on sick notes. The GP assumed that her mental health diagnosis would be unacceptable.

Case study 11.6

It was Ann's psychiatrist who instigated investigations for diabetes (a correct diagnosis) when her tiredness had been dismissed by her GP as caused by her mental distress. On the other hand, a detained patient's complaints of chest pains were written off as anxiety, when in fact she had sustained two broken ribs when she was forcibly transported to hospital.

Case study 11.7

Patrick, a high achiever all his life, found making contact with other people well nigh impossible after a long in-patient stay. He was helped by coaching from his psychiatrist to value very small steps which he had previously denigrated and seen as failure.

schizophrenia without being a 'schizophrenic'. For the person with mental health issues to take control of their life and to say what they need to get better is important. People have to take risks to improve their situation. Too often the mental condition itself can be a way of life and give one a self-image of being ill.

My recovery, I related to the equivalent of leaving prison. It was going into the wide world full of challenges to be faced. A change from my comforting, yes, comforting, depression, which kept me away from the problems of living and gave me a dependency on others, especially the medical profession. My recovery has been so life-changing that people find me a totally different person from the one they knew 4 years ago, including my wife of 40 years. I am outgoing and warm compared with withdrawn and cold and this shows in my volunteering work and social life. I have many friends compared with none in the past.

The recovery occurred quite rapidly. It followed a year off work with depression and being in a day hospital and I believe it was due to a combination of things: time at a day hospital and then going to a day centre. A new and first-class psychiatrist and a first-time excellent mental health key worker played an important role. I found that they gave me hope and saw something good in me. I also had meaningful activity and mixed with people with similar problems. I came to realise that I could help people and be a leader. Peer support made a big difference and my new friends boosted my ego, especially when I was voted top in the day centre election for representatives at the business meetings. Help and understanding by my peers played a large role in my recovery. I blossomed and 'found myself', by small changes to my lifestyle and vast changes to my ways of thinking. An amount of cognitive–behavioural therapy (CBT) helped a lot with my feelings of paranoia.

Joining the involvement team as a volunteer at the local mental health trust made a big difference. I found that I had a flair for speaking and playing a role in meetings, interviewing, training and making speeches. Another ego boost was being appointed as a service user consultant. I work closely with the executive director of nursing and I am treated equally with frontline staff. I am a member of many strategic steering groups including national groups representing the trust. I also work nationally as a quality reviewer for the Mind charity. I still attend the day centre; have the same key worker and a psychiatrist. I still take medication, so that recovery in the literal sense is not complete. However, fulfilment and contentment are.

Psychiatrists have always understood people, but often the relationship and communication skills have left something to be desired. But now, I believe that things are a lot better, especially respect and listening skills. Health services for the people with mental health problems are improving. New schemes have emerged, like New Ways of Working, where you see the right person at the right time. Often a social worker can give better help during an illness, or sometimes an occupational therapist is the right person to aid recovery. A psychiatrist is always there for medical matters and the nurse is there to take care and nurture. A new scheme, Releasing Time to Care, should be valuable to the service user – the logistics of the wards and staff time spent away from the patient is to be assessed and reduced, thus giving staff more time to spend with the service users, which is a valuable requirement if people are to improve more speedily.

Inclusion is a very important step towards recovery. The chance to take part in everyday activities with those who are well is one of the main ways of getting better. How can we integrate if we never get the chance or encouragement to do so? There should be every effort made for social inclusion, not only by all of society, especially those staff working in mental health, but by the service users themselves. We must all battle against stigma and exclusion in all its forms.

Susan: A long view

Moving from a position of social exclusion to one of inclusion is intended to be the door through which making recovery a reality passes. Historically within conventional mental health services, doors are talked about as being locked – blocking people from leaving the system or blocking them returning to support and safety after discharge – or revolving, giving recurrent re-entry to the system without the possibility of recovery. But surely, the future for fully functioning social inclusion is not having a systematic door between reality and mental ill health. This is the first point of exclusion, a sense of otherness, being one of them and not one of us. Social inclusion is, after all, about tolerance, embracing our differences, individual realities within the reality of social cohesion. This may be exacerbated by the split that we make between mental health and physical health. A good start to removing the barriers between physical and mental health is already starting to happen, with the current and continuing training of GPs about mental health problems, and with CBT being available in GPs surgeries, making anxieties and depression an acceptable part of what have been perceived as centres for only physical healthcare.

This acceptance makes more tangible the essence of respect that social inclusion requires. If people with mental health problems are to be valued rather than seen as worthless, appreciated rather than considered a burden and a problem, believed in rather than doubted, seen as adding to society rather than a threat to it, then self-worth will rise along with confidence. To believe that this level of acceptance is the goal of social inclusion, colours and brings to life black and white statements such as 'individuals can be helped and supported to define and find new roles and learn to live well even in the face of significant illness or impairment' (see Chapter 14, p. 295).

In our modern world, holding on to the idea of returning people with mental health problems to 'normality within reality' is very old fashioned. These days freedom of thought and its expression is so broad in mainstream life there is even chatter about 'things having gone too far'. Yet, living with mental health difficulties often means living with public fear and judgement, being unfairly scrutinised in every action, every word, in an effort of monitoring risk and public discomfort rather than being about individual health and well-being. This is the straightjacket of discrimination. The inequalities and lack of opportunities for women have long been discussed in terms of coming up against the glass ceiling, but the inequalities of mental health discrimination is too often experienced as coming up against a 'brick floor' – and one that has something of the damp and musty smell of the Middle Ages. Examples of this abound: parents of husband of service user asking if diagnosis was grounds for divorce, forever having memories doubted, never being allowed to express opinions forcefully without it being seen as a sign of illness, at a family planning clinic being asked *sotto voce*, 'Do you have a boyfriend then?'.

Discrimination and exclusion can be so ingrained as to be invisible, even to some with the broadest, most intelligent, non-prejudicial and kindly of minds. Even though society may be seen to live with greater freedoms than ever before, it still feels the need for social cohesion. It cannot continue to heap all its fears on people with diagnosed mental health conditions and deny psycho-phobia exists. A civilised society cannot expect 'us' to be more normal than 'them'. What a disappointment to grow up, being educated to work and live in a system that tries to push people into the shapes, sizes and colours of some future corresponding hole. Life is not as simple as child's play, the early learning toy of shapes and sizes fitting corresponding holes, static, fixed, unchanging, pre-destined. Living in a civilised society means change and choice, and those living with a mental health condition need to accept that inclusiveness can be a change for the better rather than the worse.

Though the essence of social inclusion lies in the civilising power of shared respect, the humanity of tolerance and difference, it has to battle with, class, position, power, education and upbringing. In this respect, social inclusion seems to be more about power and acquisition and less about humanity. In today's society, money matters and the nature of what it is to be human has become distorted, by the same mechanism that ensured survival. Currently, the financial world is in meltdown, the markets are falling off the cliff, assets are devaluing and unemployment is rising. This was preceded by unprecedented levels of work-related stress in a 24/7 society. What might this mean for the inclusion of people with mental health problems, and the role of work for people with health-related unemployment and others in their health and well-being journey to recovery and inclusion?

For professionals, accountability to the service user has to be balanced 'against accountability to others (employing agency, wider community and professional body)' (see Chapter 14, p. 301). If linked with discrimination, these few words may scupper a lot of hope for 'negotiating achievable and meaningful goals' (p. 302). But, if accountability without unfair discrimination is used wisely, then the current changes society is going through, re-evaluating its sense of self, could be the opportunity social inclusion for users of mental health services has been waiting for. For this to happen, it is important that the socially inclusive practice does not mean the psychiatrist will use his or her position of authority to give an impression of respect and equality for the individual service users that is, in truth, to their disadvantage. Consider the service user at the first presentation to mental health services. It takes many years to become an expert patient by experience, perhaps not an accolade to which a person before their illness might aspire to, but one nonetheless earned through contact with services and through the experience of dealing with ill health.

On the one hand, experience of mental health problems can educate you – this takes time and people do not have this 'expertise by experience' when they first encounter their own problems. On the other, it is almost inevitable that service users become experts by experience because once part of the mental health system, they may have contact for a long time, sometimes unfortunately because they are not able to leave mental health services as there is nowhere to go once outside the door (the revolving door syndrome). It can also be because some mental health conditions take a long time to unravel and to come to terms with, beginning a recovery journey. With mental health services placing increasing emphasis on social inclusion and recovery, there is likely to be an increasing recognition that there are fundamental flaws in the existing system. Recovery is not cure, it is a life journey, and service users need, and should expect to be, supported in this. Early intervention for people with psychoses may be hampered by public attitudes to recognising and declaring experiences of mental ill health, but with less public prejudice and more empathy with the stresses of life there should be less reason for this. Intervening early in what may be a life-changing crisis may hasten the recovery, improve the expertise by experience and reduce the likelihood of enduring contact with services.

Recovery and social inclusion are matters that are recognised, sensed and felt by the service user – they concern a sense of well-being, of having value, a sense of being valued, of being respected. This may not easily fit with the bureaucratic and institutional restrictions of mental health services – the planning, the doing, having a timetable with goals and targets and outcomes to be assessed and ticked. There may be a lack of continuity in a person's care, team members can change, and the service user's medical notes may be inadequate to provide sufficient understanding of the person. The service user has to fit into the process, rather than the process fitting the service user. The person new to services does not know how things work, and even expert patients by experience may have difficulties, especially with services undergoing change.

There may be some perverse effects of making the system more recovery-oriented. We all want to see an end to people with glazed expressions sitting around pointlessly in daytime television lounges, yet the opportunity to not feel rushed, not urged to plan and participate, can be therapeutic. It can be important to have time out, a chance to stand and stare, a retreat to be able to listen to that still, small voice within oneself, not to be rushed and pushed and squashed into re-engaging or processed through constant assessments chanced on by signposting or finding a leaflet that might lead somewhere because the system is now 'socially inclusive'. There needs to be a space for self-discovery, unhindered by the negative values of others, to not learn the fear of being feared. It is helpful to allow service users to explore means of help for themselves, to find approaches that are not part of standard healthcare and other models for maintaining their health, and moving forward in their own time. A lifetime on strong antipsychotic medications may be seen as damaging by patients and some may prefer to explore alternative forms of therapy. Socially inclusive practice needs to recognise that there is no quick-fix cure and that experiencing social exclusion may have lifelong consequences.

My views on drug treatment and its alternatives have been influenced by my own experience and my 30-year recovery. I have never been sectioned or spent time on an in-patient ward. My GP, who was also trained as a doctor of homeopathy and yoga teacher, was helpful and introduced me to visualisation and meditation. As I was already interested in alternative lifestyles, I followed this natural interest. My experience of schizophrenia taught me mindfulness. A friend told me about a physician, Richard Mackarness, who had written two books about allergies and mental health (Mackarness, 1976, 1980) and I became interested in following a wheat-free (not gluten-free) diet. However, it was many years before I tried to follow this advice, and it was so helpful I wish I had done so earlier. I started it when I had good self-awareness and was able to observe my own reactions. I avoided wheat totally, with the same strictness as in a gluten-free diet, for several years. Then I tried to eat wheat occasionally. At first I had a violent digestive reaction and experienced anxiety and panic. My GP agreed to refer me to a homeopathic hospital to discuss wheat avoidance for mental health. I persevered and continue to avoid wheat, perhaps eating it only occasionally. I have always lived in the country, and was a fan of Richard Mabey's *Food for Free* (1972), so I was delighted when he brought out a book chronicling his recovery from depression, *Nature Cure* (2005).

I chanced on all these things after deciding to stop attending out-patients for monthly depot injections. It was fully expected I would fall flat on my face and need picking up and putting together again with those injections. I wanted to stop medication because of its side-effects of tremors and weight gain. I had experienced such severe shaking I could not hold a pen to write and I had difficulty brushing my teeth. I was given something to control the shaking, but the side-effect of this was to experience depression. Although I was given something for depression, it did not help much. I had thought I was depressed because I was having difficulty coming to terms with having schizophrenia. My weight had increased from 7 st 10 lb to 10 st 2 lb.

I continued to have severe disabling psychosis over several months at a time, for many years, which would eventually resolve spontaneously. Unfortunately, or rather perhaps, fortunately, my first marriage fell apart, but I had always had the love and support of my parents and went on to meet someone else who respected me for who I was rather than seeing me as someone with schizophrenia.

After several years without injections I tried unsuccessfully to be prescribed medication in tablet form, as I wanted to take medications in short sharp doses and quickly reduce from high to low doses then stop again. This refusal might have been because of how I wanted to use the medication, or because of comments of my ex-husband which were recorded in my notes, which I only requested to read in recent years. It would have been a great help to me if I had been able to quietly and politely ask for help when I felt I needed it, rather than be faced with an attitude of, 'if you are well enough to ask, you are too well to need it', then becoming so unwell it becomes impossible to ask – it is a Catch-22 situation. I was eventually prescribed antipsychotics in tablet form when I told a psychiatrist I was waiting to have surgery and was more scared of a mental health relapse while in hospital than I was of knowing that the surgery involved high risk. I continue to get antipsychotics in tablet form on prescription and find them very helpful for avoiding disabling relapse, and continue to take them occasionally as I choose. As requested by a psychiatrist, I have tried the more modern antipsychotics, the ones that are supposed to perk you up a bit, making you less of a couch potato, but the withdrawal side-effects are too severe, distressingly close to the onset of psychosis.

Following surgery, I have received Bowen therapy for pain relief offered through NHS physiotherapy. It is a holistic treatment which is also very calming mentally and spiritually. Regrettably, it is no longer offered by the NHS and I have to continue treatment privately. In recent years I have been able to get support from the community mental health team (CMHT), occupational therapist and the charity Rethink, and through this I have been introduced to my local service user involvement network which in turn led to my being invited to join the National Social Inclusion Programme Reference Group. I was enabled to attend by taking my assistance/support dog (work is being done for them to achieve the same status and access as guide dogs). Through the service user and carer network, I have met other service users and carers who follow and believe in alternative treatments and less dependency on the medical model. I have always eaten healthily, mostly taking organic foods and avoiding processed foods, and after reading recommended books by Patrick Holford (1997, 2003) and Stephanie Marohn (2003), I take daily vitamin and mineral supplements. I have tried to return to work several times, but find it impossible to sustain my health for long periods. I would like to work part time but the benefits system is not helpful. I find all the form filling for accessibility and eligibility benefits regressive and negative, and this is also true for all forms needed to access support and treatments. I believe that had I continued with the monthly injections, the side-effects of shaking would have made it impossible for me to continue using my skills, abilities and training for my lifelong quality of life interests. Although I very much appreciate my opinions being sought through the involvement work, I find it draining and often traumatising. Yet, at the same time, thanks to the interest and respect of kind professionalism I have gained in confidence and self-esteem.

As understanding and acceptance of people with mental health difficulties develops, public misconceptions of risk for their safety should change to public awareness of the possible vulnerability of others – a vulnerability that needs sheltering and taking care of to allow as full a life as possible, rather than a vulnerability to be exploited and abused. Recovery through social inclusion begins as an essence of an idea, a kernel, a seed of change, and it is important that its porosity, its intangibility, is not suffocated in a flotsam of meetings, job descriptions, agendas and training, washed in on the latest tide and drowned in all the dry words of procedure used to explain what an evolutionary concept it is. Because as a concept, it will have to evolve, social inclusion by the procedure of social engineering – and it needs guiding from every direction, by psychiatrists, patients, family and friends, and all other professional carers.

Rosemary: My life, my choice; your facilitation, your example

Social inclusion is about choice: choosing with whom I associate, what I do with my time, how I solve my difficulties. It is about being given the information to find the support I need in the way that I want. When I have the capacity to do so, it is about choice of treatment of my mental health difficulties in the same way that I make choices about treatment for physical conditions. But is that the choice I am given? On many occasions it has not felt like that within a service that is under-funded and under-staffed to the point that exhausted and demoralised staff fail to recognise our common humanity, fail to treat me with empathy and respect as a person with my own expertise and aspirations, and with the same right to change my mind, make mistakes and learn from them.

> Am I normal…? NO!!!
> Normal is just a setting on a washing machine
>
> Messages on greetings cards

I was 46 when a significant life event brought the poor state of my mental health to the fore. Following a family argument my eldest son, then 18, left home and refused all overtures of reconciliation. I quickly fell into a deep depression and within 3 months was admitted to an acute psychiatric ward where I spent over 12 of the next 18 months spread over three admissions. It became clear that my son's departure had triggered deep-set fears of rejection and abandonment which had been present since infancy. Once released these proved intractable and the years since then have seen repeated periods of severe distress and recurrent admissions despite largely unimpeachable ongoing care and a wide range of treatments, from electroconvulsive therapy to a 5-year psychodynamic therapy, from what feels like an entire pharmacopoeia to CBT. In my experience the practice of psychiatry has not just been a science, it has also been a creative art.

> I see the service as offering you a safe place to fall apart so that reconstruction can begin.
>
> Consultant psychiatrist (personal communication, 1994)

So for me social inclusion has had little to do with the physical setting where I carry out my daily activities. It has been relearning the tasks of infancy while carrying out the tasks and bearing the responsibilities of a woman in her fifties. I can go to the gym, go to church, attend college, do a job and still exclude myself or be socially excluded by others because of my thought patterns and responses. Social exclusion is the product of, firstly and most importantly, what I believe about myself, then – and this deeply affects what I believe about myself – how I am treated, what other people believe about me, whether they engage with me and include me, whether in effect I have equal opportunities to do as other people do. It is whether my adulthood is regarded and respected, whether I have autonomy, whether I am consulted and my opinions valued and respected, whether I am, despite my mental health issues, a person of equal value in their eyes.

Mental health professionals need to model with me an example of a good relationship, where my equality and adulthood are recognised and valued to reframe past experience of the bullying or unhelpful relationships that have coloured my life. They need to demonstrate patience, understanding and respect so that I can give them in return. What happens behind closed doors in consultations will colour my whole experience of the service and how I respond to it. Clinicians may not recognise the power they hold, but it is true. 'My psychiatrist said… or did…' features in the spoken words and thoughts of people who use services. We hold them in our minds and memories and bring out their words and actions to reflect on and puzzle over, long after they have forgotten us.

Probably the most effective treatment I have received has been throughout a consistent display of respect for me and my decisions about my life and a refusal to give up hope on the part of my mental health team. They have grown to see me as an individual like them, with strengths and weaknesses, a woman with strong views and a personal morality that cannot be ignored, but can be worked with, a woman with a host of experiences before she met them and a host of experiences to meet in the future. Getting to know me as a person takes time and is hindered if I am only seen in the context of the consulting room, as these examples show:

> 3 years in…
>
> Me: I want to do a course.
> Consultant psychiatrist 1: That's a good idea. How about cake-icing? (I had baked cakes for the team)

Me: I want to use my brain!
I went away and enrolled in a course on moral philosophy.

10 years in…

Consultant psychiatrist 2: My colleague attended your CPD training…(and then in tones of utmost surprise)…He said you were really good!
Me: Yes, I am good at my job.

16 years in and three thick volumes of notes…

Me: I have real difficulties forming more than superficial relationships.
Consultant psychiatrist 3: Really? I didn't know. You appear so confident and at ease when you are delivering training.

I was well known to each psychiatrist. They were all professional, dedicated people, who gave me time and worked hard with me. But each of them made unfounded assumptions based on the little they knew of me. The person who presents in the consulting room bears little resemblance to the person others, or I myself, see. It is a different persona; sometimes I may trust my psychiatrist enough to show my pain and despair which is veiled outside, at other times I may be presenting her or him with a competent front to cover up my inward sense of inadequacy. Largely you see what I choose to reveal and that is never the full picture.

As I achieve the work of becoming fully adult, so the work of physical social inclusion can be successful. The team then need new skills. Can they tell me what the local voluntary sector has to offer and, indeed, 'sell' it to me? What leisure opportunities there are? Does the CMHT have links with the National Institute for Adult Continuing Education (NIACE) and local colleges, or with the Citizens Advice Bureau and benefits advisors? Is there someone to coordinate volunteering opportunities? Do they liaise with the disability officer at Jobcentre Plus? They need to know their area or at least know where they can find this information for me, because my motivation is still low and the likelihood of finding it for myself is not high; for example, I have been on enhanced care programme approach (CPA) since 1993 but only in 2008 did I apply for Disability Living Allowance. The CMHT needs to work as a team with other service providers.

Nevertheless, the psychiatrist's first role is to manage the symptoms I display and experience that make my inclusion by the community difficult and lead to my self-exclusion because I am 'different'. That management will usually be through medication. Although I have my own expertise, this is not it; I do not hold the necessary body of knowledge, the psychiatrist does. But mine is the hand that will put the tablets into my mouth and mine is the decision whether to raise that hand, so the team will have to take time to persuade me that I should.

Not long ago I spent May Day holiday with thousands of others at London Zoo. Social inclusion in practice, one might say, facilitated in part by the Zoo's policy of, with proof of evidence, admitting an 'essential' companion – my adult son – free. Once past the entry point there was nothing to distinguish me from any of the other thousands of visitors and my son and

I joked about his caring role in the context of a zoo. Still it was not a good choice, despite the joy of spending it with him. Did the animals, undoubtedly healthy, well-cared for and protected from predators, feel content with their lives, I wondered? Would they have preferred to live a free life in their natural habitat, with all its concomitant risks and dangers but also pleasures and successes? Did they like the intrusion into their privacy? Some may scorn this anthropomorphism, but it was a metaphor for my own experience of mental health services: well-cared for and safe, but living in a cage for everyone to look at, comment on and direct my life. Not social inclusion at all, because this is not an experience shared with most adults. I am different (some might say 'deviant'), and yet that level of care keeps me alive and outwardly functioning to a high level. Therein lies the inner tension.

Recognising that I will never achieve full inclusion, given the long-standing nature of my difficulties, my exclusion can nevertheless be minimised: the physical exclusion through admission to hospital – with all that may entail in terms of police involvement, physical restraint, locked wards and the subsequent reverberations in my life at home – and the more insidious exclusion that I inflict upon myself in terms of guilt and shame.

Happily, with the support of a good CMHT, my experience has changed.

Compare and contrast the management of two very similar episodes presenting the same level of risk and distress. The first episode, in 2004, resulted in an emergency assessment, an involuntary 'voluntary' 6-week admission to a ward 25 miles away, management by a team to whom I was unknown, and three further months off work, leaving me with a sense of humiliation and degradation that led to three further admissions within the space of 6 months:

> I was invited to a CPA meeting on the ward where I was an in-patient. I had made it clear that I required the attendance of a member of my own CMHT, some 25 miles away. I refused to attend because nobody had been invited. 'We thought it might distress you to have someone there', I was told.

In the latest crisis, in 2009, despite pressure from accident and emergency colleagues that I be compulsorily admitted under the Mental Health Act, I was managed in the community by my own local team (including my GP) and within 3 weeks I was back at work, travelling up to London and presenting to a large audience of strangers.

This success was achieved first by the work the team had done over the 16 years I have used services. Perhaps mine is an unusual experience, but I have had the good fortune to have been treated by a very stable team. Ever since my care has been largely community-based (some 12 years) I have had only three care coordinators and two responsible medical officers, so there has been plenty of time to build relationships of trust, explore my strengths and weaknesses, my hopes and aspirations with a trusted other, learn from the role-modelling and practise the coping strategies they helped me develop. Earlier I mentioned trust, which we will not get far without, but I am distrustful and suspicious and it falls to those who work with me to exercise their interpersonal skills to build a relationship of trust, by listening, giving me time, learning about my inner and outer world and then using what they have learnt to help me. The art of communication and relationship-building is core to good psychiatry. After a recent user-led session on communication skills for trainee psychiatrists one of the participants' evaluation comments revealed an inner tension: 'I hope we will not sacrifice the science of psychiatry to the art of communication'. You cannot, I believe, have one without the other.

These processes lie at the heart of an evaluation scheme commonly called WRAP (Wellness and Recovery Action Plan). Sometimes people are sent for a course of 'WRAP training' in the mistaken belief that it is a quick fix. The reality is different – it is a long, slow process based on trust in people who demonstrate that they want you to recover, believe you can recover, show you how to recover – a relationship with someone who can remind, reinforce, encourage and forgive. We all know that there are no quick fixes in mental health. It is a process based on hope, hope in the true sense, not just a wish, but a steadfast belief that something will happen.

There have been times when my dealings with mental health professionals have been instantly revealing and have switched on a light in my mind. I think of the Muslim duty senior house officer called out in the middle of the night to the ward, who, breaking protocol, said, 'Rosemary, can you not leave it in the hands of God?' I felt less alone, not just because I recognised the presence of God, but because I stood in Her presence with another Believer, albeit from a different Faith. Or the time my care coordinator said exactly the wrong thing and when I reproached her, instead of reacting defensively, she responded with: 'Rosemary, I am so sorry, that was unforgivable', thus role-modelling for me that it was OK to make mistakes, apologise and be forgiven, an essential lesson for me given that at times of distress I lose all my social skills. But for the most part it is the long, hard struggle of a person who has learnt not to trust and not to be open to build lasting relationships that has brought me this far. Recognising this I checked out that my new 'back-up' GP, who is not a practice partner, was going to be around for a long time: 'It won't work, if you are not...', and her unquestioning acceptance that I had the right to ask cemented the relationship.

In 2005, following a full-blown pin-down incident involving inflicted pain and full de-escalation techniques on a strange ward, I made it very clear that voluntary admission was impossible and there followed a high level of partnership-working on the part of myself, my informal supporters, my mental health team and my GP surgery between 2005 and 2008. It was very far from the tokenistic gesture I have heard so often of 'What would you like us to do?' – tokenistic because on one level what I would like is impossible: 'Just take the pain away', and more practically because I have turned to the professionals for their expertise and I do not know what the treatment options are. In contrast to my previous experience of services, this was a realistic consideration of the problems and the possible solutions. The validity of my expertise in myself and my condition was recognised by those who worked with me, who acknowledged that often my risk assessment was better than theirs, that I did know what would help or hinder my recovery and that the most important factor was being given control.

First, there was consideration of how we could avoid that high level of distress that required admission. Funding was found for me for 3 years to access 16 nights of respite care at a Christian retreat healing house where I could access alternative therapies and counselling, make real friendships and receive unlimited, loving care. During that time, because I had chosen to be open about my use of mental health services, I was encouraged to draw up a very personal relapse signature which included what I recognised, what the team who worked with me recognised and, probably crucially, what my social network recognised. It was not an easy or quick piece of work; I do not relish the prospect of relapse and do my best to hide the signs from everyone, including myself, so it involved facing some uncomfortable truths. I was used to the comfortable role of victim, now I had to take responsibility.

Consultant psychiatrist: Why can't you tell us before you overdose, Rosemary?

I had to confront my difficult behaviour with professionals at times of crisis, when I lose all the interpersonal skills that are so important to me. I had to recognise my inability to stand and face my distress, my pattern of running away. Possibly the most difficult part was that I had to decide whom I could trust to be honest and open with me without embarrassment on their part or a sense of stigmatisation on mine. Throughout the process I was given encouragement and reassurance, my fears of being rejected and my tears, buckets of them, at being a 'bad' person were openly addressed. The team role-modelled to me that I remained acceptable to others even when the dark side of me was made apparent. Only once in the whole 16 years has a (very junior) doctor threatened to withdraw treatment because I was 'non-compliant', but I have always been afraid that they would. I grew in confidence and openly asked people to tell me if they witnessed the signs they and others had identified, and gave a few trusted others permission to contact the team directly if I was unreceptive.

The second stage was to draw up and disseminate a crisis plan for anyone who might be involved professionally in my care (including, importantly, my GP practice) to which all were signed up. It identified trigger factors in professional behaviour to be avoided as far as possible, how I would like to treated, where I might want to meet, how I would react to attempts at 'assertiveness', what treatment options I would find acceptable, who should be contacted for information and advice, who it would be best to involve in my care. Deputies for my care teams in both primary and secondary care were identified to cover absences and relationships of trust with them established in periods of wellness. There are few people whom I dare to trust when I am unwell.

Crucially, this work was all undertaken in periods of wellness; there was none of the sense I had had before that, once recovered, the experiences of the distress would be carefully ignored and swept under the carpet as unfortunate occurrences, leaving me with such an intolerable sense of shame and guilt that I feared rejection was inevitable. The proof of the pudding was in the eating; the crisis plan worked and I felt in control of events throughout rather than being a piece of flotsam tossed at whim by a sea of professional interventions. 'Rosemary does not believe we work as a team', was recorded in my notes as early as 1994, a belief that appeared to me to be evidence-backed and had persisted for 10 or more years.

But probably the crucial factor was that, rather than being admitted, I stayed at home, where I was able to use my own personal coping strategies and access support from a wide range of people (mostly by email) at all sorts of levels. Everyone was supportive; no one rejected me, though when I am removed from contact with them, with no evidence at all, I believe that they all hate me. Even my dog and cat played a part by insisting that their needs had to be met, but also by offering unconditional love. And once again there was the role-modelling. Although I was a risk to myself, the team demonstrated that they trusted me to keep safe. Most of the day I was alone, although I had open phone contact.

Compare that with the experience of constant observations and locked doors. Because people were concerned that in my distress I would harm myself, a nurse stayed within touching distance, dogged my every footstep, even into the lavatory, and stayed next to my bed. For them the experience was limited to a single half hour, for me the torment was prolonged. At a time when my need for personal space was at its highest, I could barely tolerate someone being in the same room. 'How do you expect me to close my eyes and sleep with a strange man within a foot of me?!' I screamed. And then there were the windows that only opened a crack, the doors that were locked to prevent my leaving unnoticed, all clear evidence to my disturbed mind that I was out of control and too bad to be trusted. It was never voiced, but it did not need to be: 'But it's just like home, Rosemary. You lock the door there'. But at home I can unlock the door whenever I choose. At that time the role-modelling was that I was not trustworthy or honest enough to be consulted; nobody ever asked whether I could manage the distress without these restrictions, just 'We are concerned about your mental state so this is what will happen...', and I responded appropriately as a naughty child, seizing every opportunity to go AWOL or overdose, demonstrating how ineffectual their decisions were. I never told them why.

The success of our forward-planning and partnership work has given me more confidence to be open about my needs at times of distress because I know that I will be heard and my words will carry weight. I carried this positive experience forward into other areas of my life. When I went back to the gym after the most recent episode, I told them what had happened. Because I was open, they were able to ask me what they could do to help, and because I was quite matter-of-fact about it all, it did not give rise to the furtive whispers and gossip that are so painful.

The quick response with appropriate treatment that I get from the team (which includes my GPs) allows me to hold down a job as a mental health trainer educating from the user perspective and working with clinicians, students, service users and the wider public, something essential to my sense of inclusion. But the job has to be in keeping with my intellectual ability and one that I personally feel is worthwhile, not a job for a job's sake, not a job where I am marginalised or discriminated against by colleagues. Social inclusion is not about driving people unwillingly to take up jobs or join gyms and clubs, but about offering them guidance and encouragement to pursue the life they find fulfilling. It is not about 'getting me off benefits' to save the tax payers' money or even seeing any form of work as good for my own self-esteem. I have to believe my work is benefiting society, not that society is being kind to (or indeed exploiting) a poor victim. Supporting me to sustain employment involves the team in other tasks such as ensuring that any side-effects of medication are minimised as I need to drive, I need on occasion to be on top form at 9 am, and I need to sleep. It means being flexible around our time and manner of contact, accepting that I may initiate that contact by phone or email. I need support to access any benefits I am entitled to so that I do not have to work dangerously long hours (I have never achieved more than a 3-day week without becoming unwell). The team may offer, with my consent, general information to my employer so that we can negotiate reasonable adjustments while respecting my confidentiality, perhaps negotiating with me around the need for openness in the workplace, checking out proactively that all is still well at work and exploring any concerns. Perhaps most importantly, they may help to keep my feet on the ground, not allowing me to be catastrophic when things go wrong, reiterating the value of what I do, giving me courage to carry on but also encouraging me to take a step back at times, offering me quite simply traditional supervision and being a critical friend.

As my need for the crisis support of the mental health team comes to an end, I see a need to return to work as this aids my recovery. But it is essential that the team's input continues alongside my return to work, especially in the early stages. In fact, it is a time of huge risk, when I need increased input as I adjust to the fast tempo of the working world. I have been working for 10 years, but still require at times a high level of support. My team counts it worth it; they see the success of a woman who had previously begged to be allowed to live her life out, if she had to live at all, on a 'rehabilitation' ward.

Some 25 years have passed since the phasing out of the large mental hospitals, with their high walls, protecting 'them' from me and me from 'them'. But it is only now that we, the professionals and the people who use services alike, are beginning to take down the same high walls in our heads. And some of those barriers are higher in the heads of mental health professionals than in mine. It was service providers who taught me, despite their assurances that it was an illness like any other, to feel ashamed and fear disclosure: 'Are you sure you want to reveal that you have been a detained patient, Rosemary?' It was mental health services who taught me that I was dangerous to others, with their locked doors and cameras and openly displayed notices that emergency bleeps were to be carried at all times. (Did they think I could not read, or did they just not care?) It was mental health services that demonstrated that I was of less value than other people and so did not have the same rights, by pinning me down in the dirt and deliberately inflicting pain, all because I wanted to sit in an enclosed garden. But throughout there have also been those professionals who demonstrated that they did value me and did care whether I lived or died, summed up in this conversation on a ward corridor with my consultant:

> Me: There is no hope, Julie. Don't prolong the agony. Let me go.
>
> Psychiatrist: I can see that you feel hopeless now. We will carry the hope for you until you are ready to take it back.

I saw her then, as I see her now at the bad times, holding the candle of hope steady in her hand, but her hand is outstretched, ready to give it back as soon as I can lift my hand to take it. I look forward to a time when her skill and sensitivity are the norm, when every mental health professional sees me as an equal and treats me with the respect due to our common humanity, when instead of 'them' and 'us', it is just 'us' pooling our different expertise to work in partnership.

> We all have a mental health problem.
>
> Publicity from Shift, the government-funded anti-stigma campaign

Conclusion

Social inclusion and recovery are inextricably linked, if we understand that

> Recovery is the process of moving on to more empowering and meaningful ways of being (Mind, 2008).

As we get on with life, so we find ourselves part of a social network and, living in community, our well-being improves. This in turn lifts our self-esteem, so that we focus less on our distress and what we cannot do and more on what we can achieve and aspire to. The outlook is brighter and we are more energised. But it is for many of us a long, slow and winding path with setbacks and obstacles to be overcome. We need teachers, guides, enablers, accompanists along the way and that is where mental health teams come in, because to find that level of understanding and expertise within one's social network is rare indeed. Until people come face to face with severe mental distress, they are largely oblivious to it, so that the confrontation is a shock which can give rise to all sorts of emotions, including fear, guilt, embarrassment and anger, rather than empathy and encouragement. Our society is slowly becoming more accepting as more people disclose, but 'coming out' is still a risk, one that is perhaps overemphasised by service providers, so that it becomes difficult to say:

'This is part of me, it is not something to hide. It does not negate who I was before or who I may become, nor is it a matter of shame. I am still me.'

Yet the focus of mental healthcare has been on seeking a 'cure', correcting the dysfunction, minimising the symptoms, rather than enabling people to find a *modus vivendi* that allows them to live *with* rather than *in spite of* their distress and encourages family and friends to do the same. And so, where the world sees danger and shuns us, people in mental healthcare see vulnerability, victims in need of care and protection, when what we need is to be recognised as still responsible, although different or diverse, as adults, capable most of the time, even in periods of heightened distress, of making choices and decisions that will be to our benefit. Mental health services can be designed to foster recovery and promote inclusion and we offer some suggestions as to what may be considered as useful components of such services (Box 11.1).

Some people who experience mental distress have a long history of difficult relationships that discourage them from getting close to people or being socially included. Too often systems within mental health services replicate these difficult relationships by the exercise of power together with a lack of communication. We may have had little experience of building positive relationships but like everyone else we can learn by example. If mental health teams can role-model good relationships, good communication and good negotiation skills and share responsibility with us, we will learn these

---

Box 11.1   Some components of a socially inclusive mental health service

- builds on strengths
- allows informed choice
- builds and develops coping strategies
- works towards the person's aspirations
- encourages person to take responsibility
- encourages the building of social networks
- respects individuals
- lets people learn from mistakes
- lets go when appropriate
- educates for personal development
- responds to the person's needs
- encourages their staff not to hide their own current or past mental health problems
- acknowledges its own mistakes
- listens and responds to concerns
- encourages the person to engage in activity that is meaningful to them
- sees the person in the context of their life and the life of the community
- educates the community to look after their own mental health
- educates the community to understand mental distress and respond to it appropriately

skills and be able to put them into practice. Like every other learner we will, however capable, make mistakes and we will learn from the experience and grow; overprotection leads us to stultification, leaving us too petrified to move in any direction for fear of the consequences. Some behaviours of mental health services can facilitate inclusion and recovery (Box 11.2) and we would recommend an approach based on choice rather than imposition (Box 11.3). It is perhaps not surprising that many of the capabilities that Michael, Rosemary and others have valued in practitioners who have worked with them or alongside them echo those set out in the *Capabilities for Inclusive Practice* document (Department of Health, 2007): partnership, difference, equality, recovery, responding to individual needs and strengths and promoting positive risk-taking.

If we find clinicians wanting to hear about our aspirations and valuing our strengths, we too will come to recognise their worth. If we are trusted and supported to exercise control over our lives, we will do so, but if every choice is made for us or if we are not given the information necessary for informed choice we will become dependent on the judgement of others. Relapse signatures and crisis plans properly undertaken demand all the important life skills; their reward is a better quality of life for all who take part. Mental health services are a microcosm of society, which can allow us

---

Box 11.2   Mental health services – behaviours that facilitate inclusion

- challenging stigma and discrimination wherever it occurs, but especially in health services
- fostering trust and basing enduring relationships on this
- setting an example of belief in and hope for the person's future
- working with people during the 'good times', not just in periods of acute distress
- recognising and valuing diversity in all its forms
- recognising and valuing the life that came before and the life that will come after
- seeing the person in the context of their close relationships and their wider community
- promoting independence and autonomy
- responding to the person's individual hopes and aspirations
- teaching and developing coping strategies
- encouraging reasonable risk-taking and supporting people through failure
- allowing people to grow in confidence by practising in a safe environment...
- ...then facilitate opportunities in the community
- working to minimise the side-effects of treatment
- addressing concerns about confidentiality
- supporting those who choose to find employment appropriate to their needs, aspirations and capabilities
- supporting others to access activities in the community that will offer them fulfilled lives

---

Box 11.3 Social inclusion as choice or imposition

Choice emerges from:

- giving encouragement, not imposing direction
- allowing responsibility to rest with the person
- tailoring the service to the individual
- encouraging goals and plans to be defined by service users
- understanding a 'two steps forward, one step (or even two) steps back' approach
- offering a range of activities not restricted to mental health services, such as libraries as well as gyms, classical choirs as well as bands
- offering easy access to information about many local activities in one place to address problem of poor motivation
- independence encouraged, for instance use of public transport (no dreaded labelled mini-buses)
- allowing the timing of re-engagement with the community to be led by person
- recognising that people have different aspirations, strengths and susceptibilities
- support that does not identify the person as 'less' than others (unobtrusive, behind the scenes)
- peer support
- support based on common interest rather than one person's need.

Imposition emerges from:

- failing to negotiate care or action plans
- withdrawing a valued service unilaterally
- withdrawing services if person is not socially included
- offering inappropriate services based on unilateral professional decisions
- withdrawing support after set periods (rather than when needs are met)
- limiting opportunities
- failure to negotiate risk management.

to practise safely what society expects of its members. If little is what we are believed capable of, little will be taught us and, in turn, we will learn little and take little out into society. Society will then see us as a burden and the responsibility of professional others rather than as people to be valued for the contribution they can make.

It is important that staff reflect on and retain the image of the people we were before our contact with them, in the same way that people caring for the very old are encouraged to look at photos of the person in their heyday, and to consider what we have the capability to become following their intervention, to nurture those capabilities and to hold our aspirations up before us as attainable targets. In other words, to create an environment of 'can' rather than 'can't', an environment of ability not disability. Michael emphasises the need for better education for the community around mental health issues, reflecting on how people become excluded because their behaviour is misunderstood or because of the failure to recognise distress as a 'real illness'. Susan stresses the right to not be rushed, pushed and processed through a system, the right to choose alternative treatments and/ or medication; she points to the failures of an over-stressed 24/7 society.

Essentially, the social inclusion of people who experience mental illness is about justice and equality. All people are born equal; few would challenge the validity of the premise. Equal, but diverse. As we grow through life each of us needs to be encouraged to celebrate and make the most of our own particular gifts and strengths, but we must also learn to confront our flaws and difficulties, be they physical, emotional or mental. We need to be supported to work as a team with others to develop strategies to overcome them. Why should those of us who experience mental illness be judged incapable: assumptions made that lifelong someone else will have to make judgements on our behalf, exclude us from decision-making, narrow our opportunities by risk aversion? We are not like those animals at the zoo described by Rosemary; we are adult people, who most of the time have capacity to make their own life decisions. We need to develop our own crisis plans and relapse signatures, we need to be supported to be open about our individual needs. In other words we need to build our own safety nets, because almost certainly we will fall through, cut a hole in, or jump out of the one that you have created for us but without us.

Until you, as clinicians, socially include us by modelling adult interaction with us, by displaying attitudes of value and respect, by acknowledging our own expertise in ourselves, by positively encouraging choice and allowing us to take responsibility for the risks our choice entails, social inclusion in the wider society will be no more than a hollow mockery, because we will know that deep down we are not valued.

Celebrating our uniqueness, our diversity, our intrinsic value, that is social inclusion.

Facilitating social inclusion means offering people opportunities to practise social skills, both emotional and physical, in a safe, nurturing environment and then offering encouragement and choice to take those skills out into the community on an equal footing with everyone else. It is recognising that we all have different perceptions of what social inclusion means to us: one person might put employment high on the list (Box 11.4), another emphasises a satisfying relationship, others see as important the opportunity to engage with other people with similar spiritual beliefs or the same passion for sport. Social inclusion is believing that there are no insuperable barriers to doing whatever fosters your sense of well-being. Facilitating social inclusion is identifying the barriers within both the person and the community, be they beliefs, attitudes, health, skills or opportunities, and then working in partnership to demolish them.[1]

---

1   The unattributed quotes in this chapter have been taken from a range of people who use mental health services and who we have spoken to over the years. They have been willing to share their life experiences, but anonymously.

Box 11.4   The potential value and limitations of employment for service users

The value of employment:

- actualisation – using experience to benefit others
- a route to (financial) independence
- improving the material quality of life
- building self-worth
- building confidence
- extending a social network
- a focus away from one's distress
- providing structure and motivation
- rewriting past negative experience
- focus on 'can', not 'can't' – evidence of one's strengths
- escape from tedium and boredom
- reality check that proves positive
- challenging negative assumptions (one's own and other people's)
- an area of life not 'directed' by mental health professionals.

The limitations of employment:

- a job that does not match abilities or expectations
- boredom
- stigma and discrimination in the workplace
- isolation in the workplace
- repeating past negative experience
- earning an income lower than on previous benefits
- uncertainty of income (fear of redundancy, dismissal, relapse)
- overwork from a sense of guilt
- focus on 'can't' compared with previous employment
- work life over-directed by mental health professionals
- reality check that proves negative
- no time or energy to focus on work towards other aspects of recovery
- loss of support from mental health services.

Summary

The accounts of experiences by three service users emphasise the multifaceted aspects of exclusion, the variety of experiences and the range of priorities and needs. They highlight the importance of relationships, choice, hope, control over one's life, opportunity and a respect of differences. The value of work and activity is underlined, as is the need for space and time to recover. While acknowledging the need for political and social change to reduce exclusion, these accounts focus mainly on the role of mental health services and professionals in facilitating recovery and exclusion. To be considered as socially inclusive and recovery-oriented, mental health services and professionals need to change and several suggestions for improvements are proposed.

References

Department of Health (2007) *Capabilities for Inclusive Practice*. Department of Health.

Holford, P. (1997) *The Optimum Nutrition Bible*. Piatkus.

Holford, P. (2003) *Optimum Nutrition for the Mind*. Piatkus.

Mabey, R. (1972) *Food for Free*. Collins.

Mabey, R. (2005) *Nature Cure*. Chatto & Windus.

Mackarness, R. (1976) *Not All In the Mind*. Pan Books.

Mackarness, R. (1980) *Chemical Victims*. Pan Books.

Marohn, S. (2003) *The Natural Medicine Guide to Schizophrenia*. Hampton Roads.

Mind (2008) *Life and Times of a Supermodel: The Recovery Paradigm for Mental Health* (MindThink Report 3). Mind.

CHAPTER 12

Social inclusion from the carer's perspective

David Chang, Michael Osborne, Rosemary Wilson
and Susan Brook

We are all members of the National Social Inclusion Programme's Reference Group and here we reflect on our experiences of carers or of being a carer for people with severe and enduring mental health problems. David and Rosemary have family members with mental health problems and Rosemary also uses mental health services herself; Michael works as a volunteer with carers and Susan is a carer of her elderly mother; they both also have experience of mental health services. Our experiences are both similar and distinct and reflect the differences between carer and service user viewpoints. For people who act as carers, particularly those who have family members with mental health problems, there is more than one individual who experiences exclusion and the journey of recovery. The four perspectives here reflect this and illustrate the potential tensions that engagement with services and the desire for different outcomes and choices can engender. Admittedly, many of the causes and solutions to exclusion involve political and social changes, but we will be concentrating on how mental health professionals and services can help in facilitating inclusion or how they may hinder the process of recovery.

David: Caring for a spouse

I have been a carer to my spouse who suffers from bipolar disorder for the past 15 years. She has not had an in-patient episode for over 7 years and we both have learnt to manage the condition and our lives. As our situation became more stable and we began to enjoy more of a 'normal' life again, I began to realise that our recovery was intimately linked to increasing experiences of social inclusion, and that much of our distress was exacerbated, even caused, by our experience of exclusion. This exclusion was experienced in many ways and for me was a reflection of my personal needs and altered personal relationships, my experiences of employment and financial difficulties, the increasing isolation from people and social contacts, my experience of health services and my need for information on matters about which I was previously ignorant.

Thinking back to my wife's first admission, it strikes me how alone and vulnerable I was. To be fair, there were people around, so I was not technically alone, but I was very lonely. The loneliness was due to the fact that the people around me were focused on her condition and needs, and not taking into account what was happening to me, and what my needs might be. I need to emphasise that almost everyone tried hard to sympathise and be helpful, but in the end I was left to figure out for myself how to sort everything out. In these circumstances it would have helped me greatly if I had been guided to know how to care not only for my wife but also for myself in the aftermath of her episode.

For example, no one included me in discharge planning (if indeed there was any). My wife was simply sent home and I was left to care for her, as well as to manage the household and continue working. It was not until after her second in-patient experience some 2 years later that, because I noticed the acronym 'CPN' on the clinic bulletin board, I enquired with the psychiatrist, 'What is a CPN?' We eventually did get a CPN (community psychiatric nurse), but I still wonder why we were not offered one after the first episode, when we (including me as a carer) could have benefited greatly from their support. In these circumstances it would have helped to include me in the planning of my wife's discharge from hospital and if my own needs had been taken into account. In addition, a mental health worker's assistance early on to navigate the months following my wife's episode would have helped.

The relationship between carers and their cared-for often undergoes undesirable changes. Parents find they must exert more influence on their once independent adult children. Spouses find their once mutual dynamic becomes more like a parent–child one. Parents are distressed by this unwelcome change, but the carer-spouse feels especially isolated because the cared-for spouse is not able to be the source of mutual support like before. Although we both knew the parent–child dynamic was unhealthy, we were unable to prevent ourselves from falling into it after my wife's episodes. Besides being damaging to our relationship, it also affected us socially because we did not function as the normal couple we once were. We were even referred to a marriage counsellor, which did not help much. Much later, after a long wait, we received cognitive–behavioural therapy (CBT) from a psychologist who understood the caring and cared-for dilemma, and so we were able to begin rebuilding a more healthy marital relationship, as well as extract ourselves from hypervigilance and anxiety. It would have been a relief if I had been more supported as a carer by professionals who could steer me away from falling into the 'parent' trap and if we both had received counselling much earlier, or even at the very beginning, from someone who understood the trap of the parent–child dynamic.

Another distressing aspect of my wife's mental health problem that feeds into the parent–child trap is her loss of memories. Besides losing some of her ability to remember everyday things such as conversations, my wife has also lost memories of many events of our years together. Sometimes I even find myself doubting whether my memories are accurate because she draws a total blank. It is a surreal and distressing experience to feel like I am the only one to remember these experiences. We are compromised socially because she may not remember having met people before, or may forget what we had previously done together. For example, in one awkward incident, my wife asked friends where they had obtained their piano, only to find out that she herself had chosen it for them only weeks earlier. Initiating social engagements with friends may not occur to her, simply because they do not come to mind. Ironically, when she attended a memory clinic, she received no practical help, and they even told her there was no evidence that the bipolar condition or its medications had any negative effect on memory. These problems were perhaps less predictable but it would have helped to have received more guidance as a carer on how to deal with loss of memory.

Employment is a crucial issue both for carers and many service users. Our situation was particularly fraught with difficulties as we were invited jointly from abroad to work in a charity. Although our line managers were initially supportive, several months later we got the news that they no longer wanted us because of my wife's 'unsuitability'. This was in spite of the fact that the work we had accomplished up until then was more than satisfactory. From the employer's point of view, my wife's mental health problems had made us both liabilities and unemployable. But despite this, we are still continuing in the same kind of work 13 years later. We were treated as inconvenient liabilities rather than as potential assets to the workforce. It would have helped me greatly if we had been given an opportunity to negotiate employment conditions to help us both stay in work at the charity or negotiate a less abrupt dismissal, so that we had had more time to recover and plan for the future.

Throughout my wife's three in-patient admissions and subsequent discharges no one asked about how unsuitable employment (or unemployment) made her unstable or how suitable employment could aid her recovery. As a carer, my employment issues were never addressed. A carer's assessment was never offered to me, rather it was up to me to request one after I saw an information leaflet. However, after three lengthy interviews, all that could be offered was a bit of money for a carer's respite break, which was wholly unsuitable for my needs. What I felt I needed at the time was coaching for employment and training to be a better (and healthier) carer, neither of which fit into what was then the 'carer's allowance'. Subsequently, my wife developed a full-time private music teaching practice in which she thrives and which now plays a large part in keeping her healthy. I have also branched into additional self-employment, including work as a carer trainer in mental health. At that time, employment support and counselling for both me and my wife would have been hugely beneficial, as would training to help me be a better, healthier carer, receiving a carer's assessment at the beginning and if the budget had been more flexible to meet my needs.

Although carers should, in theory, be able to access further education like anyone else, in practice there are invisible barriers to overcome.

The National Extension College and The Princess Royal Trust for Carers sponsored a joint programme offering carers a selection of courses with specially trained support staff, tutors and bursaries. The programme took seriously the particular needs of carers, such as lack of time, low confidence, need for flexibility and financial aid.

Closely related to employment, the matter of adequate finances is a major factor affecting social inclusion. We lived below the poverty line for many years because of a large drop in income. We survived by being undemanding, frugal and creative, for example by foregoing a TV license and dining out, or volunteering for medical trials, until we later obtained more stable income through self-employment. Finding stable housing was also a major stressor and barrier to our participation. After my wife's first episode, we had to move homes at a very stressful time. More recently, we got stuck in a housing gap and had to move 21 times in 8 months. We got through that, but it was not without impact on our mental health.

Social isolation has been an ongoing issue for me as a carer. Aside from the isolation that stemmed from people focusing only on my wife's needs, there are other layers, such as family members and colleagues hinting that I am part of the cause of my wife's mental illness. Because of what happened when we disclosed my wife's illness to our supervisors (we later discovered other charity workers who had mental health problems but did not say anything), we decided as a general rule not to tell many people about it. Yet as much as disclosure can have consequences, so does not disclosing. For example, we have learnt to plan social engagements only 2 days in advance, because when we tried to do otherwise, we would often have to cancel owing to my wife's fluctuating condition. Since these friends did not know about my wife's condition, we just appeared unsociable and not interested in getting together. Hence, our social circle has become very limited. Moreover, even close friends cannot easily relate to how bipolar disorder affects us. As my best friend once poignantly put it, even after visiting us and reading about it, 'We just don't get it'. I believe that I also impose some self-stigma on our situation. Regardless of whether others stigmatise us, I cannot help myself *perceiving* that they do. I wish I could be totally honest and open about my wife's condition and how it affects me, but in the instances where I have done so the consequences have often been negative. At this point in our journey to recovery, the consequences of stigma, and our fear of those consequences, affect us far more adversely than the condition itself. As a carer I need support in dealing with self-stigma.

In the past we holidayed with friends, which was very enjoyable and deepened our relationships. Nowadays, although we can manage holidays on a fairly regular basis, we go alone. Our choice of destination is quite restricted as we must avoid early or late flights and crossing time zones, because disturbed sleep has triggered episodes. My wife tires easily and as she rises late and retires early it is difficult to fit in with social activities – we tried and eventually gave up. For the same reasons, we do not often offer to have friends (or even family) stay over. Recently we felt pressure and anxiety when close friends requested to stay at our house for their holiday: we wanted to be with them, but could not sustain this for any length of time. In the end we limited the time spent with them, to our own disappointment and probably theirs too. Situations like these make me realise that my social life is compromised in small and big ways owing to being a carer. I suppose a simple solution would be to arrange social activities without my wife. On rare occasions I have taken trips alone, for example to visit my family, but on the whole I feel uncomfortable (and guilty) since we are a couple and the 'normal' mode would be to travel together. In addition, others wonder why she is not with me, which becomes awkward socially. In the end, I often do not bother at all, which is not a good solution. We are grateful for the friendship and kindness extended to us in our times of need. Disappointingly, I usually find myself with such low reserves emotionally and physically (my wife similarly) that we cannot reciprocate in kind, whether it be a meal or, more regretfully, when they are in need themselves. I have come to realise that our relationships and social life as such have been quite limited.

Sometimes faith communities may be unwilling or unprepared to be inclusive of people with mental health problems. Thankfully, our faith community has been crucial support for us. We now realise that they have the rare combination of avoiding two extremes: focusing on 'problem people' (such as us with mental health difficulties) as 'projects', or ignoring the issue altogether. One psychiatrist I know about proactively asks patients, 'Do you have a faith that helps you in times of crisis?' Health professionals are not always willing or able to give a sense of hope to patients and carers, so it would lead to better outcomes if they worked in collaboration with faith communities and opened discussions about how they and the faith community could work together for better recovery. Luckily in our case our faith community leaders understood mental health issues.

A major factor blocking social inclusion is the low expectations (coupled with risk aversion) of health professionals. In our case, the focus has been on disease containment, rather than any move towards recovery of a normal life. A doctor advised our sponsor that we should not continue working and living in the UK as my wife may have more episodes. This did not fit with what we desired, so why this conclusion? I think it reflected the doctor's low expectations of my wife's abilities and his own aversion of risk. On another occasion, she happily prepared a solo piano concert, but the GP scolded her because it would be 'too stressful' to perform. We have found, however, that performing is not stressful for her, but it was all too easy for the GP to project personal anxieties and assumptions on her. With encouragement from me to take a little risk, she has successfully managed many solo performances to large audiences and produced three CDs. Most importantly, these have played a significant role in keeping her healthy and widened her participation. Another example of clinicians' risk aversion occurred when my wife complained to her psychiatrist that medications were making her sleep 16 hours a day and the psychiatrist's response was that this was preferable to having anxiety. But, from our perspective, it would have been preferable to work with her to try reducing the medications and take an informed risk. On another occasion, when my wife had an episode and entered hospital, I decided to take a holiday alone as I knew she was safe and being cared for. I realised that I needed the break in order to better care for her when she was discharged. As one can imagine, the professionals did not support the idea as they felt it too risky, but I decided to take the risk of leaving her, which turned out to be a good decision. In general, however, I am probably more reluctant to take risks than I should be because of the trauma we have endured. I would like professionals to guide me to consider more risks like that holiday, both for my own and my wife's good. Normal life includes having reasonable expectations and taking appropriate risks on a daily basis. Yet, health professionals constantly deny these to mental health patients and their carers. There was never an openness to discuss risks and options with my wife, much less with me as a carer. It would have helped me greatly if professionals openly discussed the expectations and hopes of the patient and carer for recovery, rather than focusing on their own low expectations and risk aversion.

Michael: Experience of carers

I am not a carer, but I have had my wife as a carer for 40 years. I have observed and have sympathised with her role, but closeness has precluded a clear insight. Also, through my time as a service user, I have come into contact with many carers of my fellow sufferers in hospitals, day hospitals and day centres. This has given me a clearer focus.

Through my recovery and my voluntary work with the local mental health NHS trust, I have talked to carers on wards and in day centres and have become very aware of their problems and concerns. I have cooperated with carers in many meetings and as a member of the community mental health team committee; I have links with the local carers' council and I have worked on my trust's confidentiality procedure with carers. I have great sympathy with the carers' difficulties but I am also aware of their commitment and heroism in dealing with the ones they care for.

Inclusion is an important and very serious need of the carer. Their concern for the improvement in the health and well-being of the person they care for is often overwhelming. A life beyond mental health services is the wish of all carers. To see the one that they care for well and not needing the service any more is their greatest desire. There is always the worry of a relapse and both the carers and service users are on their guard for quite a long while after the illness has dispersed. So there are still worries to contend with even after the illness is no longer present. If the patient's illness is under control with medication, there can be trouble with side-effects. There is always the fear that the patient will decide to stop taking the medication.

Some carers are told that the illness will never go away, which is often a great shock to them, with the immediate impact that it can mean a life sentence of distress and heartbreak for the family. This is dispiriting and is not always true. Some have been told that the service user will never work again, which can be drastic, especially if they are the breadwinner. This kind of statement attempts to predict what cannot be predicted and is demoralising because it suggests inevitable deterioration and exclusion. More thought and understanding should go into providing realistic hope for the future. The carer's need for information on a diagnosis, the illness and a prognosis is paramount. To be excluded from knowledge about the health of the person they care for can be soul-destroying not only for the immediate carer but for all the family and friends. Too often clinicians take no time to explain the situation to a carer when their relative or friend is admitted to an in-patient unit. They only deal with the service user and exclude the carer from all involvement. This may be correct procedure as it is important that the immediate needs of the patient are met. However, it is important that carers should be included, consulted and informed as early as possible, especially after a first admission. Instead, often they are sent home knowing no more about the illness or what is happening to the loved one than they did at the start of the crisis.

Psychiatrists and other mental health workers quote the need for confidentiality as a reason for excluding the carer. It is important that the service user's wish for privacy is respected and that they may wish to exclude the carer. However, matters such as medication, information about the illness including a prognosis should be considered as not coming under the confidentiality banner unless specifically prohibited by the service user. Otherwise the carer is dependent on information about the illness from the internet or library, which can be painful to them or emphasise the worst aspects of the illness, whereas the benefits that medication and therapy can give to the condition are not always mentioned. Information from a psychiatrist is more related to the service user's actual degree of illness and can be related in a caring manner and in a supportive environment.

Matters of confidentiality can cause conflict between service users and carers. The service user may not want the carer to know about their illness. This is sometimes because they believe that the carer will use the information to interfere in their life. It is often a case where the service user does not want people telling them to do things and fussing but wants to be left in peace. Sometimes they want information to be held back to save the carer from distress. They do not want them to know of suicidal thoughts or other unpleasant matters. The carer cannot understand why the person will not let them know the information. They want to help but feel helpless. The carer believes that if they know how the person feels they can help or give advice. The carer can also feel that if they know about the symptoms they can spot when the person is going to be ill again. The person in turn does not want them to know this as they believe that they will use it to get them back into hospital. The psychiatrist is often at the centre of these disputes.

For the carer, inclusion can be measured to some degree in the provision of knowledge about all aspects of the illness, care and medication. They have a strong desire to help with improving the service user's health and well-being. They want to be able to tell someone and get help when the cared one's health is deteriorating. They are experts in many aspects of the person's mental condition and at spotting warning signs. A clinician who can satisfy all these needs will have gone a long way towards fulfilling the carer's need for inclusion. The fulfilment of these needs can lead to a form of recovery of the carer, which may be closely tied up with the recovery of the service user. The concepts of recovery and the use of a wellness recovery action plan can have a most beneficial effect on the service user and if the carer can help to inspire them on the way to recovery it is beneficial to both. Seeing the patient coming to terms with their illness and achieving small steps to living a better life gives the carer hope and fulfilment in being a part of this. A working partnership can only be beneficial, with more understanding and closeness between carer and service user.

Exclusion can occur if the carer has to give up their employment. This is often because they are afraid or cannot leave the cared one on their own. Giving up a job means leaving all their work friends, who often do not keep in contact because of fear of getting 'involved' or 'interfering'. It also means lack of income, which limits going out to or taking part in social activities. Attendance allowance does not compensate. Carers become isolated and their sole interest becomes the person they are caring for, sometimes watching every move for fear of a relapse. In this situation carers can easily become anxious and depressed. Lack of finance has an effect on their physical health; attendance at a gym can be an expense, as is the cost of a healthier diet.

To assist in participation, it is beneficial if carers can be signposted to a carers' organisation. These sometimes have a support worker but mainly the benefit comes from the help, knowledge and inspiration of other carers. If a person is a lone carer the support of other carers and possibly Social Services is important. Carers need to carry on with their lives in a usual manner as before. Work and play can take their mind off their worries and it should be encouraged. Carers are entitled to a carers' assessment and this should be produced with the need for social inclusion very much taken into account. There should also be provision of a complaints procedure. It is very difficult to treat the carer as a whole person because they are attached to the one they are caring for, but both have to be treated as whole people. There is often more than one carer, for example mother and father, sometimes several where a whole family are involved. This can be difficult for the clinician and it needs careful consideration. It can be the best policy in these cases to choose the 'main carer' and make them aware that they should pass on information to the others. A caring clinician will try to accommodate as many as be reasonably expected.

There is often a lot of difficulty for the carer in the early stages of the cared one's illness. Sometimes the ill person will not go to a GP or will not admit that they are ill. The carer's only way to prevent a crisis is to approach the GP themselves, but many GPs give the carer short shrift and refuse to attend a patient unless the patient asks for it. This puts the carer into a very painful and debilitating position. They can only cajole and nag the person, but this can cause anger and conflict and make their condition worse. The carer often can only await a crisis and hope that it does not end in tragedy. The impact of crisis resolution home treatment teams is very beneficial but many carers do not know that they exist. There must be some thought as to how a carer can initiate early treatment when a loved one will not take part. A requirement that a GP should visit the home when a person does not engage would help immensely. After the first crisis access may be improved by taking care to provide the carer with relevant contact details.

It is rare for psychiatrists to encourage the patient to come off medication. Sometimes there is a grudging reduction after a request by the patient, but rarely in response to a carer's request. Sometimes the carer asks for an increase in medication, which may not be accepted by a doctor. A carer can never accept that the cared one is fully better until they go a long time without relapse or medication. This is also true of a patient. The carer can be very helpful in getting the patient to adopt the ideas of recovery as well as in encouraging and praising the patient in their steps to recovery. They can also suggest the small steps necessary and play a part in the building of a wellness recovery action plan. They can also help the person to recognise the warning signs of illness. However, it must be recognised that the service user is the one making their recovery journey. The carer can only be a supporter and encourager, which can be a frustrating role.

The most satisfying outcome, other than independence from services, is the acceptance of the person's 'illness', with both carer and cared one learning to live with the illness throughout each phase of wellness and illness. This takes some strength of character but can, and should, be helped by the allocated mental health practitioners. For the carer to be included in the whole business of the other person's illness is of benefit to all concerned, including the mental health team. The prevention of unnecessary distress to the carer is an essential requirement of good medical practice. Good communication between all parties will improve the situation. This will also result in a learning process that will give a greater understanding of each other's situation. There should also be some thought given by clinicians to the mental and physical health of the carer. It is hoped that the service user will also understand the needs of the carer, which are often overlooked. If the carer is well in mind and body it is all to the good of the service user and medical profession, as there is evidence that many carers become mentally unwell in their turn because of the stress of the caring role.

Service users may blame the carer for their situation, as, in some circumstances, do friends and relations. The medical profession can be sympathetic to this view. This can be destructive to the carer and have a drastic effect on their self-esteem. The service user should take the responsibility for their illness and lifestyle. In my opinion, carers have only the good of the one cared for at heart. They are usually viewed as being very necessary to the well-being of the service user and play a vital role in combating the effects of mental health problems. The well-being of the carer should be of high importance to the medical profession, themselves and indeed to the service user, as if the carer becomes unwell the service user loses their informal support. They should be made aware of their own need for social inclusion. The carer should be given the support that they need to continue their valuable care of the service user and themselves.

Rosemary: The family and caring for others

As I write this I am in crisis. As usual at these times I am making my family's life very difficult. In my case 'the family' are two adult children, aged 31 and 23 years, who live some distance from me, have full-time jobs and their own lives to lead. At the time of my admission via accident and emergency department I was adamant that they were not to be contacted and gave my care coordinator's name and contact number in place of my next of kin, saying that she would be the intermediary who would contact my children if necessary. When I discharged myself the following morning, a nurse used information stored from a previous episode to contact my daughter on her mobile phone and ask whether I had 'arrived home'.

I am sure this situation has been witnessed countless times. I wanted them to be spared distress, but they are caused more distress by my exclusion of them and by the well-meaning intervention of a third party who knows none of us. Bridges laboriously built up over years have been torn down.

You will notice that I have not described my children as my carers – they are not. We have always had a mutually loving and supportive relationship, not a one-sided carer and cared-for relationship. I have worked hard to let them get on with their adult lives without guilt. I have seen too many families where children have felt obliged to set their own aspirations on one side and become informal carers to their parent and this is seen as normal and acceptable by services (witness the nurse who assumed that my daughter lived with me).

They now feel themselves responsible for my safety and well-being; they have established rotas to check up on me, asked people to 'drop in' to see how I am and to report back; they have become my gaolers. I have taken to parking my car away from my house, so that people will assume I am not in; I let the telephone go to answerphone so that I can choose whether to respond or not. I tell them I am fine and add to my distress the guilt of lying to those I love best. They know that they can contact my care coordinator for information and that she has my permission to be open with them, but that is not enough. They feel rejected and I feel torn by my need for privacy and autonomy and their need to know. I feel that I have enough to contend with already in my distress without having to take on board theirs. They feel that somehow they have failed me, that they ought to know how to make it better. So how should clinicians respond to this? I wish I had an answer, but during a crisis there is little they can do. I am in no mood for compromise and neither are my children. But later on, when I am well, there is plenty they could do to help us to understand what has happened and why. Except that once the crisis has passed, they will have to devote their time and energies to someone else's crisis. This may reflect one of the current inadequacies of mental health services, which are to all intents and purposes crisis response services. Perhaps this is because of pressures, perhaps because of inadequate design or because there is insufficient funding for anything more, but whichever it is, it does reflect a limitation that must change to make them responsive to the needs of service users and carers.

Social inclusion for my children is doing the normal activities of young adulthood: going away to university, finding a job and place to live, building relationships outside the safety of the family. In other words breaking the ties of childhood and becoming independent, while knowing that I am there to turn to and fall back on at times of need. This is tough for every young person, but for those with a parent with health problems it is tougher and they need support to do so – support that professionals can provide in the form of advice and counselling, in reassurance that they are available to talk through difficulties, but most importantly by ensuring that the young person has confidence that the care formal services can provide is sufficient. I count it as my mental health team's success that we have accomplished this, that my children both left home at 18 to pursue their own chosen paths, that both now live in another city and that I visit them there or they come here at will.

People who use mental health services may also find themselves in the role of carer and circumstances have dictated that I am also the main supporter of another family member, my nephew Jack (not his real name) who experiences periods of psychosis. At the onset of Jack's first episode, when his mother was still alive, we would have liked a responsive primary care team who knew enough psychiatry or worked in partnership with a mental health team to understand that a person in psychosis probably does not recognise that there is anything amiss and is not going to present at the surgery, so they will have to listen to other people's concerns rather than saying that because the person is an adult only they can speak to them, so the parent needs to bring them to the surgery. You cannot expect a young man in his twenties to respond favourably to the suggestion. A home visit is eventually much less painful than having to call an emergency duty team, who will have had no previous contact with the family, with the concomitant expectations of admission under the Mental Health Act. Perhaps it was because my sister lacked knowledge of the appropriate jargon and talked about her son 'saying and doing strange things' rather than using the term 'in psychosis', but it took a month before anyone would take her concerns seriously, although early intervention has far more chance of a good outcome. Even when he was seen by a GP and immediately referred to the mental health team, the assessing psychiatrist asked us to explain to him the need for admission and transfer him to the hospital, leaving him, as so many young service users have been left, with a grievance against their relatives for conspiring with the mental health professionals. We all know how difficult the task of parenting young adults is at the best of times and dealing with someone in psychosis is certainly not that.

My position as a person with her own mental health problems having family responsibility for another family member is not uncommon. Often it is the result of a deep, loving sexual relationship that has developed post-diagnosis because here is a significant other who understands. But each person is entitled to their privacy. A very successful move for Jack and me was to allocate us to different teams, which gave both us and the teams clear boundaries. When I am concerned about Jack I raise the matter with his team not with mine, except insofar as it has an impact on my own well-being.

Jack does not live with me, although he frequently hints that he would like to. Perhaps I am fortunate in this in that I have the support of my team to resist the temptation to give in lest my own mental health suffers. I feel guilty enough about it although he is not my child, but for a parent it must be horrendous. One's instinct is to protect one's offspring, to curtail one's own life to keep them from harm, to keep on forgiving transgressions of boundaries because the 'child', however adult in years, is sick. 'They cannot help it' and the prophecy is self-fulfilling because the 'sick child' never has to take responsibility for themselves and 'help it'. I know of a man in his mid-forties who is taken and fetched from his workplace by his mother, although he demonstrates at work that he is quite capable of independent life and would greatly benefit from the opportunities it would bring him.

By gently encouraging families to let go, mental health teams can benefit the social inclusion of all concerned. It will not be a quick process; it requires a lot of strength and understanding to be able to stand back, let go and allow people to make their own mistakes with what sometimes feel like life-shattering consequences. Part of the being able to let go, being at arm's length, is having the confidence that your concerns will be listened to. I know that most trusts employ a carers' support worker, but in my view, their needs are often minimalised in the effort to look after the 'real' service user. It might be a good move if, at the point of assessment, the family's needs were assessed and met. At present, carers can request an assessment but there is no obligation to meet the assessed needs. Too often it is assumed that family members will set their own needs aside; but for them it feels like, and can be, a life sentence. Perhaps services need to recognise that where there is a long-term condition, they need to engage with the whole family. Too much healthcare is undertaken in isolation, away from real life, in the privacy of the consulting room.

The mental health team can also build confidence by teaching the family about: what the diagnosis means in the short and the long term; what family and friends can do to support the person's recovery; what the likelihood of relapse is; how they might respond in a crisis; and when in crisis, who should be informed, whether they should tell the person what they are going to do first, how quick a response they can expect. All this may seem very obvious, but when you are worried and frightened or when in the relief of discharge you have promised the person they will never be sent into hospital again (especially where a family member, as the nearest relative, has consented to compulsory admission), then knowing that you have been sanctioned to behave in a certain way by a mental health professional can be an enormous relief as the responsibility is then shared.

Six months after Jack's mother's, my sister's, death, we spent the following Christmas at Center Parcs as it was simply too painful to have a big extended family celebration at home as we usually did. Jack was just coming out of a psychotic episode, probably occasioned by his mother's death and then moving out of the erstwhile family home into an independent flat. While we were away I was given open access to Jack's psychiatrist and was able to ask him to speak to the medical team on site when Jack appeared to be hearing voices. The result was positive and Jack was able to continue his holiday. Given the public's fear of mental distress and their confusion that children might be at risk, we might have been asked to leave. It was the forward planning on the part of the team that made that holiday, a very obvious example of social inclusion, viable. I was also able to demonstrate to the medical team at the site that I was knowledgeable about psychosis and my refusal to get excited about it. All supporters need to know enough to appear competent and in control of the situation.

To allow Jack the freedom he needs to be socially included by his own age group, I must not appear to be 'supervising'. I need to feel confident that someone will contact me if he is not attending appointments and there are concerns about him. Clearly this needs Jack's informed consent and I hope that the team would be proactive in negotiating this. He also needs coordinated support and encouragement to undertake meaningful activity when he is not actively unwell to help him get his life on track. He uses cannabis because he is lonely and bored.

After his mother's death Jack needed a psychiatrist who knew the family, one who would have been willing to support his solicitor and family, who knew how easily his good nature could be abused by others, to see that he could not be exploited by 'friends' when he inherited money. In fact he got through more than my annual income in less than 6 months by 'lending' large sums to friends. With no apparent consultation his locum consultant psychiatrist declared that he was competent to manage his money and made the family feel they were actually trying to defraud him.

In the family's view the mental health team needed to work in cooperation with the police and other Social Service teams to protect Jack from exploitation as a vulnerable adult. He has alienated both family and friends by allowing two men, both known to police and Social Services, to live in his flat and cause a public nuisance by their lifestyle and behaviour. One of the men, known to be violent and dishonest, was being encouraged by his learning disabilities social work team to stay with Jack. It was not until I insisted on seeing them as Jack's responsible adult (I knew the jargon they would respond to) that they understood Jack's position. They told me that they had not done a home visit because they feared for their own safety. Apparently Jack's safety was not a relevant issue.

From the different accounts, the reader will identify that it is easy to say what the 'carer' wants. It is easy to say what the 'service user' wants too, but I would find many of the issues that I have raised above difficult to accept and would regard them as interference in my situation as a person who uses services. Finding a way to an outcome that is satisfactory to both parties requires huge interpersonal skills, skills in partnership working and the skill to bring issues never usually discussed out into the open. But are those not exactly the skills required of a mental health worker?

Susan: Shifting roles

Ambivalence, having mixed feelings – those are appropriate words to introduce a service user writing about social inclusion and carers. In the big world out there, caring is not a one way street and the boundaries of carer and cared-for are intertwined. I write from the perspective of a service user experiencing change, from being primarily cared for to being a carer. I now have to provide some care for an ageing mother who has cared for me during some of my periods of illness. My transition has not been an easy one, and I now support the frailties and vulnerabilities of old age. I have become increasingly relied upon as a main carer by a parent growing older who is relinquishing their own responsibility as a carer. I would like to reflect on the situation that I am now in and contrast two people who have begun to alter their roles.

Throughout our lives most of us will provide care and be cared for. Yet being the main carer for any illness arrives unexpectedly, and is a test of patience, fortitude and thoughtfulness. Whatever the mental health difficulties, carers need the strength for a marathon and need to sprint in a crisis. But perhaps in a system with more socially inclusive practice, even being a carer for someone with a serious and enduring mental health condition or problems in old age should become a gentler relay.

There are commonalities between being a carer and a service user: loneliness and isolation, uncertainties, having a poor quality of life, poverty and not being gainfully employed. The shock and fear of a family member developing mental health difficulties are perhaps not the same as for one growing older, because old age may be an experience for everyone and to some extent can be anticipated and planned for. One similarity between the needs of people who are ageing and those with mental health problems is the need for decorum, for being circumspect. While some may want to let it all out, some may want privacy, for various reasons, and both professionals and carers need to be aware of this difference. Although unlike age-related problems, mental health service users need to know when to reciprocate respect, to understand how both parties feel about disclosure or non-disclosure of a mental illness. It is not something to be decided in a hurry

– it needs individual choice and discussion when some stability has been achieved.

My own experiences suggest that mental health services may learn from the practices of general medicine in the care of the elderly, as could carers of people who use mental health services, particularly in the discussion of diagnosis, the respect for confidentiality and in the process of discharge from hospital. With the frailties and illnesses of old age, even with high levels of incapacity, the patient is the focus and is respected. This has seemed to me to be almost automatic. Illnesses are diagnosed in vague terms until there has been a round of appointments and tests. Carers' hospital visits have to be timed to the rounds of the medical staff, and if they have any questions these are asked and replied to through the patient and with the patient's permission. Confidentiality is assured. The carer is conferred with about discharge if there is doubt about the patient being able to manage on their own. Nevertheless, the patient is still discharged on the medical criteria of the hospital. If they are not fit to go home, and if no support can be put in place to aid the patient and carer, then the patient has to go to alternative care, possibly for rehabilitation, before being able to return home.

Other common experiences of service users and carers are those of people changing, of loss, of the unknown, and the emotional reactions to these. Distress, fear, shock, apprehensiveness, guilt and embarrassment are all emotions carers and service users particularly recognise. Carers, service users and professionals all need to be able to talk through their fears without being negative or clichéd, and without prejudice. Clear communication can change perception, and help all three groups recognise and own their own emotions, and recognise where they are coming from. Carers may find that if they are able to develop an emotional resilience to adjust to change and disappointment, they can work through and gain strength in seemingly negative transitions. My own experience suggests that a good way to influence the outcomes of change is for carers to find ways of effective personal development. By helping themselves, they will also help the professional and the person they care for.

Currently there are many changes being put in place for the delivery of mental health services – improving access, promoting recovery, creating greater availability of talking therapies, individual budgets to be offered as part of the personalisation of care. These potentially socially inclusive improvements for the service user should help and support carers better too. As service users use self-directed support to fund alternatives outside conventional services, so too must carers consider continuing to look to self-help. There are bound to be gaps during the transformation to getting these new services running smoothly, so carers still need self-reliance and need to support each other.

It is a difficult standpoint to write from, being both service user and carer, and perhaps because the caring is from child to parent. What I have found helpful is a self-help workshop that talked 'the language of loss', something that has been useful to many people overwhelmed by chaos.

This programme started as 'The Stepping Stones to Unrecognised Grieving' and is now called 'Emotional Logic' (www.emotionallogiccentre.org.uk). It deals with loss and grief, shock, denial, anger, guilt, yearning, emptiness, sadness. For many carers and service users there is often a sense of loss for what might have been. To be able to communicate clearly when life seems to be falling apart is a great gift.

Conclusion

It is apparent that people identified as carers struggle just as much, although often in different areas, as the person formally identified by mental health services as in need of care – 'the patient'. The potential for carers to experience significant mental health issues of their own as a result of the pressures put upon them has long been recognised and it is clear that carers as well as people with direct experience need access to available services when required.

Family members are not exempt from the stigma that surrounds mental ill health. This may be by association (not wanting to be in the presence of someone diagnosed as mentally ill); it may take the form of blame for the person's condition (we have probably all heard the comment 'What could you expect with a mother/father like that?'); it may be the expectation that the carer will become an unreliable employee, putting family before work. Whatever the causes, the reduced social support network comes at the worst possible time, when the family is struggling to come to terms with an unfamiliar and distressing situation, one that they had not expected to face, one to which they may themselves have adopted a stigmatising approach in the past. Serious mental health problems are something that most people believe happens only to other families, not their own. The reducing social network becomes a vicious circle: as the family spends more time addressing the needs of the 'sick' person, they spend less time with their friends, whereas friendship requires careful nurturing to survive let alone flourish. The carers spend more time seeking explanations and solutions to the problems they face and run the danger of being seen as preoccupied and 'boring' to friends and colleagues.

There is a very clear message in this chapter that informal carers need easy access to good-quality information about mental health problems in a range of formats from the first assessment onwards. They need balanced information about the condition written straightforwardly and lucidly in layperson's language; they need contact details for appropriate national voluntary sector groups for both themselves and the person they care for; they need information about the different treatments available. All of this is general information and can be easily accessed by the appropriate service within the trust. Then there is the information on what is available within the locality; what services and support the person and family can expect from the local statutory and voluntary health and social services. As services tend to cover wide localities, this information is perhaps more difficult to make appropriate to the individual, but will be worth its weight in gold in promoting the inclusion of the whole family.

Hope, it has become clear, is not just a fundamental necessity for the service user. Carers also need to have hope: hope that the person they care for will be restored to a full and satisfying life, even if periods of relapse occur, hope that the carer will be able to retain their usual life, including employment, safe in the knowledge that the person they care for will receive the requisite attention, hope that they will learn to adjust to and value the new relationship with the person.

The sensitive problem of sharing confidential information about the direct service user is raised. Service users may wish to withhold consent, for example, consent to the sharing of information about how they are behaving and interacting with the team, what they are saying about their problems, the sharing of care plans and their physical whereabouts. The mental health team needs to consider how they can manage and attempt to resolve the conflict. How can the direct service user's privacy and the family's need to understand the situation be reconciled?

It is not just good-quality information about the condition that is required. We have drawn attention to the drop in the family's income, the increased costs of medical care, travel, looking after the house, holidays. Families need to know how to negotiate the new situation they find themselves in with their employers so that the employee gains support and the employer retains a valued member of the workforce. They need to know how to find the best advice on possible benefits entitlements and travel passes for the person they are caring for and possibly for themselves, how to access advocacy and possible charitable funding for respite care or activities for young carers. Often this sort of information is available to people on income-related benefits, but others, whose incomes are also reduced, are unaware that they, too, can access help.

The four contributors have made it clear that carers require emotional support as well as practical help. This may come from many sources: carers' support workers, other informal carers in support groups, counsellors, carers' centres. However, it seems that attention is not always drawn to these support networks; rather the carer stumbles on them by chance. We talk about clear patient pathways, but we forget that carers need the same clarity and guidance. Within general practice in the UK, there are targets to be met about regular physical health checks for people with mental health issues; perhaps we need the same for people who are main informal carers.

Carers want education and training: first, about the condition, prognosis, treatment and support available to the person they are caring for, but then, too, about how far they should involve themselves in the treatment regime, how far they should learn to demonstrate their love by letting go, how to maintain their own well-being by leading a balanced life rather than one that revolves around the direct service user. All this needs to be encouraged from the outset; too many carers have found themselves trapped in the cocoon they have themselves woven only to end up feeling either bitter and resentful or making martyrdom the excuse for increasingly unproductive and unfulfilled lives. As service users observed in Chapter 11, victimhood is a surprisingly comfortable role. Taking responsibility for yourself and positive risk-taking are hard, but equally hard is the handing over of responsibility and the promotion of risk-taking. Both parties need support and guidance.

Just as mental health teams promote the opening up and examination of difficult thoughts and beliefs in the service user, so, too, they need to do with the carer. Many families struggle with the fear that somehow they were responsible for the illness, but often this remains unvoiced unless a professional is willing to make the opening move.

We need to move towards a mental health service that works holistically, not just with the service user but with their family, where from the first assessment the needs of both are recorded and addressed, a system that brings the shadowy figure of the carer into equal focus with the person cared for.

Summary

In these accounts by carers and service users, several common threads emerge:

- the experience of stigma by carers
- the importance of being given assessments, information and help at an early stage
- the need for realistic hope – blaming of carers is destructive
- employment – preventing drop in income and lack of financial security
- the problems of a retracting social circle
- disclosure and clarity about confidentiality
- dealing with conflict between service users and carers – and with tensions that may inhibit risk-taking or greater participation
- looking at the separate needs of users and carers, as well as their overlapping problems and dynamics
- the physical and mental health of the carer.

Part 3

Working towards inclusive psychiatry

CHAPTER 13

Social inclusion: research and evidence-based practice

Geoff Shepherd, Michael Parsonage and Tom Scharf

As we have seen in earlier chapters, social inclusion is a complex concept which overlaps with several other important ideas in social and community psychiatry and which has potentially wide applicability to a range of individuals and groups.

In this chapter we will discuss some of the key methodological issues and research outcomes relating to research in social exclusion and mental ill health. Throughout, we will be concerned with research that addresses both social exclusion and mental illness, not with either alone, although they are clearly related. Given the breadth of this field, our review will be selective, aiming to give a general overview of the literature, rather than a comprehensive account.

Measurement

Conceptual and methodological issues

Measures of social inclusion fall into two broad categories, individual level and societal level (Berman & Phillips, 2000):

1 individual-level measures reflect the situation and life experience of people belonging to socially excluded groups (in this case people with mental health problems); they are usually of more interest to mental health practitioners and clinically-oriented researchers

2 societal-level measures, also sometimes referred to as a 'social indicators' approach, rely on existing data sources that characterise levels of participation in larger community samples – examples of this are employment rates as assessed in the annual Labour Force Survey (Department for Work and Pensions, 2007) and the number of rough sleepers as calculated by local authorities (Palmer et al, 2007); this approach tends to be of more interest to planners, politicians and social policy-makers.

Notwithstanding the importance of reliability, any measurement tool for social inclusion must also have validity. Thus, it must 'converge' with other instruments measuring similar concepts, such as poverty, citizenship, social capital, 'quality of life'. However, it must also 'diverge' (discriminate) between social inclusion and these related concepts. For example, social inclusion combines aspects of poverty (e.g. income, welfare benefits, exclusion from the labour market) but also elements of social participation. Similarly, it includes aspects of social capital (e.g. membership of social networks, community groups and civic participation) but adds in poverty and stigma and discrimination. It also overlaps with quality of life measures in terms of both objective and subjective indicators. Any comprehensive measure of social inclusion must therefore meet these challenges to content and discriminant validity.

The measurement of social inclusion must be built around a set of principles that assume it to be (Burchardt, 2000):

- relative (to a given society, place and time)
- multidimensional (whether those dimensions are conceived of in terms of rights or activities)
- dynamic (because inclusion is a process, rather than a state; individuals can move in and out of inclusion through the life course)
- multi-layered (in the sense that it operates at an individual, familial, communal, societal – even global – level).

This is a daunting list of requirements. Technical reports reviewing the area (Huxley *et al*, 2006, personal communication; Morgan *et al*, 2006, personal communication) have concluded that, although there is considerable methodological work on both the objective indicators of social inclusion and subjective measures of quality of life, no satisfactory, widely accepted measure of social inclusion yet exists.

Indicators

Despite the lack of a comprehensive measure of social inclusion currently available, there are a number of indicators that consistently recur through the literature. These have been covered in earlier chapters and include:

- income (poverty)
- employment (labour market participation)
- social activity (friendships, networks of social support)
- participation in family life
- participation in leisure activities
- participation in political and civic activities
- community integration (involvement in 'mainstream' community activities)
- access to education and training
- access to physical healthcare services
- access to mental healthcare services
- access to adequate housing (including safe neighbourhoods)
- involvement with the criminal justice system
- use of the benefits system
- use of transport.

The extent of exclusion or inclusion in relation to these indicators is not a simple binary – being 'included' is not simply the opposite of being 'excluded'. Each indicator therefore needs to be measured on a graded dimension of participation.

Huxley *et al* (personal communication, 2006) also suggest that each indicator should be rated in terms of:

- opportunities for access (safeguards to ensure equity and provide support for access if required, e.g. in legislation)
- perceived ease of access (notwithstanding the formal social structures)
- actual level of participation
- perceived benefit
- perceived desire for further participation.

They argue that the person can only be properly regarded as 'socially excluded' if it is objectively difficult for them to access certain opportunities, they recognise these barriers exist and their choices are restricted as a result of factors outside their control. In these circumstances one would expect that they would also feel excluded from a potential set of benefits and would want to increase their participation if possible. These last two caveats are necessary to account for individuals who may appear to be excluded, but do not appear to be concerned.

Measures of a person's subjective sense of 'exclusion' – the perceived importance of not being able to access the benefits of inclusion and the desire for more (or less) participation – are more difficult to quantify. The subjective component of quality of life ratings (Gaite *et al*, 2006) is relevant here, but more work needs to be done to develop these measures specifically in relation to social exclusion.

Interventions – can social exclusion be prevented?

Primary prevention

When considering the concept of prevention, it is useful to distinguish between 'primary', 'secondary' and 'tertiary' prevention.

Primary prevention refers to efforts to intervene, usually at a population level, to reduce the incidence of new problems arising. Secondary prevention refers to the process of 'early intervention', usually with high-risk groups, in order to reduce prevalence (i.e. duration of illness episodes). Tertiary prevention refers to the delivery of effective treatment and management interventions to reduce symptoms and disabilities – it is not 'prevention' in the sense that most people would understand the term, it is simply effective treatment and management. We will therefore omit it from further discussion.

In the field of social exclusion (and mental ill health) primary prevention has always been regarded as the Holy Grail: desirable, but probably mythical. Social exclusion and associated mental health problems are over-determined and, as indicated in Chapter 10, we know little about the causal mechanisms leading to their emergence. It is therefore unrealistic to think about primary prevention at this stage of knowledge.

Whereas primary prevention may be difficult, early intervention and secondary prevention are much more feasible. We will now review the available research evidence in relation to the effectiveness and cost-effectiveness of mental health-based interventions that aim to identify groups who are at high risk of social exclusion (and/or the development of mental health problems) and to deliver interventions that might interrupt – or at least slow – the processes of social exclusion (and decrease risk of mental health problems).

We will consider evidence in three areas:

1 interventions aimed at young children who are already identified as having emotional and behavioural problems and family disadvantage
2 interventions aimed at young adults with first episodes of psychosis
3 interventions aimed at improving social inclusion via employment for working-age adults with severe mental health problems.

Children and young people

Longitudinal studies undertaken both in the UK and in other countries indicate a high degree of persistence (continuity) between adverse mental states in childhood and those in adult life (Kim-Cohen et al, 2003). For example, the most common mental health problem in childhood is conduct disorder, affecting nearly 6% of all children between the ages of 5 and 16 (Green et al, 2005). Longitudinal data suggest that these disorders persist into adulthood in about 40% of cases and they are particularly associated with family disadvantage in early life.

Childhood conduct disorder is also strongly predictive of a range of poor outcomes in adult life, including criminal behaviour, substance misuse, poor educational and labour market performance and disrupted personal relationships (Stewart-Brown, 2004). These are all major risk factors for social exclusion.

The social and economic costs of conduct disorder are also high, with one study suggesting that by age 28 the costs incurred by the public sector for individuals with conduct disorder were about ten times higher than for those with no problems, with an average cumulative cost since childhood of around £70 000 per person (Scott et al, 2001). Nearly two-thirds of the costs for those with conduct disorder were borne by the criminal justice system; those falling on the NHS were a relatively small proportion of the total.

A broader-based, but less detailed, study drawing on a range of secondary sources has suggested that the lifetime costs of childhood conduct disorder (relative to individuals with no conduct problems) may be in the order of £200 000–250 000 per case, taking into account such factors as reduced lifetime earnings, poorer health outcomes and the costs of crime incurred by victims as well as the criminal justice system (Friedli & Parsonage, 2007).

The main form of intervention aimed at addressing conduct disorder and related emotional and behavioural problems in early childhood has been pre-school parenting programmes. Drawing on recent meta-analytic reviews (Nelson *et al*, 2003; Dretzke *et al*, 2005), some of the key findings on the effectiveness of these interventions are summarised in Box 13.1. Dretzke *et al* (2005) also concluded that the costs of intervention are relatively low, at around £6000 per child for a home-based individual programme and £1350 per child for a community-based group programme (allowing in each case for a refresher course a year after the original intervention).

When set against the estimated lifetime costs of conduct disorder given above, the effectiveness of these programmes therefore justifies investment in these interventions on a significant scale.

A new family intervention that builds on early intervention to improve parenting skills is known as multisystemic therapy. This is a multi-faceted, short-term, home- and community-based intervention for families where there are children and/or adolescents (aged 10–17) with severe psychosocial and behavioural problems (Henggeler *et al*, 1998).

Littell *et al* (2005) have conducted a meta-analysis of the available randomised controlled trials relating to multisystemic therapy (eight trials) and concluded that there was insufficient evidence regarding its effectiveness compared with alternatives to come to any definitive conclusions. Results were 'inconsistent across studies that vary in quality and context' (Littell *et al*, 2005: p. 4). There was no evidence that the therapy had harmful effects. A more selective review commissioned by the Cabinet Office covered similar ground but suggested that there were positive results

---

Box 13.1   Key findings on the effectiveness of pre-school parenting programmes for conduct disorder and related emotional and behavioural problems in early childhood

- Parenting skills training improves the mental health and behaviour of children, measured on a range of clinical scales, and many of the beneficial effects persist into adulthood, subject to some attenuation as children pass through adolescence into adult life.
- The long-term benefits include both higher earnings for programme participants and savings for the wider community, mainly in the form of reduced welfare and crime-related costs and higher taxation associated with higher earnings.
- Children brought up in the worst conditions in terms of economic deprivation and related environmental stressors benefit most.
- Follow-up in primary school significantly improves long-term outcomes.
- The evidence confirms the importance of intervening early: 'Like it or not, the most important mental and behavioural patterns, once established, are difficult to change once children enter school' (James Heckman, quoted in Cabinet Office, 2006: p. 48).

demonstrating reduced adult offending in a 13-year follow-up compared with individual therapy (Utting *et al*, 2007).

There remain a number of questions regarding the effectiveness of multisystemic therapy. Which of its several facets contribute most to favourable outcomes? Is it related to the specific therapies employed, or is it just a reflection of the intensity of the intervention (24 hours a day, 7 days a week, available for 12 weeks)? How durable are any long-term effects? Is the therapy cost-effective? Admittedly, it is a very intensive intervention, but if the long-term effects are replicated, then there are likely to be very considerable cost savings in terms of the demands on other health, social and criminal justice services by these young people later in their lives. These questions wait to be answered before one could make evidence-based policy recommendations.

Notwithstanding these questions, the UK government now does seem very eager to implement multisystemic therapy and has recently funded ten pilot sites in addition to two already existing sites (http://www.cabinetoffice.gov.uk/social_exclusion_task_force/multi_systemic.aspx). It is also contemplating a randomised controlled trial.

Young people with psychosis

Each year in the UK about 7500 people develop a first episode of psychosis and in about 80% of cases the onset occurs in young people (those aged 16–30). Psychosis can lead to long-term, even lifetime, problems, putting those affected at particularly high risk of social exclusion (Chapter 8).

The case for early intervention rests on clear evidence that late treatment results in poor long-term outcomes. The cognitive and psychosocial damage caused by psychosis occurs mainly during the early stages of the illness (up to 5 years after onset), after which a plateau of disability is reached that then predicts the level of disability at 15 years (Harrison *et al*, 2001). The greater the delay in providing treatment, the greater the risk that individuals will experience more long-term problems, including decreased probability of complete remission, increased resistance to conventional treatments, unemployment, impoverished social networks and loss of self-esteem (Marshall *et al*, 2005). Suicide is also a significant risk in the early phase of illness: one in ten people with psychosis die by suicide and two-thirds of these deaths occur within the first 5 years (Department of Health, 2001).

In addition, delay in treatment for some people with first-episode psychosis can lead to a distressing and coercive first contact with mental health services, often following a crisis and sometimes involving the police and involuntary admission to hospital. People from Black and minority ethnic groups appear particularly likely to follow this route. One consequence of this experience is subsequent disengagement with services, with 50% of patients being lost to services within 12 months (McGovern *et al*, 1994).

Research studies from a number of countries now provide evidence that early intervention after first onset, based on quicker detection and treatment by specialist teams, is not only feasible but also cost-effective. Compared with standard mental healthcare, early intervention services report shorter durations of untreated psychosis, lower relapse rates, lower use of legal detention, reduced hospital admissions, better service engagement, higher user/carer satisfaction and lower suicide rates (Addington, 2007). In many studies these benefits are demonstrated only over a relatively short period of time (1 or 2 years), but there is now increasing evidence to suggest that at least some of the gains persist into the longer term.

There is also some evidence that intervention in the prodromal (pre-psychotic) phase of illness, based on the identification of very high-risk individuals, can delay or even prevent the onset of first-episode psychosis (McGorry *et al*, 2002; Morrison *et al*, 2004; McGorry *et al*, 2007; Morrison *et al* 2007).

Evidence for cost-effectiveness comes from a study carried out at the Early Psychosis Prevention and Intervention Centre (EPPIC) in Melbourne. The study found that health service costs per patient were reduced by about a third over the first 12 months of treatment compared with the previous model of care (Mihalopoulos *et al*, 1999). A subsequent 8-year follow-up has found that over a longer period the EPPIC sample incurred only about half the costs of the pre-EPPIC group (McGorry *et al*, 2007). Most of the savings resulted from lower use of in-patient services. Positive clinical outcomes for the EPPIC sample were also maintained over the 8-year follow-up, indicating that early intervention was both more effective and less costly than standard care. Economic analyses of early intervention services in London broadly confirm the findings of the EPPIC study (McCrone *et al*, 2007, personal communication).

This evidence clearly justifies a policy of early intervention ('secondary prevention') for young people with first-episode psychosis on clinical, social and economic grounds.

Employment

Not having a job is perhaps the single most important cause of social exclusion among adults of working age, most obviously because it is usually associated with low income, which has a determining influence on social isolation and lowered self-esteem (Chapters 7 and 8). In addition, prolonged unemployment is linked to worsening mental and physical health, including an increased risk of suicide and premature death. Conversely, having a job can lead to a reduction in symptoms among people with mental health problems, fewer hospital admissions and reduced service use, in addition to the benefits of increased income, social contact and sense of purpose. In short, 'work is good for you' (Waddell & Burton, 2006).

Despite these benefits, people with long-term mental health problems have the lowest employment rate of any of the main groups of disabled people (Chapter 7). This is not generally because of an unwillingness to work, as survey evidence indicates that between 70% and 90% of people with mental health problems in the community want to gain or return to work (Rinaldi & Hill, 2000; Secker *et al*, 2001). Other barriers seem to be more important, including negative attitudes among employers and, as is the case for the domains of life in which exclusion is experienced, the low expectations that are frequently held by mental health professionals (Social Exclusion Unit, 2004).

The low employment rate may also reflect shortcomings in traditional methods of rehabilitation for people with mental health problems, particularly the emphasis on extended preparatory training before engagement with the labour market. This approach has had little success and many patients find employment only in sheltered workshops (Lehman *et al*, 2004). Pre-vocational training and sheltered employment continue to play a leading role in the provision of vocational services for people with severe mental health problems in the UK, despite the fact that there is now a substantial body of evidence to demonstrate that much better outcomes can be achieved by the alternative individual placement and support (IPS) models (Rinaldi & Perkins, 2007; Drake, 2008) (Box 13.2). Such models emphasise rapid placement in work and ongoing support after placement ('place-and-train'), as opposed to the traditional 'train-and-place' models which focus on a prolonged period of assessment and preparatory training.

The individual placement and support model has been most extensively developed and evaluated in the USA, where a number of randomised controlled trials have demonstrated its effectiveness compared with traditional approaches to vocational rehabilitation. A Cochrane review of this evidence concluded that the IPS model was more effective than all

---

Box 13.2 Key principles of the individual placement and support model and the evidence supporting it

There is strong evidence that:
- services should be focused on competitive employment, with a primary goal of integration into the general workforce
- eligibility should be based on the individual's preferences
- programmes should involve rapid job search and minimal pre-vocational training.

There is moderately strong evidence that:
- vocational services should be integrated into the work of the clinical team
- attention to personal preferences is important
- support should be available for an unlimited period and tailored to the individual's needs.

There is weak evidence that:
- benefits counselling should be provided to help people claim the welfare benefits to which they are entitled.

Source: Bond (2004)

other approaches in helping people with severe mental health problems to gain and retain employment (Crowther *et al*, 2001). The model has also demonstrated its effectiveness under randomised controlled trial conditions in Canada (Latimer *et al*, 2006) and in a multicentre European trial covering sites in England, the Netherlands, Germany, Italy, Bulgaria and Switzerland (Burns *et al*, 2007). It has also been successfully deployed in routine clinical practice in some NHS trusts, notably South West London and St George's Mental Health Trust (Rinaldi & Perkins, 2007).

In general, employment rates for people who are helped to find and sustain open employment through IPS average 30–40%, compared with 10–12% for other approaches. Those supported by IPS also work significantly more hours per month, have higher earnings and have a better job tenure. There is no evidence to show that the higher rates of employment resulting from IPS have an adverse effect on clinical well-being and relapse. Indeed, in the European trial mentioned earlier (Burns *et al*, 2007), IPS was associated with reduced rates of psychiatric admission and less time spent in hospital. Follow-up studies conducted after 8–12 years confirm that the greater effectiveness of IPS is sustained over the longer term (Salyers *et al*, 2004; Becker *et al*, 2007).

These positive findings on effectiveness are generally supported by the evidence on cost-effectiveness. Thus, it has been suggested that IPS is generally less expensive to implement than alternative methods of vocational support and also that there are some indications of overall cost savings in terms of reduced mental health service use and reduced reliance on welfare benefits. This is mitigated by the fact that most service users take up part-time positions, so limiting the scope for benefit savings (E. Latimer, personal communication, 2008). The cost-effectiveness of IPS is likely to emerge more strongly as more evidence becomes available on long-term outcomes.

On this basis, there is very strong evidence to recommend implementation of IPS as routine practice for specialist mental health services that aim to improve the employment rate (and thereby social inclusion) of people with long-term mental health problems who are currently unemployed. This could be funded by the closure of existing 'non-IPS' work and day services which do not deliver comparable employment outcomes.

Problems in the conduct of research

We have already explored some of the methodological challenges arising from the contested nature of social exclusion. Measuring concepts where there is little consensus and no agreed definition of its component parts is obviously problematic. Notwithstanding these difficulties, there are a number of other methodological problems associated with the conduct of research with socially excluded individuals and groups. We will now review these and suggest some approaches to overcome them.

Methodological difficulties

The most obvious problem is that people who experience one or more forms of social exclusion may be very difficult to include in empirical studies, especially in quantitative study designs. By virtue of their personal characteristics, their location or place of residence they may be overlooked and prove hard to involve. This may occur for a number of reasons. For example, many research designs automatically exclude people with certain types of (mental) health condition (e.g. forms of dementia), and people living in certain types of settings (e.g. institutional care, rough sleepers). Other designs may exclude people affected by mental health conditions in less obvious ways. For example, people with irregular routines might be disproportionately classed as 'non-contactable' in surveys. In addition, people with poor literacy or language skills may be excluded because they may feel unable to complete a self-administered questionnaire.

In research terms, this 'exclusion of the excluded' means that a specific perspective is not being included, further increasing the risk of marginalisation of such people. The absence of the 'voice' of excluded groups, including those with mental health conditions, could also potentially lead to inappropriate and ill-founded policy outcomes for these groups.

How can we counteract these problems? Two areas are: sampling and recruitment and the use of alternative research designs.

Sampling and recruitment

We must pay particular attention to generating suitable samples, but this is not straightforward. Although a range of potential sampling frames are available, each tends to have its own difficulties and limitations. For example, GP patient registers might be used. Such lists have major advantages for researchers as the overwhelming majority of citizens are registered with a GP, providing the necessary data-set for generating a representative sample. Registers also contain most of the relevant information on age, gender, ethnicity, etc., and thereby hold the potential to generate stratified or purposive samples. Finally, registers are generally kept reasonably up to date.

Given the personal nature of the information contained within GP registers, a number of restrictions are also (necessarily) placed on their use and access to patient registers is safeguarded by a system of ethical and governance processes. Local research ethics committees tend to favour a recruitment approach that is based on potential research participants opting in to the study (often in writing). This is perfectly understandable, but, for all the reasons given above, those choosing to opt in may not be representative of the wider population of disadvantaged people.

Opt-in procedures also tend to generate samples composed of people from higher socioeconomic groups, with better levels of education, better physical and mental health and who belong to majority ethnic groups. Conversely, they tend to exclude the socially disadvantaged, those of lower social status and lower levels of education, people in poorer health, and those belonging to specific Black and minority ethnic groups. In some cases, researchers seeking to study the socially excluded may therefore need to argue robustly with ethics committees for the acceptance of a sampling strategy and recruitment methods that fail to conform to conventional practice.

Alternative sampling frames, such as electoral registers or postcode address files, provide potential access to other representative population samples, but they do not allow researchers to target individuals with mental health conditions and may therefore be unsuitable for some forms of research. Moreover, electoral registers are often incomplete (requiring individuals to add themselves to the register) and a person can remove their details from the publicly available register. People who move frequently are also unlikely to be contactable through electoral registers or postcode address files.

As a result of such difficulties, it may be necessary to supplement standard sampling frames with 'booster samples' composed of groups known to be under-represented in the sampling frame (e.g. McCrystal et al, 2003; Scharf, 2005; Hickman et al, 2007). Depending on the research aims, this might involve purposive sampling strategies and recruitment of additional participants from particular age groups or geographic areas, or individuals with specific characteristics (health condition or ethnic background). Clearly, this represents a compromise between the desire for generalisability on the one hand, and the need to include specific, marginalised groups on the other.

An alternative, and on occasion complementary, strategy is the 'pooling' of data from successive years or waves of a longitudinal or panel survey (as undertaken by Evandrou, 2000; Morris et al, 2005). This can ensure that adequate numbers of participants with the key characteristics are included.

Alternative research designs

Rather than seeking to identify generalisable findings using survey or experimental methods in quantitative designs, it is also possible to develop more qualitative approaches, which aim to disentangle some of the complexities of individuals' social exclusion by direct interviewing or the use of observational techniques. Such approaches lend themselves especially well to the analysis of the circumstances of particularly marginalised groups, such as rough sleepers, people from ethnic or religious minorities, gypsies and travellers, etc.

If designed appropriately, qualitative methodologies may also be better able to explore individual change over time, potentially elucidating causality in relation to the onset of mental ill health, and providing valuable insights into the ways in which an individual's exclusion is influenced simultaneously by a variety of factors. The following approaches lend themselves particularly well to the study of exclusion in relation to mental health conditions:

- biographical/narrative interviews, in which the researcher encourages the research participant to give an account of their lives, and in which the participant sets the agenda for the interview (e.g. Chamberlayne, 2004; Dinos *et al* 2004; Cook & Nunkoosing 2008)
- (participatory) action research, in which participants help in setting the agenda for the research programme and can be involved in all aspects of data collection and analysis and in a range of dissemination activities (e.g. Triese & Shepherd, 2006; Restall & Strutt 2008; Thompson *et al* 2008)
- focus groups, an approach that is increasingly used within the social sciences, and has proved effective in exploring a diverse range of themes and reaching shared understandings of potentially complex topics (such as exclusion/inclusion) (e.g. Lester & Tritter 2005; Connor & Wilson, 2006; Bradby *et al* 2007).

It is also increasingly common for studies to adopt a combination of such qualitative methods. For example, Whitley & Prince's (2005) study of links between common mental disorder and social capital in a London neighbourhood drew effectively on in-depth interviews, focus groups and participant observation.

Although the data yielded by these approaches may be 'richer' than those obtained by traditional quantitative methods, the sampling problems and limitations on generalisability may still remain.

Ethical issues

All research should take account of key ethical concerns relating to such issues as securing informed consent, maintaining confidentiality and anonymity, and the avoidance of harm. When conducting research with marginalised groups, such concerns gain added weight and it is therefore essential that researchers understand and abide by relevant professional guidelines on research ethics (e.g. the British Sociological Association's *Statement of Ethical Practice*, 2002). Researchers should also be aware of the potential risks that arise when conducting fieldwork and be familiar with the Social Research Association's *Ethical Guidelines* (2003).

In relation to people with mental health conditions, there may be particular concerns around the capacity of individuals to understand what taking part in a research study entails and therefore to be able to give informed consent. Individuals may also not fully appreciate their right to withdraw from the research at any stage, especially if there seems to be a connection between the research study and any medical or welfare support the individual is receiving. Ethical committees usually insist that this information is set out clearly in the consent forms.

Other ethical issues include: problems with using proxies to collect information on behalf of someone with a mental health condition; the potential disclosure of information that might be relevant to criminal proceedings; and the ways in which data are stored and the period for which they are kept. These issues apply to the full range of enquiry and evaluation research designs, whether using quantitative or qualitative techniques.

We have argued in this chapter that considerable weight is to be attached to accommodating people who are vulnerable to social exclusion within research designs. This also entails paying sufficient attention to the ethical concerns outlined here. Although securing ethical approval for a particular research approach is frequently regarded as an unavoidable nuisance, when dealing with the issue of social inclusion, ethical concerns require careful consideration at each stage of the research process.

Summary

Measures of exclusion may be individual level, reflecting the situation and life experience of people belonging to socially excluded groups, or societal level ('social indicators'), which rely on existing data sources that characterise levels of participation in larger community samples.

The evaluative evidence regarding interventions that aim to improve social inclusion and/or mental health is reviewed in the context of prevention. The evidence comes from family interventions for conduct disorder and related behavioural disorders in children, early intervention in first-episode psychosis, and supported employment for people with schizophrenia.

There are some general problems associated with the conduct of research in this area, including those with sampling and recruitment and the choice of research design.

References

Addington, J. (2007) The promise of early intervention. *Early Intervention in Psychiatry*, **1**, 294–307.

Becker, D., Whitley, R., Bailey, E., *et al* (2007) Long term employment trajectories amongst participants with severe mental illness in supported employment. *Psychiatric Services*, **58**, 922–928.

Berman, Y. & Phillips, D. (2000) Indicators of social quality and social exclusion at national and community level. *Social Indicators Research*, **50**, 329–350.

Bond, G. (2004) Supported employment: evidence for an evidence-based practice. *Psychiatric Rehabilitation Journal*, **27**, 345–359.

Bradby, H., Varyani, M., Oglethorpe, R., *et al* (2007) British Asian families and the use of child and adolescent mental health services: a qualitative study of a hard to reach group. *Social Science and Medicine*, **65**, 2413–2424.

British Sociological Association (2002) *Statement of Ethical Practice for the British Sociological Association*. British Sociological Association (http://www.britsoc.co.uk/equality/Statement+Ethical+Practice.htm).

Burchardt, T. (2000) Social exclusion. In *The Blackwell Encyclopaedia of Social Work* (ed. M. Davies). Blackwell.

Burns, T., Catty, J., Becker, T., *et al* (2007) The effectiveness of supported employment for people with severe mental illness: a randomised controlled trial. *Lancet*, **370**, 1146–1152.

Cabinet Office (2006) *Reaching Out: An Action Plan on Social Exclusion*. Cabinet Office.

Chamberlayne, P. (2004) Emotional retreat and social exclusion: towards biographical methods in professional training. *Journal of Social Work Practice*, **18**, 337–350.

Connor, S. L. & Wilson, R. (2006) It's important that they learn from us for mental health to progress. *Journal of Mental Health*, **15**, 461–474.

Cook, K. & Nunkoosing, K. (2008) Maintaining dignity and managing stigma in the interview encounter: the challenge of paid-for participation. *Qualitative Health Research*, **18**, 418–427.

Crowther, R. E, Marshall, M., Bond, G. R., *et al* (2001) Helping people with severe mental illness to obtain work: systematic review. *BMJ*, **322**, 204–208.

Department of Health (2001) *The Mental Health Policy Implementation Guide*. Department of Health.

Department for Work and Pensions (2007) *Opportunity for All: Indicators Update 2007*. Department for Work and Pensions (http://www.dwp.gov.uk/docs/opportunityforall2007.pdf).

Dinos, S., Stevens, S., Serfaty, M., *et al* (2004) Stigma: the feelings and experiences of 46 people with mental illness: qualitative study. *British Journal of Psychiatry*, **184**, 176–181.

Drake, R. (2008) *Future of Supported Employment*. Sainsbury Centre Lecture, March 2008 (http://www.scmh.org.uk/employment/ips_resources.aspx).

Dretzke, J., Frew, E., Davenport, C., *et al* (2005) The effectiveness and cost-effectiveness of parent training/education programmes for the treatment of conduct disorder, including oppositional defiant disorder, in children. *Health Technology Assessment*, **9**, 1–250.

Evandrou, M. (2000) Social inequalities in later life: the socio-economic position of older people from ethnic minority groups in Britain. *Population Trends*, **101**, Autumn, 11–18.

Friedli, L. & Parsonage, M. (2007) Building an economic case for mental health promotion. *Journal of Public Mental Health*, **6**, 14–23.

Gaite, L., Vazquez-Barquero, J. L., Oliver, J., *et al* (2006) The Lancashire Quality of Life Profile – European version. In *International Outcome Measures in Mental Health: Quality of Life, Needs, Service Satisfaction, Costs and Impact on Carers* (eds G. Thornicroft, T. Becker, M. Knapp, *et al*). Gaskell.

Green, H., McGinnity, A., Meltzer, H., *et al* (2005) *Mental Health of Children and Young People in Great Britain, 2004*. Office for National Statistics.

Harrison, G., Hopper, K., Craig, T., *et al* (2001) Recovery from psychotic illness: a 15- and 25-year international follow-up study. *British Journal of Psychiatry*, **178**, 506–517.

Henggeler, S. W., Mihalic, S. F., Rone, L., *et al* (1998) *Multisystemic Therapy: Blueprints for Violence Prevention, Book Six*. Blueprints for Violence Prevention Series (series ed. D. S. Elliott). Center for the Study and Prevention of Violence, Institute of Behavioral Science, University of Colorado.

Hickman, M., Vickerman, P., Macleod, J., *et al* (2007) Cannabis and schizophrenia: model projections of the impact of the rise in cannabis use on historical and future trends in schizophrenia in England and Wales. *Addiction*, **102**, 597–606.

Kim-Cohen, J., Caspi, A., Moffitt, T., *et al* (2003) Prior juvenile diagnosis in adults with mental disorder. *Archives of General Psychiatry*, **60**, 709–717.

Labour Force Survey (2005) *Labour Force Survey*. Office for National Statistics.

Latimer, E. A., Lecomte, T., Becker, D. R., *et al* (2006) Generalisability of the individual placement and support model of supported employment: results of a Canadian randomised controlled trial. *British Journal of Psychiatry*, **189**, 65–73.

Lehman, A. F., Kreyenbuhl, J., Buchanan, R. W., *et al* (2004) The Schizophrenia Patient Outcomes Research Team (PORT): updated treatment recommendation 2003. *Schizophrenia Bulletin*, **30**, 193–217.

Lester, H. & Tritter, J. Q. (2005) 'Listen to my madness': understanding the experiences of people with serious mental illness. *Sociology of Health and Illness*, **27**, 649–669.

Littell, J., Popa, M. & Forsythe, B. (2005) Multisystemic Therapy for social, emotional and behavioural problems in youth aged 10–17. *Cochrane Database of Systematic Reviews*, issue 3, article no.: CD004797.

Marshall, M., Lewis, S., Lockwood, A., *et al* (2005) Association between duration of untreated psychosis and outcome in cohorts of first-episode patients: a systematic review. *Archives of General Psychiatry*, **62**, 975–983.

McCrystal, P., Higgins, K., Percy, A., *et al* (2003) Emerging patterns in adolescent drug use in Northern Ireland: The Belfast youth development study 2002. *Child Care in Practice*, **9**, 73–83.

McGorry, P., Yung, A. R., Phillips, L. J., *et al* (2002) Randomised controlled trial of interventions designed to reduce the risk of progression to first episode psychosis in a clinical sample with sub-threshold symptoms. *Archives of General Psychiatry*, **59**, 921–928.

McGorry, P. D., Purcell, R., Hickie, I. B., *et al* (2007) Investing in youth mental health is a best buy. *Medical Journal of Australia*, **187**, s5–7.

McGovern, D., Hemmings, P. & Cope, R. (1994) Long-term follow-up of young Afro-Caribbean Britons and White Britons with a first admission diagnosis of schizophrenia. *Social Psychiatry and Psychiatric Epidemiology*, **29**, 8–19.

Mihalopoulos, C., McGorry, P. & Carter, R. (1999) Is phase-specific, community-oriented treatment of early psychosis an economically viable method of improving outcome? *Acta Psychiatrica Scandinavica*, **100**, 47–55.

Morris, S., Sutton, M. & Gravelle, H. (2005) Inequity and inequality in the use of health care in England: an empirical investigation. *Social Science and Medicine*, **60**, 1251–1266.

Morrison, A. P., French, P., Walford, L., *et al* (2004) Cognitive therapy for the prevention of psychosis in people at ultra-high risk: randomised controlled trial. *British Journal of Psychiatry*, **185**, 291–297.

Morrison, A. P., French, P., Parker, S., *et al* (2007) Three-year follow-up of a randomized controlled trial of cognitive therapy for the prevention of psychosis in people at ultrahigh risk. *Schizophrenia Bulletin*, **33**, 682–687.

Nelson, G., Westhues, A. & Macleod, J. (2003) A meta-analysis of longitudinal research on preschool prevention programs for children. *Prevention and Treatment*, **6**, article 31.

Palmer, G., MacInnes, T. & Kenway, P. (2007) Monitoring Poverty and Social Exclusion 2007. Joseph Rowntree Foundation and New Policy Institute.

Restall, G. & Strutt, C. (2008) Participation in planning and evaluating mental health services: building capacity. *Psychiatric Rehabilitation Journal*, **31**, 234–238.

Rinaldi, M. & Hill, R. (2000) *Insufficient Concern: The Experiences, Attitudes and Perceptions of Disabled People and Employers towards Open Employment in one London Borough*. Merton Mind.

Rinaldi, M. & Perkins, R. (2007) Comparing employment outcomes for two vocational services: individual placement and support and non-integrated pre-vocational services in the UK. *Journal of Vocational Rehabilitation*, **27**, 21–27.

Salyers, M., Becker, D., Drake, R., *et al* (2004) A ten-year follow-up of a supported employment program. *Psychiatric Services*, **55**, 302–308.

Scharf, T. (2005) Recruiting older research participants: lessons from deprived neighbourhoods. In *Recruitment and Sampling: Qualitative Research with Older People* (ed. C. Holland): pp. 29–43. Centre for Policy on Ageing.

Scott, S., Knapp, M., Henderson, J., *et al* (2001) Financial cost of social exclusion: follow-up study of antisocial children into adulthood. *BMJ*, **323**, 194.

Secker, J., Grove, B. & Seebohm, P. (2001) Challenging barriers to employment, training and education for mental health clients: the clients' perspective. *Journal of Mental Health*, **10**, 395–404.

Social Exclusion Unit (2004) *Mental Health and Social Exclusion*. Office of the Deputy Prime Minister.

Social Research Association (2003) *Ethical Guidelines*. Social Research Association (www.the-sra.org.uk/documents/pdfs/ethics03.pdf).

Stewart-Brown, S. (2004) Mental health promotion: childhood holds the key? *Public Health Medicine*, **5**, 8–17.

Thompson, N. C., Hunter, E. E., Murray, L., *et al* (2008) The experience of living with chronic mental illness: a photovoice study. *Perspectives in Psychiatric Care*, **44**, 14–24.

Triese, C. & Shepherd, G. (2006) Developing Mental Health Services for Gypsy Travellers – an exploratory study. *Clinical Psychology Forum*, **163**, 16–19.

Utting, D., Monteiro, H. & Ghate, D. (2007) *Interventions for Children at Risk of Developing Antisocial Personality Disorder: Report to the Department of Health and Prime Minister's Strategy Unit.* Policy Research Bureau (http://www.prb.org.uk/publications/P182%20and%20 P188%20Report.pdf).

Waddell, G. & Burton, A. (2006) *Is Work Good for Your Health and Well-Being?* TSO (The Stationery Office).

Whitley, R. & Prince, M. (2005) Is there a link between rates of common mental disorder and deficits in social capital in Gospel Oak, London? Results from a qualitative study. *Health and Place*, **11**, 237–248.

CHAPTER 14

Implications of social inclusion for individual practice

Alan Currie

> If you can't get listened to in a ward round you don't believe that you have
> a chance of getting what you want in the outside world.
>
> Pauline, service user

The preceding chapters confirm what psychiatrists already know from their daily practice – that the people they see experience exclusion and lack access to a wealth of opportunities including employment, housing and education and that this exacerbates their mental health problems.

Psychiatric training, with its long and repeated exposure to direct clinical contact and involvement in the lives of patients equips practitioners to see the importance of social disadvantage. Psychiatrists are well able to see that social disadvantages are both a cause and a consequence of mental illness (Horwitz & Scheid, 1999), that these disadvantages do not necessarily stem simply from a lack of material resources (Morgan *et al*, 2007), and that those with mental health problems are often excluded in multiple ways (e.g. low income, poor housing). Psychiatry has a long tradition of highlighting the disadvantages that service users face and of working to increase their control and empowerment.

To address the social exclusion experienced by users of mental health services practitioners need skills, knowledge and values that recognise not only the damaging effects of exclusion, but also the benefits of inclusion. Improving the breadth and quality of opportunities afforded not only benefits a person's mental health, it allows people to make positive contributions to their communities and to society and restores the hope for them and their families that they can adapt to the constraints that may be enforced by illness or disability.

These themes overlap significantly with the idea of recovery as applied to psychiatry (Chapter 3). Central to this is the hope that individuals can be helped and supported to define and find new roles and learn to live well even in the face of significant illness or impairment. Empowering individuals to describe their own new roles, to support them in finding or rediscovering opportunities and, where possible, equipping and allowing them to direct and manage their own care, are all important if socially inclusive practice is to become the norm (Case study 14.1). Acquiring the skills for both recovery-oriented practice and to support self-care is a necessary stepping stone for practitioners who aspire to genuine socially inclusive practice.

Recovery-oriented practice

Three principle uses of the term recovery have been described (Ralph & Corrigan, 2005). In a medical context, recovery is first, the spontaneous resolution of symptoms, and second, resolution as a consequence of treatment/intervention. A third definition moves beyond the mere giving or receiving of treatment towards the experience of personal recovery in the context of continuing symptoms and/or disability.

The aim of practice that is oriented towards recovery is to support patients to 'live a satisfying, hopeful and contributing life, even with the limitations caused by illness' (Anthony, 1993). A 'contributing life' is one where opportunities are available and sought and where a service user's roles (and functioning in them) are as important as their symptoms (Case study 14.2). Social exclusion therefore becomes a significant barrier to recovery and social inclusion a step towards a life lived well in the face of illness and disability.

Central to the practice of socially inclusive psychiatry is the role of the psychiatrist. A consultation that is focused on the service user, clarifying their strengths and aspirations, collaborating to empower them to make choices about their care and empowering them to manage their own situation is based on ideas that have much in common with the concept of recovery. The role of the psychiatrist who adopts recovery-oriented practice is that of 'offering professional skills and knowledge while learning and valuing from the patient who is an expert by experience' (Roberts & Wolfson, 2004). If the patient is an expert by experience, the psychiatrist's parallel expertise is in making available knowledge in support of collaborative treatment decisions and viewing effective treatment as a lever towards self-defined recovery rather than as an end in itself (Case study 14.3).

Recovery-oriented practitioners

The components of recovery, described in Chapter 3, relate directly to the process of recovery, which includes: finding new hope; re-establishing a positive identity; building a new and meaningful life which incorporates illness; developing efficacy and feeling in control of an illness; and having the opportunities to participate. Hope, agency and opportunity are all relevant considerations during the journey to recovery.

Recovery-oriented practitioners (Borg & Kristiansen, 2004), those best placed to support the patient's journey, should display: openness, collaboration as equals, a focus on the individual's inner resources, reciprocity, and a willingness to 'go the extra mile'. These defining practitioner qualities should be allied to general therapeutic skills such as empathy, acceptance and mutual affirmation, where positive risk-taking

Case study 14.1   Chloe: the benefits of social inclusion

Chloe has consulted two psychiatrists who have helped her to be more socially included. The first encouraged her to focus on writing poetry and suggested local groups she could join to pursue this. The second encouraged her to join sports clubs. She feels that both psychiatrists took an interest in her and obviously listened to what she was saying as they suggested things that would interest her. As a result she got out of the house and met new people and now regularly goes to Pilates and yoga. Because of their approach, Chloe has had an effective working relationship with both doctors and is able take on board their other suggestions about treatment and medication.

Case study 14.2   A patient with a life

When my psychiatrist writes reports to my GP after we've had a review, he always includes a bit about how I'm doing at work. He says it's important to see me as a person with a life and not just a patient with a mental illness.

Case study 14.3   Natasha

I felt I had finally been listened to. I felt that I was no longer a lost cause, someone doomed to spend their life fighting for help and struggling to survive. I now have a diagnosis that makes sense and know there is a treatment to help me recover and be able to live life to the full. This includes being able to work full time, socialise – all the things that many people take for granted. I feel I have become a part of society, instead of someone on the outside, not knowing why I continually ended up depressed and isolated.

is encouraged and where hope and optimism are reflected in a positive expectation for the future.

The role of therapeutic hope is emphasised as an important central belief for mental health practitioners (Royal College of Psychiatrists *et al*, 2007). The role that doctors' expectations play in shaping outcomes in schizophrenia has been described by others (Warner, 2004). The practitioner's role moves beyond merely offering treatments, to incorporate concern about how treatments are delivered. Optimistic doctors are responsible for increased recovery rates and better outcomes (Boardman & Walters, 2009).

Shepherd *et al* (2008) have described ten top tips for practising in a manner that best supports recovery (Box 14.1). For mental health professionals, including psychiatrists, these points may form the basis of their day-to-day recovery-oriented practice. They could provide a set of standards for individual clinicians and could be used to assess performance.

Understanding the concept of recovery is central to helping service users find identity and meaning in their lives that incorporates their mental health problems and allows them to participate as fully as possible in the life of their community. Creating collaborative relationships is one way of turning this understanding into action. Knowing how to collaborate

Box 14.1 Ten top tips for recovery-oriented practice

Understand recovery

1 Actively listen to help the person make sense of their mental health problems.
2 Help the person identify and prioritise their personal goals for recovery (not the professional's goals).
3 Demonstrate a belief in the person's existing strengths in relation to the pursuit of these goals.
4 Be able to identify examples from your own lived experience, or that of other service users, which inspire and validate hope.
5 Accept that the future is uncertain and that setbacks will occur, but continue to express support for the possibility of achieving the person's self-defined goals, maintaining hope and positive expectations.

Know how to collaborate

6 Encourage self-management of mental health problems (by providing information, reinforcing existing coping strategies, etc.).
7 Discuss what the person wants in terms of therapeutic interventions, whether they want psychosocial treatments, alternative therapies, joint crisis planning, etc. Show that you have listened.
8 Behave at all times so as to convey an attitude of respect for the person and a desire for an equal partnership in working together, indicating a willingness to 'go the extra mile'.

Have a broad view

9 Pay particular attention to the importance of goals that take the person out of the traditional sick role and enable them to serve and help others.
10 Identify non-mental health resources – friends, contacts, organisations – relevant to the achievement of these goals.

Adapted from Shepherd *et al* (2008)

is a key quality for all doctors. It is reflected in the most recent General Medical Council (2006) guidance on the roles of doctors and is a central pillar in the development of self-care skills. Clinicians need to understand the patient's situation in all its breadth. This may be facilitated by a genuine biopsychosocial model that is already incorporated in psychiatric training and practice. This model values not only the signs and symptoms of a traditional biomedical model but also their context.

Self-care, self-management and self-directed care

To support the experience of personal recovery and to escape the constraints of roles defined by illness it is important to allow the development of skills in self-care, self management and self-directed care.

Self-care means individuals taking responsibility for their own health and well-being and involves adopting a lifestyle that promotes mental and physical health. Self-management is a related term and refers specifically to those who are adapting to a long-term illness. This entails developing the ability to manage not only symptoms and treatment but also the physical and psychological consequences and lifestyle changes that can be inherent in living with a chronic condition. Practitioners need to be familiar with the evidence base that supports self-care, self-management and self-directed care. For example, the Cochrane database now contains systematic reviews of aspects of self-management in bipolar disorder (Morriss *et al*, 2007) and eating disorders (Perkins *et al*, 2006).

Empowerment and enablement are important elements of clinical encounters, as emphasised in *Vulnerable Patients, Safe Doctors* (Royal College of Psychiatrists, 2007). The guideline outlines good practice in clinical relationships and describes empowerment as allowing patients to assume control of their treatment facilitated by information from experts and a consultation style that favours collaboration. In its position statement, the American Psychiatric Association (2005) also emphasises the importance of practising in a manner that enables patients to define the goals of their treatment (both pharmacological and psychosocial).

Supporting patients in self-directed care means embracing the concept of collaborative decisions. Practitioners may have detailed technical knowledge and be expected to help patients interpret this but the active participation of patients in all decisions would be the expected norm. This approach also requires a high level of jargon-free communication skills in sharing professional knowledge with patients and their families in ways that they will retain and understand. A competent psychiatrist will be able to explore the treatment choices available to an individual and work with them to weigh up the evidence in support of different therapeutic options (Case study 14.4). This will also extend to being able to support the development of advance agreements and crisis plans.

Care plans can serve as useful tools for detailing the components of self-management and self-directed care, including patient-determined contingency plans and advance directives. Direct payments can additionally serve as a very clear means by which individuals are self-determining in respect of their treatment and care. Competent practitioners need to be familiar with both approaches.

Finally, individuals need to be free to leave services. This requires knowledge of how to negotiate ceasing treatments and stepping down supports once they are no longer needed, with an understanding of how overprovision of treatment or support can promote an unproductive dependency and be an impediment to self-care.

Capabilities for socially inclusive practice

The National Social Inclusion Programme (NSIP) in collaboration with the professional colleges, including the Royal College of Psychiatrists, has developed a profile of the capabilities necessary for inclusive practice across all professions (Royal College of Psychiatrists *et al*, 2007).

Case study 14.4   Pauline: treatment choices

Over the years Pauline's consultant has suggested many different medications, none of which seemed to work. Once he prescribed a drug that made her severely tired and feel almost like a 'zombie', so she stopped taking it. Later at her clinic appointment his response was, 'OK. We need to work with this. What can we do?' She was relieved that he was not accusatory and listened to why she had stopped the medication.

Using the *Ten Essential Shared Capabilities* (Department of Health, 2004) as a framework, the NSIP capabilities profile describes distinctive skills that explicitly promote inclusive practice. The intention is that this acts as a resource to: support staff selection, job design and planning, appraisal processes, and recognition of good practice; influence the research agenda; and contribute to a shared vision of the local community through engaging with key individuals and organisations. The NSIP capabilities are listed in Box 14.2 and show significant overlap with the features of recovery described in Box 14.1. The principles of socially inclusive practice are for everyone and not to be triaged out to 'inclusion specialists'.

Working in partnership

Practitioners should expect to work in teams that are capable of developing and maintaining links with community networks. The nature of these networks goes some way beyond the kind of knowledge of local services possessed by a community mental health team (CMHT) or other sector team. Practitioners should see themselves as belonging to the local community and should expect to inform and support the developing mental health knowledge of that community.

Box 14.2   Ten Essential Shared Capabilities

1 Working in partnership
2 Respecting diversity
3 Practising ethically
4 Challenging inequality
5 Promoting recovery
6 Identifying people's needs and strengths
7 Providing service user-centred care
8 Making a difference
9 Promoting safety and positive risk-taking
10 Personal development and learning

Source: Royal College of Psychiatrists (2007)

Networks would include any organisation able to provide access to valued community roles for service users. The capable practitioner would expect to understand how community organisations work and be able to identify and challenge discriminatory practices. Naturally, a high level of communication skills is a prerequisite to dialogue with others in the network.

Respecting diversity

The ability to respect diversity sits alongside the ability to understand the impact of discrimination and prejudice. Exclusion requires compensatory behaviours from practitioners and necessitates a commitment to reaching out to the excluded. Knowledge of the wide range of cultural norms allows sensitive communication as well as a deeper understanding of the lived experience of the service user.

Practising ethically

An ethical practitioner recognises the power differential that can exist in a help-seeking relationship and takes steps to minimise this. User-defined outcomes (and ultimately recovery) are not possible without empowerment within the consultation. Moreover, services that are difficult to leave can be disempowering.

The ethical practitioner recognises their accountability to the service user and balances this against accountability to others (employing agency, wider community and professional body). Ethical practice means working positively with the tensions present when legal powers are exercised and striving to allow the service user to make choices and exercise control wherever this is possible. Practitioners recognise their own values and how these influence others and are transparent in their actions.

Challenging inequality

Inclusive practitioners understand what drives stigma and discrimination in communities and how systems can create inequality and deny opportunities. Furthermore, they understand the emotional impact of these experiences. The impact of inequality necessitates efforts to (re)create opportunity, challenge stigma and support individuals to develop and maintain valued social roles. This extends to advocating for excluded individuals and groups within the community and challenging myths, misconceptions and misunderstandings where they occur.

Promoting recovery

The skills to empower individuals, to clarify their aspirations and determine their strengths are core to the concept of recovery. Resilience is necessary to sustain hope and optimism as individuals are helped to plan their recovery journey. Flexibility is required to ensure that care plans are tailored and that it is individuals who are matched with the opportunities they seek and not vice versa. Knowledge of the opportunities available in the community can only lead to a good match and genuine personal choice if this knowledge is broad.

Identifying people's needs and strengths

Collaborative practitioners are able to work in a way that acknowledges the personal, social, cultural and spiritual strengths of an individual. Strengths are harnessed to inspire the confidence necessary for individuals to define and direct their own care. Central to this is the ability to provide 'just enough support' (Case study 14.5).

Providing service user-centred care

Centring care on the service user means using the perspective of the user as the primary determinant when negotiating achievable and meaningful goals.

The practitioner needs to be able to clarify who is in a position to assist in pursuit of these goals and to do so needs not only a breadth of knowledge on the range of community supports but also a depth of relationship with these supporters. The practitioner needs skills as a broker or intermediary, especially with community partners who are not specifically providers of mental health services, to be effective in supporting the supporters.

Making a difference

Practitioners need to be familiar with both the evidence base and the values base that underpin quality health and social care. Collecting evidence of what works for an individual is an important ongoing task. Making a difference also means being aware of a person's strengths, the areas of their lives where they are already included and working to sustain these.

Promoting safety and positive risk-taking

All practitioners need a comprehensive knowledge and skills base in the identification and management of risk. Wherever possible, individuals

---

Case study 14.5   Sian: 'What I want from my psychiatrists'

To truly believe that it's not a weakness or your fault but an illness, and to not feel sorry for or pity you. To give you a good kick up the arse when you need it but also to believe in you, support you and know when you can't take any more pushing! Also not trying to be your best mate, i.e. keeping things professional and at a safe distance. To believe in you and believe you can do it when almost no one else does.

should be empowered to decide the level of risk that they are prepared to take for themselves and positive-risk taking means being able to support others in making difficult decisions. When collaborating to decide on the most appropriate way of managing a risk it can be helpful to consider both the concept of 'least restrictive alternative' alongside 'most inclusive alternative'. Positive risk-taking is promoted in a manner that encourages user-defined recovery and learning by experience.

Personal development and learning

The personal development plans (or their equivalent) of individual practitioners must be driven by the values of socially inclusive practice. This is a means to ensure that all practitioners possess a high level of ability to collaborate with individuals, to identify their strengths and define their aspirations and from there to sustain hope and optimism as they are supported to pursue these aims. For this to be effective, organisational support from, for example, the employing provider trust is needed alongside effective governance arrangements (Chapter 15).

Perceived obstacles to socially inclusive practice

Practitioners may be concerned that socially inclusive practice may have untoward effects on their working practices. A series of potential obstacles to recovery-oriented and socially inclusive practice have been described (Box 14.3) (Davidson *et al*, 2006; Shepherd *et al*, 2008), some of which are discussed here. There are many important counter-arguments to these concerns.

- *Extra-work*. Many practitioners have understandable concerns that a new way of practising will add to an already considerable workload. However, the proposition is that working in this way replaces (rather than adds to) traditional assessment–treatment–cure ideologies. In any event, the biopsychosocial paradigms that prevail in psychiatric practice are well placed to receive the principles of recovery-oriented and socially inclusive practice.
- *'Recovery' means that the person is cured*. A misunderstanding of the meaning that is accorded to the word recovery would represent a significant obstacle to collaborating with patients towards living well within the constraints of illness. Recovery refers to the individual and their life and, by extension, their adaptation to new circumstances. This understanding of recovery aspires to develop new opportunities to live life well in changed circumstances (illness). Cure may describe what happens to the illness, where recovery describes what happens to the individual who is ill.
- *Professional roles are devalued*. Professionals remain key sources of knowledge, advice and support, and for patients, they may be the most important 'holders of hope' (Glover, 2002). Working to support self-defined recovery and promote social inclusion does, however, mean

---

Box 14.3 Ten top concerns about recovery in serious mental illness

1 Recovery is old news
   'What's all the hype? We've been doing recovery for years'
2 Recovery-oriented care adds to the burden of mental health professionals who are already stretched thin by demands that exceed their resources
   'You mean that I not only have to care for and treat people, but now I have to do recovery too?'
3 Recovery means that the person is cured
   'What do you mean your clients are in recovery? Don't you see how disabled they still are? Isn't that a contradiction?'
4 Recovery happens for very few people with serious mental illness
   'You're not talking about the people I see. They're too disabled. Recovery is not possible for them'.
5 Recovery in mental health is an irresponsible fad
   'This is just the latest flavour of the month and one that sets people up for failure.'
6 Recovery only happens after, and as a result of, active treatment and the cultivation of insight
   'My patients won't even acknowledge that they're sick. How can I talk to them about recovery when they have no insight about being ill?'
7 Recovery can be implemented only through the introduction of new services
   'Sure, we'll be happy to do recovery, just give us the money it will take to start a (new) recovery programme.'
8 Recovery services are neither reimbursable nor evidence-based
   'First it was managed care, then it was evidence-based practice, and now it's recovery. But recovery is neither cost-effective nor evidence-based'
9 Recovery approaches devalue the role of professional intervention
   'Why did I just spend 10 years training if someone else with no training is going to make all the decisions?'
10 Recovery increases providers' exposure to risk and liability
   'If recovery is the person's responsibility, then how come I get the blame when things go wrong?

Source: Davidson *et al* (2006) & Shepherd *et al* (2008).

---

that professional expertise is not given automatic hegemony over the views of the patient, necessitating a high level of skill in open and collaborative working.

- *Exposure to risk and liability is increased.* In some instances risk may be increased, but usually in the context of an agreement that aims to facilitate personal growth and learning. Risks that are agreed collaboratively are also shared risks and it is not helpful for either party if professionals feel that they carry sole responsibility for how people live their lives. If an individual chooses to ignore clearly documented, professional advice, then they carry the burden of risk, whereas a professional who acts to contravene his 'duty of care' is responsible for what he does.

Moving to socially inclusive practice

The caricature of the medical model applied to psychiatric practice is that it is 'a reductionist, mechanistic, disability-enhancing approach taken by powerful doctors towards patients' (Shah & Mountain, 2007). More generously, perhaps, it can be seen as a scientific process of observation to identify symptoms, ascribe illness or disease, and prescribe treatment (Clare, 1980). If practising psychiatrists are indeed wedded to the caricatured medical model, then it would seem a major task to move to practising in a socially inclusive manner.

However, current psychiatric practice is some way from the caricature and contains much that will support the practice of social inclusion. A biopsychosocial model of understanding is familiar to most mental health workers. It is an approach that combines the scientific and the humanistic (recognising the pitfalls of biomedical reductionism), and that privileges the patient and their context over diagnostic categorisation (Pilgrim, 2002). Consider also the emphasis in current practice that is placed on service user-defined aims and aspirations, the focus on identifying strengths in an atmosphere of hope, and the need to collaborate as a facilitating mentor rather than a paternalistic (albeit wise) giver of advice to passive or compliant listeners.

Recovery-oriented practice does not mean abandoning traditional skills and techniques. For example, a high level of technical expertise in psychological and pharmacological therapies is still central and to be valued highly. Their application in helping individuals to live well within the confines of illness and to define their own goals and aspirations is an adaptation of existing practice based on a collaborative therapeutic relationship. Collaboration is central in current General Medical Council guidelines issued in November 2006, emphasising both new duties and new themes for all doctors. These include:

- support patients in caring for themselves to promote and maintain their health
- work in partnership with patients
- take patients' views into account when assessing their condition
- encourage patients to use knowledge about their condition when making decisions about their care, and
- support self-care.

Detailed guidance on non-discrimination, equality and diversity is also included.

The nature of this type of doctor–patient relationship (probably more accurately called a 'partnership') is a firm footing on which to support recovery and, in turn, social inclusion.

In contrast to the caricatured 'medical' model, a humanistic understanding of the unique history and personhood of patients, locating this in a genuinely biopsychosocial context, acknowledging the contribution that social exclusion makes to mental ill health and then practising in a way that supports collaboration and self-care already puts most psychiatrists in a strong position to practice in a socially inclusive manner.

Subspecialty perspectives in psychiatric practice

Just as recovery is not exclusive to specialist rehabilitation services, so socially inclusive practice is not exclusive to any specific branch of psychiatry. Indeed, there may be much to gain by advocating wide adoption of the principles of socially inclusive practice and it can be illuminating to look at what this might mean for particular subspecialties.

There are some areas in psychiatric practice where the adoption of practices that support social inclusion might seem at best difficult and at worst impossible. For example, how can an indefinitely detained patient be able to exercise choice? How can an individual with markedly diminished decision-making capacity be said to collaborate in treatment choices?

Forensic psychiatry

There is a fundamental tension to practising in a socially inclusive manner in a clinical setting that is defined by the application of restriction and coercion. This tension is magnified if the surrounding sociopolitical structure is one dominated by the primary aim of public protection and management of risk by exclusion.

Of course, some may argue that forensic psychiatric patients have forfeited at least some rights to be fully socially included both because of what they have done and because of the need to reduce future risk to others. Many criminal convictions will result in the individual being automatically excluded from certain types of accommodation, employment and interpersonal interactions with family or others considered at risk.

Although the need to manage risk to the public may sometimes appear to 'trump' the patient's wishes or preferences with regard to treatment, this does not mean that their wishes should not be sought, considered and respected wherever possible. A collaborative relationship between patient and clinician is important. Re-conceptualising restrictions as necessary to allow the patient to engage with rehabilitation and reduce the risk of their offending – the so-called 'therapeutic use of security' – can be helpful for clinicians and service users alike.

Patients in forensic psychiatry settings are likely to have experienced social exclusion even before their engagement with mental health services. The socioeconomic and cultural indicators of deprivation and disadvantage are all over-represented in this group, with educational and vocational drop-out and failure, and little lifetime experience of mature, intimate or non-abusive relations.

In some respects forensic patients may have most to gain from socially inclusive practice because of their high levels of disadvantage, social deprivation and stigma. Practitioners need to consider how best to identify and assess social deficits and impairments and how to address skills deficits with targeted interventions. Needs in respect of social inclusion (and how these needs will be addressed) can and should be explicitly included in individual care plans.

Child and adolescent psychiatry

All children are socially excluded to an extent. To varying degrees they are inherently dependent on adults for guidance and protection. By reason of their age they are specifically excluded from directly influencing social policy (e.g. voting) and from other activities such as opening a bank account and serving in the armed forces.

Children who experience poverty (an indicator of social exclusion) are more likely to develop mental health problems than children from more affluent families and there are important psychological and neurobiological correlates of growing up in deprivation and social exclusion. Living with parents who are unable to instil a sense of security in their children is not conducive to normal emotional development and such parents themselves often come from backgrounds of childhood adversity.

In the face of generational 'cycles of deprivation' it is indeed a challenge to foster the hope and optimism that are central to recovery-oriented practice and to help create the opportunities to actively participate in community life that are integral to socially inclusive practice.

Learning disability

Those who use learning disability services by definition have impaired intellectual function and almost invariably this is accompanied by impairments in social functioning. They experience lifetime risks of low expectations, low self-esteem, lower levels of physical and mental well-being, and at times the risk of abuse and neglect. Most have long-term dependencies on family and other carers, with associated disempowerment, and are exposed to social exclusion in multiple and enduring ways.

Such people have much to gain if social inclusion is an aspiration and seen as integral to their care. It is realistic for service users to aspire to choice in daily life and inclusion in local communities. This can include choices (which they help to define) in areas such as adult (including sexual) relationships, housing and paid employment. The principles of socially inclusive practice and an orientation towards user-defined recovery are powerful means by which this can be achieved.

Psychiatry of old age

Recovery-oriented practice seeks to facilitate access to the opportunities to be part of a community and to be valued by that community. For older people this task is compounded by age discrimination, by the change of roles inherent in ageing, such as widowhood and retirement, and by the narrowing of social networks that can accompany this. It may require considerable efforts on the part of practitioners to overcome a seemingly inevitable pessimism about outcome and to restore hope and optimism that a life can be lived well within the confines of illness and ageing.

Life-changing events raise the challenge of finding a new sense of self, meaning and purpose in life. When the life change is the prospect of a relentlessly progressive condition that is likely to result in impaired decision-making capacity (e.g. dementia) it is still possible for psychiatrists to practise in a manner that allows patients to exercise their own choices much of the time. Supporting patients in making their own choices and valuing the contributions they can make increases the prospect of living a satisfying and contributing life even within the limitations caused by illness.

Social inclusion and carers

Carers provide help on a voluntary basis for people with disabilities. Some carers will be supporting an adult to live independently, whereas others will be meeting all or most of the needs of a care recipient living in the same home.

Carers may find their role to be rewarding and a source of great personal satisfaction and may have their own support network of friends and family. Others may have fewer supports of their own to draw on, may be isolated by their role and may have difficulty coping with the burden of care.

Caring can be physically and emotionally draining and tasks may vary during the trajectory of the care recipient's mental health problems. The loss of the care recipient's health can lead to significant changes in carer's and care recipient's respective roles and significantly alter the relationship. Carers may experience poor physical and mental health, especially elderly carers and those with pre-existing physical health conditions (Cormac & Tihanyi, 2006). Certain forms of behaviour in the care recipient, such as poor self-care, shouting and incontinence, may be especially difficult to cope with.

Carers often have to make major changes to their own lifestyle. They may be unable to participate in full-time employment or in education and may have difficulty pursuing previously valued activities. They may withdraw from family and social contacts. Isolation and poverty can increase the burden of care. Carers, too, experience social exclusion and this, in turn, contributes to the exclusion experienced by the care recipient.

Simple measures may make a significant difference to carers, for example payment for a professional carer to allow short periods of respite to see friends, go shopping, etc. If this is arranged regularly, the carer may even be able to sustain more regular commitments and roles such as part-time employment or education. Personal care tasks can be especially demanding and support with these especially welcome. A carer who is involved in developing the care plan and who has knowledge of local services will be better able to facilitate attendance and inclusion in community activities.

Carers may seek information and support to help sustain their caring role but may themselves need assistance to access what support is available. In England and Wales, carers are entitled to an assessment of their own care needs (Carers (Equal Opportunities) Act 2004) and some carers are entitled to state benefits.

Many voluntary sector organisations provide support for carers (e.g. the Princess Royal Trust for Carers, www.carers.org). Many voluntary organisations, such as the Alzheimer's Society (www.alzheimers.org.uk), lobby for carers' rights.

Carers whose role is valued, whose needs are considered and who are given appropriate support are more able to sustain their role. They are invaluable in helping service users, as care recipients, maintain roles, relationships and activities and remain socially included.

Conclusion

Psychiatrists understand the importance of exclusion in the lives of patients. They see it every day.

In every field of medicine clinical practice is founded on the establishment of a therapeutic relationship (or partnership) whose key features are empathy, understanding, hope, optimism and a willingness to help. This is no less true in psychiatry and the importance of these elements is not diminished simply because they are hard to measure.

Despite criticism of the medical model as reductionist and purely biomedical, it is, in reality, holistic and includes both scientific and humanistic elements. It is not an obstacle to taking a broad view of a patient's condition, nor an obstacle to addressing social exclusion in mental illness.

For all these reasons the move to socially inclusive practice need not be a major shift for psychiatrists. Indeed, many clinicians will already be familiar with the necessary tools and ultimate aims of practising in this manner – even if they have yet to attach the social inclusion rubric to their work.

Summary

The knowledge, skills and values required of practitioners to support socially inclusive and recovery-oriented practice are described. Although some of these are adaptations of existing practices, many are simply those of a competent clinician and at the heart of good clinical care. Practising in a socially inclusive manner is entirely consistent with the defined duties of doctors and is not at odds with a medical approach. Furthermore, socially inclusive practice is supported by a scientific and humanistic biopsychosocial model – the prevailing orthodoxy in psychiatric practice. These ways of working can bring benefit to service users and also enhance the working life and job satisfaction of clinicians.

References

American Psychiatric Association (2005) *Use of the Concept of Recovery: Position Statement*. APA (http://www.psych.org/Departments/EDU/Library/APAOfficialDocumentsandRelated/PositionStatements/200504.aspx).

Anthony, W. A. (1993) Recovery from mental illness: the guiding vision of the mental health service system in the 1990s. *Psychosocial Rehabilitation Journal*, **16**, 11–23.

Boardman, J. & Walters, P. (2009) Managing depression in primary care: it's not only what you do, it's the way that you do it. *British Journal of General Practice*, **59**, 76–78.

Borg, M. & Kristiansen, K. (2004) Recovery oriented professionals: helping relationships in mental health services. *Journal of Mental Health*, **13**, 493–505.

Clare, A. (1980) *Psychiatry in Dissent* (2nd edn). Routledge.

Cormac, I. & Tihanyi, P. (2006) Meeting the mental and physical healthcare needs of carers. *Advances in Psychiatric Treatment*, **12**, 162–172.

Davidson, L., O'Connell, M., Tondora, J., *et al* (2006) The ten top concerns about recovery encountered in mental health system transformation. *Psychiatric Services*, **57**, 640–645.

Department of Health (2004) *The Ten Essential Shared Capabilities: A Framework for the Whole of the Mental Health Workforce*. Department of Health.

General Medical Council (2006) *Good Medical Practice*. General Medical Council.

Glover, H. (2002) *Developing a Recovery Platform for Mental Health Service Delivery for People with Mental Illness/Distress in England*. National Institute for Mental Health in England.

Horwitz, A. V. & Scheid, T. L. (eds) (1999) *A Handbook for the Study of Mental Health: Social Contexts, Theories and Systems*. Cambridge University Press.

Morgan, C., Burns, T., Fitzpatrick, R., *et al* (2007) Social exclusion and mental health: conceptual and methodological review. *British Journal of Psychiatry*, **191**, 477–483.

Morriss, R. K., Faizal, M. A., Jones, A. P., *et al* (2007) Interventions for helping people recognise early warning signs of recurrence in bipolar disorder. *Cochrane Database of Systematic Reviews*, issue 1, doi: 10.1002/14651858.CD004854.pub2.

Perkins, S. J., Murphy, R., Schmidt, U., *et al* (2006) Self-help and guided self-help for eating disorders. *Cochrane Database of Systematic Reviews*, issue 3, doi: 10.1002/14651858.CD004191.pub2.

Pilgrim, R. (2002) The biopsychosocial model in Anglo-American psychiatry: past, present and future. *Journal of Mental Health*, **11**, 585–594.

Ralph, R. & Corrigan, P. (eds) (2005) *Recovery in Mental Illness: Broadening our Understanding of Wellness*. American Psychological Association.

Roberts, G. & Wolfson, P. (2004) The rediscovery of recovery: open to all. *Advances in Psychiatric Treatment*, **10**, 37–48.

Royal College of Psychiatrists (2007) *Vulnerable Patients, Safe Doctors* (CR 146). Royal College of Psychiatrists.

Royal College of Psychiatrists, Social Care Institute for Excellence & Care Services Improvement Partnership (2007) *A Common Purpose: Recovery in Future Mental Health Services*. SCIE.

Shah, P. & Mountain, D. (2007) The medical model is dead – long live the medical model. *British Journal of Psychiatry*, **191**, 375–377.

Shepherd, G., Boardman, J. & Slade, M. (2008) *Making Recovery a Reality*. Sainsbury Centre for Mental Health.

Warner, R. (2004) *Recovery from Schizophrenia: Psychiatry and Political Economy* (3rd edn). Brunner-Routledge.

CHAPTER 15

Socially inclusive mental health services: what will they look like?

Helen Killaspy and Jed Boardman

What would a socially inclusive service look like?

The previous chapter illustrated the significant implications of recovery-oriented mental health services for partnership working with service users (Care Services Improvement Partnership, 2005). This approach encourages psychiatrists and other mental health professionals to move from a traditional compliance relationship to one of collaboration where there is negotiation in agreeing specific treatments, interventions and all other aspects of the care plan and risk assessment with service users, recognising there are two experts working in partnership, the patient and the clinician (Deegan & Drake, 2006).

Good practice also includes meaningful service user involvement in various aspects of mental health service planning since the direction taken in any new or continuing project will have an impact on the users of the services, and service users know how the system *is* working rather than how it is thought to be working. Support for this comes from NICE (2005):

> The views of patients or service users, their carers and the public matter to NICE. We want to involve them, as well as doctors, nurses, other healthcare professionals and managers in our work. By working with patients, carers, patient organisations and the public, NICE aims to produce guidance that addresses patient/carer/public issues, reflects their views and meets their healthcare needs. Our clinical guidance aims to improve the quality of care across the NHS by providing clinicians and patients with the information they need to make good decisions about treatment and care.

Although it is recognised that there is no such thing as 'the' service user view, service user input can be considered on a continuum of involvement, from user-led to collaborative and consultative. Different approaches have been used successfully to involve service users in service planning and delivery: participation in focus groups; representing users on local borough committees, on trust and health authority committees and on project teams or planning groups; training professionals; being involved in staff recruitment; being active members of mental health charities; acting as research consultants; undertaking paid work within the health system;

leading projects such as user-focused monitoring, which is probably the gold standard in this area. Carers also have a similar role to play in the planning of services.

This paradigm shift in the relationship between service users and mental health professionals has gathered momentum over the past 10 years in the UK, but has been around for much longer in the USA, Australia and New Zealand, where the recovery approach is now well established. In the USA, Liberman & Kopelowicz (2002) have suggested a number of 'markers of recovery' for service users, which were discussed in depth in Chapters 3 and 6, including: working, studying and participating in leisure activities in mainstream settings; good family relationships; living independently; having control of one's self-care, medication and money; having a social life; taking part in the local community; voting; and satisfaction with life. Many of these clearly also reflect a more 'socially included' life. Recovery is closely associated with social inclusion and being able to take on meaningful and satisfying social roles within local communities. It therefore follows that a recovery-oriented mental health service will also be a service that promotes social inclusion. This relationship between recovery approaches, socially inclusive services and improved socially inclusive outcomes is illustrated in Fig. 15.1.

The development of recovery-oriented services presents a series of challenges for mental health services (Box 15.1). The overall challenge is to embed the principles of recovery-oriented practice into all parts of the organisation, from the practices of staff, to the services provided and to the culture of the organisation. This will take time and serious commitment, and, although many mental health trusts have begun to look at ways in which they can develop a recovery orientation, there are enormous

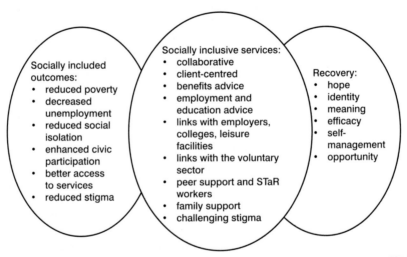

Fig. 15.1 Recovery, socially inclusive services and socially included outcomes. STaR, support, time and recovery.

Box 15.1   Making organisations more recovery-oriented: ten key organisational challenges

1   Changing the nature of day-to-day interactions and the quality of experience
2   Delivering comprehensive, service user-led education and training programme
3   Establishing a 'recovery education centre' to drive the programmes forward
4   Ensuring organisational commitment, creating the 'culture'
5   Increasing personalisation and choice
6   Changing the way we approach risk assessment and management
7   Redefining service user involvement
8   Transforming the workforce
9   Supporting staff in their recovery journey
10 Increasing opportunities for building a life beyond illness.

Source: Sainsbury Centre for Mental Health (2009)

---

variations in their commitment and progress with this agenda. A number of tools to assist clinicians with this process exist, including: the Recovery Star (www.mhpf.org.uk) for service users to monitor their own outcomes; the Wellness Recovery Action Plan (Copeland, 1999) that promotes service users to identify the interventions, supports, people and activities that aid their recovery; advance directives that can be used to plan care for times of crisis; and relapse prevention and crisis plans drawn up through collaborative and therapeutic sessions between service users and staff.

This shift in culture and operation also means making the organisation much more outward looking in order to develop its partnerships with agencies other than mental health organisations, particularly those that provide supported housing and assistance with meaningful occupation, education and employment, so that these become much more of a central focus for care planning alongside medical treatment and other interventions. Mental health services are there to help people with mental health problems live their lives. Stabilising symptoms and optimising social and everyday functioning through specific treatment and interventions are starting points to facilitate this. Supporting service users to access meaningful occupations such as education, employment and leisure must be seen as equally important and not an 'add on' to treatment. Similarly, the facilities and resources that are chosen and developed to encourage successful community living must achieve outcomes based on inclusion in the community, not just integration which may in fact mean co-existence in the same physical location.

The facilitation of service users' access to leisure, education and employment are clearly key roles for mental health services as they support service users through the acute phase(s) of their illness and beyond. Supporting family, carers and employers in order to minimise the loss of service users' valued social roles and to ensure that continuing social support remains available to them is obviously also of paramount importance. Similarly, attention to problems that service users may be experiencing in maintaining stable housing and in their receipt and management of their finances is well within the remit of mental health services. These social interventions are as important as the medical and psychological interventions that can resolve acute symptoms, yet it is easy to relegate these within the context of services that have an ever increasing focus on the management of acute crises. The evidence for interventions that promote social inclusion has been presented in Chapter 13. The capabilities of socially inclusive practice include having individual knowledge of a person's strengths, awareness of the areas of their lives where they are already 'included' and working to sustain these.

Thus, in addition to increased partnership working between individuals (professionals and service users), achieving social inclusion implies increased – and more effective – partnership working between agencies (specifically those providing mental healthcare and social care). Partnership working is essential to facilitate service users' access to socially inclusive activities and their access to services. It includes partnerships between services within the same organisation (thus minimising the chance that service users are caught in 'boundary conflicts' between services), as well as partnerships between organisations. How might this be achieved?

Improving partnership working between agencies

Promoting partnership working between mental health services and community organisations can be facilitated by mental health commissioners and primary care trusts who wish to develop joint social, recreational and employment initiatives, and to plan and oversee appropriately supported housing projects, but it needs to be informed by existing knowledge about the conditions for effective working.

The need for effective partnership working is now part of the traditional rhetoric of mental health service development. Yet, improving partnership working is seldom subjected to any kind of rigorous, academic analysis. What do we mean by it? Can it be operationally defined? How might it be improved?

Partnership working may be defined as the relationship between two or more people or agencies where they work together to achieve agreed and mutually beneficial goals. The phrase 'agreed and mutually beneficial goals' is particularly important – if the partnership does not deliver benefits to both partners it is unlikely to survive. This must be remembered when we are thinking about trying to facilitate more effective partnership working between agencies, where the power relations are often very unequal.

In terms of operationalising effective partnership working there is a substantial research and good practice literature to draw upon (Audit Commission, 2000; NHS Confederation, 2002; Peck, 2003). This suggests strongly that there are a number of key elements that are necessary for effective partnership working (Box 15.2). These may occur independently or in association. Each should therefore be regarded as a 'necessary, but not sufficient' condition.

These statements can be developed into an audit framework which can then be used to assess the quality of partnership relationships and to improve them (Shepherd, 2003).

Promoting social inclusion and combating stigma

As we have seen in Chapters 2 and 3, the concept of social exclusion has a theoretical basis that incorporates components that affect a broad range of disenfranchised social groups, not just mental health service users. The areas of exclusion that are common to all these groups include: material

---

Box 15.2   The main ingredients of effective partnership working

1   Clear, shared vision of goals and objectives
  - there is a clear written statement of overall objectives for the partnership, including identification of areas of mutual benefit
  - there are clear verbal expressions by partners of shared objectives and mutual benefit
  - there is clear evidence of 'inclusivity', i.e. all those agencies or groups that should be included are included
  - members are able to claim to be credible representatives with respect to their respective constituencies
  - there is demonstrable inclusion of minority groups or interests (e.g. ethnicity, gender, religious, cultural groups)
2   Trust and respect between partners (even when there are differences in perspectives and priorities)
  - there is a jointly agreed, written 'code of conduct' for meetings (e.g. avoidance of jargon, encouragement of inclusive participation, toleration of dissent)
  - during meetings partners report they feel that the agreed code of conduct is followed
  - there is clear commitment from all partners in terms of regular, agreed attendance at meetings
  - there is a perception among partners that disagreements are resolved fairly
  - there is an honest acknowledgement of differentials in terms of power and influence
  - there is evidence of joint commitment in terms of co-chairing of meetings.
3   Fair – and transparent – commitment of resources according to capacity
  - there is a clear understanding between the partners regarding the resources in terms of staff, time, administrative support, etc. that each will commit to the partnership
  - the commitment of resources is perceived by both partners to be 'fair' and commensurate with their organisational size and capacity

---

Box 15.2 *(contd)*

- partners are perceived to be delivering the agreed level of resources
- the agreed commitments of resources are subject to regular (e.g. every 6 months or annual) review.

4 Clear lines of accountability (both within and outside the partnership)
- there is a clear, written statement regarding the lines of accountability of the partners (e.g. to whom people report, what the mechanisms for reporting are, how frequently they report)
- there is evidence that the agreed accountabilities are operating in practice (regular reporting, annual reports)
- the workings of the partnership are characterised by clear identification of responsibilities for implementing key actions (e.g. minutes indicate who is responsible for what by when)
- there is evidence that accountabilities are subject to regular review (e.g. every 6 months or annually).

5 Agreement on realistic ways of measuring progress
- there is a clear statement of short- and medium-term objectives, with timescales
- there is a jointly agreed set of process and outcome indicators (e.g. referral patterns, waiting list rates, treatment outcomes)
- there are systems in place for the collection of these agreed indicators.

6 Use of agreed indicators to assess 'productivity' of the partnership (e.g. is it delivering the objectives?)
- the information derived from the progress indicators agreed above is used regularly (minimum annually) to assess progress in achieving objectives
- significant over- or under-achievement is analysed and there is evidence that appropriate actions are then taken.

7 Joint commitment to long-term aims and regular review
- there is a clear statement of the long-term aims of the partnership, with timescales for completion
- there is evidence of consistent commitment of partners over time
- there is evidence of regular reviews of progress and effectiveness of the partnership (e.g. annually)
- there is evidence that processes and goals are adjusted in the light of these reviews

resources (i.e. poverty); productive activity (e.g. work); social relationships (i.e. family and friends); civic activities (e.g. voting); neighbourhood support and involvement (i.e. social capital); and access to appropriate services (Chapter 8). In addition, all socially excluded groups experience stigma and discrimination to various degrees (Social Exclusion Unit, 2004).

In Chapter 14, the ten essential shared capabilities for socially inclusive practice were detailed and these include challenging inequality, stigma and discrimination in order to support individuals to gain and maintain social roles. Stigma against people with mental health problems is well documented and shows little sign of abating. Despite the existence of clear anti-discrimination legislation (for example, the Disability Discrimination

Act 2005) stigma remains a daily reality for many people struggling with the effects of symptoms and attempts to access 'socially included' goals such as employment, training opportunities and housing.

Thornicroft's (2006) distinction between three different components of stigma: ignorance (lack of knowledge or information); prejudice (negative emotional reactions); and discrimination (behaviour that tends to exclude or operate unfairly towards the stigmatised group) is helpful in this regard as it points to action needed to address all three components at both a local and national level. Remedying ignorance requires the provision of relevant information (materials and training); combating prejudice requires face-to-face contact with trained service user educators in a controlled environment; and combating discrimination requires active vigilance (monitoring), combined with appropriate legislation.

The evidence for the effectiveness of general, population-based interventions aimed at reducing stigma is weak and inconclusive. However, the evidence in favour of targeted interventions, aimed at specific groups (e.g. neighbours, employers, police) is more encouraging, although the demonstrated effects appear to be limited to changes in knowledge ('ignorance') and 'prejudice', rather than behavioural change ('discrimination') (Wolff et al, 1996).

It remains to be seen how effective the current national anti-stigma campaigns, Time to Change in England and See Me in Scotland, will be. Time to Change is led by the mental health charities Mind and Rethink and funded by the Big Lottery, whereas See Me is a government-funded initiative. Both comprise programmes of projects such as challenging negative media representations of people with mental health problems, local community based anti-stigma and health promotion projects, national anti-stigma campaigns that use high-profile celebrities and public advertising, legal test cases, training in mental health awareness for student teachers and doctors, and grassroots activism. The campaigns are subject to robust evaluation which will assess their impact and identify their most effective components.

Mental health services and social exclusion

Mental health services can themselves create socially excluding and disempowering environments. In-patient wards may necessarily socially exclude individuals in order to provide a secure environment for the containment of risk. However, they have been greatly criticised for failing to provide a therapeutic and safe environment (Quirk & Lelliott, 2001; Appleby 2003) and those that fail to attend to the recommended standards of care (Department of Health, 2002a) contribute to social exclusion by compounding the factors associated with it. A further example is that of mental health day centres, which are experienced by some as alienating environments that create dependency (Bryant et al, 2004). The National Service Framework for Mental Health (Department of Health, 1999) delineated a strategic approach to reconfigure and invest in community-based services that could deliver more individually tailored support, minimise the need for hospital admissions and therefore reduce the potential for service users to become institutionalised. Current policy highlights the need for mental health services to increase service users' access to, and participation in, the kinds of activities and occupations that the majority of society enjoys. A move away from 'buildings-based' day services and specific guidance and examples of how to do this successfully are detailed in the Care Services Improvement Partnership report *Redesigning Mental Health Day Services* (2005) and the Department of Health (2006) guidance for commissioners.

A person's opportunity to do the things that they value in life is central to their rebuilding their life with mental health problems. This means accessing those opportunities that citizens without mental health problems take for granted. One of the biggest barriers to social inclusion is the low expectations of mental health staff (Social Exclusion Unit, 2004), whereas maintaining hope and realistic expectations are central to recovery (Shepherd *et al*, 2008).

If mental health professionals believe that people with mental health problems can achieve little in life, this not only significantly lowers the expectations of the individual and those around them, it also decreases the extent to which efforts are made to provide the person with help to do the things they want to do ('What would be the point?') and has a wider impact on the expectations of people and organisations outside the mental health system. Low expectations on the part of the individual and low expectations on the part of communities combine to decrease the expectations of both individuals and communities about what people with mental health problems can achieve. Rinaldi & Perkins (2005) have described the way in which this can create a vicious cycle of low expectations that perpetuates and increases social exclusion in relation to employment, but, as noted by the Social Exclusion Unit (2004), the same principles apply to other areas of life (Fig. 15.2).

The status and esteem in which doctors are held both within and outside mental health services, and the leading role that they play in multidisciplinary teams, means that they have a central role in determining the expectations of individual service users as well as the expectations that other staff, and the service as a whole, have for service users. It is therefore extremely important that psychiatrists consider the degree to which their patients are socially excluded. Issues of employment, housing, education or engagement in social and community-based activities should be reviewed at every care programme approach meeting and the promotion of social inclusion should be incorporated into every service user's care plan. Social participation should therefore be seen as a priority from an early stage in care planning.

Holding therapeutic optimism is a critical component in recovery-oriented practice (Roberts & Wolfson, 2004) and taking calculated risks in allowing service users to explore their interest and abilities in relation

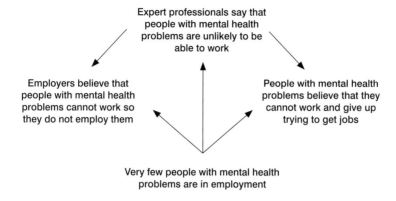

Fig. 15.2 Vicious cycle of low expectations that perpetuates and increases social exclusion. Source: Social Exclusion Unit (2004).

to different community activities may be one aspect of this. Psychiatrists may also hold an important modelling role in disseminating therapeutic optimism among other mental health professionals that people with mental health problems are capable of participation in socially inclusive activities (Bertram & Stickley, 2005).

In addition, psychosocial research has started to pay dividends for conditions such as schizophrenia and is leading to changes in service delivery. However, despite the inclusion of psychosocial and cognitive therapies in clinical practice guidelines, such as those produced by NICE in England, there remain considerable problems with implementing these new treatments. For example, family psychoeducation has an excellent evidence base but is poorly implemented in mental health services, yet engaging and supporting families to support a relative with mental health problems will obviously be of major importance in their social inclusion. Psychiatrists can play an important role in ensuring that adequate staff training is provided for all staff to feel confident about engaging families in their patient's care. They should also advocate for their local service to provide adequately trained staff to deliver family psychoeducation in keeping with NICE (2010) clinical guidelines.

Professional bodies such as the General Medical Council and the Royal College of Psychiatrists have a key role in ensuring that the competences they demand and promote are consistent with the capabilities expected of a socially inclusive psychiatrist. Guidance issued by the General Medical Council (2006) emphasises both collaborative working with service users and facilitation of their empowerment and greater self-care, all of which are consistent with recovery-oriented practice. Similarly, the Royal College of Psychiatrists' *Roles and Responsibilities of the Consultant in General Adult Psychiatry* (2006) stresses the importance of addressing social exclusion to ensure optimal outcomes, of planning healthcare in partnership with service users, of collaborating to support treatment choices (rather than

319

simply prescribing treatments), of considering multiple dimensions when evaluating problems and of a broader cultural understanding.

It follows that individual practitioners and organisations should include evidence of the promotion of socially inclusive practice and social inclusion outcomes in personal development plans, service benchmarking, audit and other forms of clinical governance.

Multidisciplinary approaches and New Ways of Working

The ten capabilities necessary to deliver socially inclusive practice (Box 14.2, pp. 302) need to be available to all those who use mental health services. However, they need not be present to the gold standard in every practitioner. It is here that the team approach advocated in the assertive outreach model (Department of Health, 2001) and in New Ways of Working (Department of Health, 2005) has potential utility. In other words, the philosophy of socially inclusive practice needs to be shared by all and seen as everybody's business, but the sharing of the skills of the team is likely to be both more efficient and more effective than expecting every member of the team to be expert in all aspects of socially inclusive practice.

New Ways of Working embodies a genuine joint and collaborative effort between a range of professionals and experts with complementary skills but similar core values, rather than allocation of separate responsibilities by delegation. It is also a further illustration of the first capability of socially inclusive practice: working in partnership. At a team and service level, to work in a way that promotes socially inclusive practice demands a significant change in ways of working for all mental health practitioners and the need for consideration of the competences and skills required to facilitate such practice. Partnership working is key to delivering socially inclusive outcomes that service users value.

All members of the multidisciplinary team play a significant role in promoting recovery and socially inclusive practice and as such this practice needs to be considered at the outset of working with service users. For example, initial assessments in teams need to include a thorough assessment of social roles, relationships and activities, with the outcomes of the assessment being meaningfully included within care plans and reviewed with the same importance as other issues in a care programme approach review. Individual care plans need to include targets relating to the maintenance of existing roles, relationships and activities for all service users.

However, the specialist skills of individual team members may be particularly relevant to some aspects of socially inclusive practice. As senior clinicians, psychiatrists can play a key role in leading, facilitating or encouraging partnership working with other statutory and non-statutory organisations, in planning new initiatives for community-based activities and supported housing, and in advocating for adequately resourced mental health teams to provide a service that is capable of promoting social inclusion. They are key in reinforcing the message that social inclusion is 'everybody's business' and in helping to define how individual team members' skills may be best used to promote social inclusion.

For example, occupational therapists have many years' experience of forming links with mainstream leisure facilities, colleges and other higher education institutions, employment agencies and other vocational rehabilitation services to facilitate service users' community activities in mainstream settings. As occupation forms an important part of each person's personal and social identity (in the eyes of the world and in our own eyes we are largely what we do), it is obvious that service users also require occupations that enable them to make a contribution to society and reward them for that contribution. Occupational therapy services often lead on partnerships with key community organisations (such as Jobcentre Plus, adult education, voluntary and leisure services), promoting socially inclusive interventions, such as job retention or preparation, re-engagement with community facilities or supporting the development of confidence and skills to take on valued roles in society again. A number of successful initiatives that have supported service users to access community activities such as sport, arts, education, volunteering and employment have been reported in *New Ways of Working for Everyone* (Department of Health, 2007), in particular in the sections describing New Ways of Working for occupational therapists and allied health professionals (relevant documents can be found at www.newwaysofworking.org.uk).

Bridge builders

Historically, addressing service users' social needs has been seen as part of the work of mental health services, but the way in which this has been implemented has a number of serious shortcomings. Individual care coordinators often lack specialist knowledge and expertise in these areas and it is not infrequently the case that qualified mental health professionals' time is spent doing practical tasks that do not require their specialist expertise and could be better performed by someone with different skills. In ensuring that each person's social needs are addressed within the initial assessment and care plans, teams need to have much closer working relationships with a whole range of mainstream organisations and services in their areas. Like a lot of change, such an approach would, at first, be perceived to add a burden onto care coordinators. Nevertheless, closer partnership working between teams and a range of mainstream agencies and organisations is essential if we are to improve individual social outcomes.

The skills and competences that are often lacking within mental health services are those that facilitate effective 'bridge building' between mental health services and local communities. Such an approach is required if service users are to access mainstream opportunities in the local area. This approach requires knowledge of what is available locally and how it works, as well as the personal links and support necessary to increase the capacity of different mainstream agencies and organisations to accommodate people with mental health problems while providing support for them to access these services. In effect there are three aspects to bridge building:

1   knowledge of mainstream community agencies/organisations within a local area

2   contacts within these agencies/organisations to help build their capacity to offer services to people with mental health problems

3   provision of support to enable people with mental health problems to access these mainstream community agencies/organisations.

Bridge building works across key life domains such as sports and leisure (including healthy living), homes, family and neighbourhood, faith and spirituality, performing and visual arts, and volunteering. A bridge builder could be any member of a multidisciplinary team who has specific knowledge, skills and experience within one or more of these domains. As well as occupational therapists, of particular note is the contribution of support, time and recovery (STaR) workers (Department of Health, 2003). They have already been shown to achieve good outcomes in terms of promoting a more individually tailored approach to the facilitation of service users' daytime activities and community integration (Davis *et al*, 2004; Department of Health, 2008).

Bridge builders may work with other members of the team to deliver different aspects of bridge building. Their role is to focus on community engagement with mainstream community agencies/organisations to effectively support a person to participate within an activity or support them through a particular social crisis. They provide practical support to help people to access different social activities. For example, they can give information about the facilities and activities that are available locally, they can organise or provide individual peer or staff support for individuals to access facilities (such as going swimming together, going to church, a club, etc.), they might set up a specialist group or session within a mainstream community setting (e.g. an introduction session at the local gym), or they might identify 'mentors' within mainstream settings who can provide informal support to individuals when they visit or attend the facility (e.g. a member of the local church, a friendly local librarian, etc.). They can also negotiate any reasonable adjustments that the person might need to access these mainstream facilities and support staff to work effectively with people with mental health problems, providing a clear point of contact if they have any difficulties (Box 15.3).

Transforming the workforce

A further means of creating inclusive mental health services would be to increase the numbers of people who have a lived experience of mental health problems in the workforce. There are two main ways by which this may be achieved: through employing people with mental health problems

---

Box 15.3 Bridge builders: examples of provision of practical assistance

Bridge builders may:

- help people to access concessionary rates for using services/facilities/transport
- help people to get all the welfare benefits to which they are entitled, either directly or by accessing other sources of expertise
- help people to access the direct payments via which they can fund the support they need to do the things they want to do
- offer support to establish, re-establish and maintain friends and close relationships
- provide a drop-in service involving volunteers and people on work experience to encourage individuals to socialise in the evenings and at weekends
- provide people with help to clean and maintain their homes
- support people to pay their rent/sort out any debts they may have
- help people to
  - liaise with housing providers when problems occur
  - resolve disputes with neighbours
  - move into new accommodation to set up home, get the things they need, buy/assemble furniture, etc.
  - negotiate moves to different accommodation should this be necessary
- help people admitted to in-patient care to make sure that their homes are fit to return to when they are discharged
- make links with people who live alone and are about to be discharged from in-patient care, making sure that they have the things they need at home, taking them home, helping them to settle in, and supporting them over the first few days.

---

in the general trust workforce and by increasing the number of peer support specialists working in mental health teams. There is already a commitment (Department of Health, 2002b) and useful guidance (e.g. Seebohm & Grove, 2006) to employing people with mental health problems in mental health services in England. The introduction of support, time and recovery workers may provide the basis for introducing peer support workers (Department of Health, 2003). Both these approaches would help in transforming the workforce, shifting the focus towards those with experience of mental health problems and possibly challenging some entrenched views of existing mental health workers and stigma.

Good examples of the employment of people with mental health problems in the NHS trusts' workforce are uncommon, but one can be seen in the South West London and St George's Mental Health NHS Trust. The Trust established a user employment programme in 1995, designed to increase access to ordinary jobs within mental health services for people who have themselves experienced mental health problems. They have achieved good rates of employment: between 1995 and 2007, 142 people were supported in 163 posts within the Trust and on 1 January 2007, 86% of these people continued to work within or outside the organisation or were engaged in professional training (Perkins *et al*, 2010). In addition, in every year between 1999 and 2006, at least 15% of new recruits within the Trust were people who had themselves experienced mental health problems.

The use of peer support workers aims to increase the number of people with lived experience who work in mental health teams and directly with service users. A model for this approach can be seen in an American mental health provider organisation, META, which has taken a radical approach to promoting recovery. A not-for-profit organisation, META recruits and trains people with lived experience to work alongside other professionals in the organisation (Ashcraft & Anthony, 2005; Hutchinson *et al*, 2006). Such people comprise at least 70% of META's workforce, working both full and part time, and by radically changing the ratio of the profession to peer-support staff they have successfully transformed the culture of the organisation. Peer support workers are engaged in all areas of service provided by META, from generic mental health services, to crisis response, to housing and employment. Importantly, META consistently meets its performance targets, competing in the tough world of independent mental health sector providers in the USA.

The use of peer support workers would require a commitment to create training schemes to be devised to support their development. A 'recovery education unit' could be set up in each trust, staffed and run by educators who are, or have been, service users and linked to the delivery of the trust's recovery strategy (Sainsbury Centre for Mental Health, 2009). Such a unit would not only train people to provide direct care as 'peer professionals' within the service, it would also train and support people with lived experience of mental health problems to tell their stories and promote awareness of recovery principles among staff and other service users. The education unit would need to work with local education providers to ensure that the training is of a high standard and to be able to offer accredited courses. A potential beneficial off-shoot of this kind of development would be the general promotion of an educational, rather than a therapeutic, model.

Community development

In considering how services may facilitate the social inclusion of people with mental health problems, it may be useful to broaden the focus of intervention from the individual to the community. Community development (Communities and Local Government, 2006) – 'a progressive intervention that helps people identify common concerns and then work together to address them, all in ways which promote equality, inclusiveness and participation' (Seebohm & Gilchrist, 2008: p. 17) – may help in this regard. Community development workers may be either paid or unpaid.

Community development has a long history (Communities and Local Government, 2006) and there is some evidence that community development workers have a role to play in empowering participation for people with mental health problems (Seebohm & Gilchrist, 2008). They may enable people with longer-term mental health problems to participate in community activities (Pozner *et al*, 2000; Sainsbury Centre for Mental Health, 2000) or share in decision-making; they may help to improve social capital (Gilchrist, 2002); assist in reducing stigma (Quinn & Knifton, 2005); foster peer support and mutual aid (Seebohm *et al*, 2005); and improve the lives of Black and minority ethnic groups (Thomas *et al*, 2006).

A qualitative study of community development workers and participants in community development projects (Seebohm & Gilchrist, 2008) found that the community development practitioners helped mental health staff to improve services for diverse communities, worked to improve awareness of mental health problems in generic services, and developed structures, processes and skills for public participation. The study concluded that 'at its best [community development] has much to offer...[it] can contribute to individual recovery and community well-being through making connections between groups and organisations. People who are often excluded can be included both as a participant and leader in their communities' (p. 58).

Such an approach clearly has a potentially valuable role in improving social inclusion for people with mental health problems and as such it needs further support and wider implementation.

How to achieve organisational change?

Both clinical leadership and management are needed for organisations to progress (Byrne, 2006). If culture and practice are to be changed, recovery and socially inclusive practice must be part of the core business of the organisation as a whole. It is important to harness the energies of mental health professionals and managers in the quest for improvements in performance that benefit service users. To succeed with this requires managers to develop a better appreciation of the organisations they are striving to change, and mental health professionals to acknowledge the need for change (Berwick, 1994). It is often assumed that changes in practice result from changes in principles and attitudes, but causality can operate in the other direction as well: changes in values and philosophy may be a consequence of changes in practice. This is where both clinical leadership and management play important roles.

The Department of Health (2006) guidance on commissioning day services, along with the report of the National Social Inclusion Programme (2008) on the reconfiguration of day services, provide some useful markers for psychiatrists who want to become involved as mediators, supporters, or even champions of change within their own organisations (Box 15.4).

Obstacles to change

Despite this helpful advice, a number of barriers can potentially impede the progress of developing more socially inclusive services. As indicated, individuals may resist changes to their usual daytime activities, particularly if they have formed an important attachment to a 'building-based' service such as a day centre. This may be a manifestation of psychopathology (e.g. personality issues such as dependency) or symptoms of psychosis such as paranoid delusions, concrete thinking or amotivation. Any of these can lead to fears and anxieties about the proposed change and subsequent inflexibility and resistance to it. However, for mental health professionals who are trained in the assessment and management of psychopathology, these factors should not be insurmountable.

Mental health professionals themselves may resist these kinds of service redesign because of their natural confidence in 'well-tried and tested' service options which provide a container for their own anxieties about

---

Box 15.4 Commissioning day services: some useful markers for psychiatrists

- Gain local support for the change
  At the outset, get explicit support for change from provider organisations and people using the service by involving them in reviewing existing service provision to ensure it better meets people's needs. This includes ensuring all views and reservations are heard and acknowledged.

- Ensure leadership from the top
  An understanding of, and commitment to, modernisation from those who hold financial responsibility, including elected officials in local authorities and those at director level in commissioning and provider organisations, is critical to seeing through service change in the face of resistance.

- Keep people involved and informed
  People using the services, carers and providers should be involved throughout the process, giving an opportunity for them to understand the issues, influence the process and take ownership of the outcomes. This should include both face-to-face and written communication and recognition that consultation is a two-way process.

- Be clear as to what is being proposed
  Often the uncertainty and lack of clarity causes as much anxiety as the proposals. Address people's fears, but also be clear and transparent about what is not known.

- Help people to visualise the modernised services
  There is often an acute sense of loss for staff and people using the service when changes are proposed. This can be mitigated by giving a clear sense of the reality of, and gains inherent in, the new model for service delivery.

- Talk to others who have been there
  Facilitating people who use the service and staff to meet with their peers in other services that have already been through a restructuring process can be very beneficial, as can visiting modernised services to see how they operate.

Sources: Department of Health (2006), National Social Inclusion Programme (2008)

---

how best to support patients. Professionals may also feel deskilled at the suggestion of more individually tailored support to facilitate service users' access to mainstream activities and occupations. They may fear that this could cause unnecessary stress, even potential relapse. Such views should not be dismissed, but need to be weighed carefully for each person, taking into account their specific level of function and abilities.

Those who work in mental health services may view the current focus on socially inclusive practice as a passing fashion that they do not need to attend to in the context of other competing demands on their time and energy. Hospital-based services may consider that social inclusion is a job for community services and they, in turn, may feel it is a job for the voluntary sector. Resistance may arise from any (or all) of these sources.

Senior service managers and clinicians therefore need to use their experience and expertise in appropriate change management to prevent these resistors from stifling socially inclusive practice. There are similarities here with the obstacles identified by Shepherd *et al* (2008) in the implementation of recovery-oriented practice (Chapter 14, Box 14.3). For example, in responding to the criticism that recovery orientation is 'an irresponsible fad', the authors highlight that recovery is in fact a convergence of an increasing emphasis in policy and practice on service user empowerment, self-management, disability rights, social inclusion and rehabilitation, and that its implementation does not require new policies or services, but a commitment to make services work more effectively in direct response to service users' needs.

Shepherd *et al* also make the very important point that, 'It is certainly not helpful if professionals think that they carry the sole responsibility for how people live their lives' (p. 7). This sentiment seems particularly pertinent not just to the recovery orientation of services and collaborative working with service users, but to the forging and maintenance of helpful partnerships with other organisations that can facilitate social inclusion of mental health service users.

What are the benefits of socially inclusive practice?

By addressing the skills and competences of recovery-oriented practice, service user involvement in service planning, bridge building and community development, people access individualised help and support based on their preferences and choice. The service focuses on community engagement with a view to building the capacity of those mainstream agencies/organisations to accommodate people with mental health problems. This approach may effectively break down the stigma and discrimination that people with mental health problems experience. A frequent finding within the literature on community engagement in relation to people with mental health problems and as identified in the *Mental Health and Social Exclusion* report (Office of the Deputy Prime Minister, 2004) is that community agencies and organisations can find relating to mental health services extremely confusing. If links are to be forged by many different teams and a lot of individual care coordinators, external agencies have difficulty in finding a consistent point of contact when a problem arises, which often results in such agencies choosing not to work with people with mental health problems. In addition, by working in closer partnership with other agencies and organisations this opens up further potential funding opportunities for services through, for example, Supporting People or the Arts Council and Sports Council funding. There are obvious benefits for carers too since a greater focus on planning and delivering a more socially inclusive package of care will inevitably increase service users' social supports and networks and potentially reduce carer burden. Clinicians, especially care coordinators, may also experience a sense of having a shared responsibility with other providers as they expand their community resource networks. In addition, they may also have the positive challenge of witnessing service users achieving in community activities that extend way beyond their original expectations.

Summary

Recovery-oriented practice plays a central role in developing socially inclusive mental health services and services should be designed to deliver 'socially in-cluded' outcomes. Ten organisational challenges are outlined for mental health services which emphasise the need to embed recovery ideas throughout the organisation. Importantly, mental health services should work in partnership with other agencies and address ignorance, prejudice and discrimination. It is important in service planning that measures are taken to increase the number of people with lived experience of mental health problems working in mental health services, to re-design day services, follow multidisciplinary approaches, introduce bridge builders and develop new forms of partnership with service users.

References

Appleby, L. (2003) So, are things getting better? *Psychiatric Bulletin*, **27**, 441–442.

Ashcraft, L. & Anthony, W. A. (2005) A story of transformation: an agency fully embraces recovery. *Behavioural Healthcare Tomorrow*, **14**, 12–22.

Audit Commission (2000) *Developing Productive Partnerships – A Bulletin*. District Audit.

Bertram, G. & Stickley, T. (2005) Mental health nurses, promoters of inclusion or perpet-uators of exclusion? *Journal of Psychiatric and Mental Health Nursing*, **12**, 387–395.

Berwick, D. (1994) Eleven worthy aims for clinical leadership of health system reform. *Journal of the American Medical Association*, **272**, 797–802.

Bryant, W., Craik, C. & McKay, E. A. (2004) Living in a glasshouse: exploring occupational alienation. *Canadian Journal of Occupational Therapy*, **71**, 282–289.

Byrne, P. (2006) A response to the Mental Health Commission's discussion paper 'Multi-disciplinary Team Working: From Theory to Practice'. *Irish Psychologist*, **32**, 323–339.

Care Services Improvement Partnership (2005) *Redesigning Mental Health Day Services: A Modernisation Toolkit for London*. Care Services Improvement Partnership.

Communities and Local Government (2006) *The Community Development Challenge*. Communities and Local Government.

Copeland, M. E. (1999) *Wellness Recovery Action Plan*. Peach Press.

Davis, F. A., Alder, S. & Jones, P. (2004) Day services modernisation and social inclusion. *A Life in the Day*, **8(3)**, 18–24.

Deegan, P. & Drake, R. E. (2006) Shared decision making and medication management in the recovery process. *Psychiatric Services*, **57**, 1636–1639.

Department of Health (1999) *National Service Framework for Mental Health*. Department of Health.

Department of Health (2001) *Mental Health Policy Implementation Guide: Assertive Community Treatment Teams*. Department of Health.

Department of Health (2002a) *Acute Adult In-Patient Care: Policy Implementation Guide*. Department of Health.

Department of Health (2002b) *Mental Health and Employment in the NHS*. Department of Health.

Department of Health (2003) *Mental Health Policy Implementation Guide: Support, Time and Recovery (STR) Workers*. Department of Health.

Department of Health (2005) *New Ways of Working for Psychiatrists. Enhancing Effective, Person-Centred Services through New Ways of Working in Multidisciplinary and Multiagency Contexts*. Department of Health.

Department of Health (2006) *From Segregation to Inclusion: Commissioning Guidance on Day Services for People with Mental Health Problems*. Department of Health.

Department of Health (2007) *Mental Health: New Ways of Working for Everyone. Developing and Sustaining a Capable and Flexible Workforce (A Progress Report)*. Department of Health.

Department of Health (2008) *Support, Time and Recovery (STR) Workers Learning from the National Implementation Programme*. Department of Health.

General Medical Council (2006) *Good Medical Practice*. General Medical Council.

Gilchrist, A. (2002) *The Well-Connected Community*. Policy Press.

Hutchinson, D. S., Anthony, W. A., Ashcraft, L., *et al* (2006) The personal and vocational impact of training and employing people with psychiatric disabilities as providers. *Psychiatric Rehabilitation Journal*, **29**, 205–213.

Liberman, R. P. & Kopelowicz, A. (2002) Recovery from schizophrenia: a challenge for the 21st century. *International Review of Psychiatry*, **14**, 245–255.

National Institute for Health and Clinical Excellence (2005) *Patient and Public Involvement Policy*. NICE (http://www.nice.org.uk/getinvolved/patientandpublicinvolvement/patientandpublicinvolvementpolicy/patient_and_public_involvement_policy.jsp).

National Institute for Health and Clinical Excellence (2010) *Core Interevntions in the Treatment and Management of Schizophrenia in Adults in Primary and Secondary Care (update)* (NCG82). British Psychological Society & Royal College of Psychiatrists.

National Social Inclusion Programme (2008) *From Segregation to Inclusion: Where Are We Now?* National Social Inclusion Programme.

NHS Confederation (2002) *Getting Closer: A Guide to Partnerships in New Health Policy*. NHS Confederation.

Office of the Deputy Prime Minister (2004) *Mental Health and Social Exclusion*. ODPM.

Peck, E. (2003) Partnership working: principles, progress and practice. *University of Birmingham, School of Public Policy, Health Services Management Centre Newsletter*, **9**, 2–3.

Perkins, R., Rinaldi, M. & Hardisty, J. (2010) Harnessing the expertise of experience: increasing access to employment within mental health services for people who have themselves experienced mental health problems. *Diversity in Health and Care*, **7**, 13–21.

Pozner, A., Hammond, J. & Ng, M. L. (2000) *Working Together: Images of Partnership*. Pavilion Publishing.

Quinn, N. & Knifton, L. (2005) Promoting recovery and addressing stigma: mental health awareness through community development in a low income area. *International Journal of Mental Health Promotion*, **7**, 37–44.

Quirk, A. & Lelliott, P. (2001) What do we know about life on acute psychiatric wards in the UK? A review of the research evidence. *Social Science and Medicine*, **53**, 1565–1574.

Rinaldi, M. & Perkins, R. (2005) Early intervention: a hand up the slippery slope. In *New Ways of Thinking about Mental Health and Employment* (eds B. Grove, J. Secker & P. Seebohm). Radcliffe Press.

Roberts, G. & Wolfson, P. (2004) The rediscovery of recovery: open to all. *Journal of Mental Health*, **10**, 37–49.

Royal College of Psychiatrists (2006) *Roles and Responsibilities of the Consultant in General Adult Psychiatry* (CR 140). Royal College of Psychiatrists.

Sainsbury Centre for Mental Health (2000) *On Your Doorstep: Community Organisations and Mental Health*. Sainsbury Centre for Mental Health.

Sainsbury Centre for Mental Health (2009) *Implementing Recovery: A New Framework for Organisational Change*. Position Paper. Sainsbury Centre for Mental Health.

Seebohm, P. & Gilchrist, A. (2008) *Connect and Include: An Exploratory Study of Community Development and Mental Health*. National Social Inclusion Programme.

Seebohm, P. & Grove, B. (2006) *Leading by Example: Making the NHS an Exemplar Employer of People with Mental Health Problems*. Sainsbury Centre for Mental Health.

Seebohm, P., Henderson, P., Munn-Giddings, C., et al (2005) *Together we will Change: Community Development, Mental Health and Diversity*. Sainsbury Centre for Mental Health.

Shepherd, G., Boardman, J. & Slade, M. (2008) *Making Recovery a Reality*. Sainsbury Centre for Mental Health.

Shepherd, G. (2003) *An Audit Framework for Partnership Working*. Cambridgeshire and Peterborough NHS Foundation Trust.

Social Exclusion Unit (2004) *Action on Mental Health: A Guide to Promoting Social Inclusion*. Office of the Deputy Prime Minister.

Thomas, P., Seebohm, P., Henderson, P., et al (2006) Tackling race inequalities: community development, mental health and diversity. *Journal of Public Mental Health*, **5**, 13–19.

Thornicroft, G. (2006) *Shunned: Discrimination against People with Mental Illness*. Oxford University Press.

Wolff, G., Pathare, S., Craig, T., et al (1996) Community attitudes to mental illness. *British Journal of Psychiatry*, **168**, 183–190.

CHAPTER 16

Training for socially inclusive practice

Jed Boardman, Alan Currie, Helen Killaspy and Gillian Mezey

In Chapters 14 and 15 we set out some of the components for the future of socially inclusive psychiatric practice and service delivery. In this chapter we examine some of the implications of this for the training of psychiatrists. It is important that the principles of social inclusion and recovery are embedded in the training of future psychiatrists, whether they be medical students or psychiatric trainees, and in the continuing professional development of consultant psychiatrists and non-consultant grades. This shift in training also applies to other mental health professionals and a consensus across these groups needs to be developed as to what is required in training and practice to deliver the shift from conventional to socially inclusive practice.

The training and policy context

Policy drivers

There have been a number of policy drivers to promote social inclusion and to reduce stigma and discrimination in mental health service users, including the recovery approach, the expert patient initiative and New Ways of Working, which we have outlined in Chapter 4. In addition, two further policies that relate to socially inclusive practice are: the Race Equality Action Plan and the Disability Discrimination Act 1995 (with 2001 and 2005 amendments) (Sayce & Boardman, 2003, 2008).

Revision of postgraduate medical training

The changes to the curriculum for trainee psychiatrists of the Royal College of Psychiatrists (2009) seen since 2000 and the move towards the acquisition of specific competences during training (knowledge, skills and behaviour) provide an opportunity to ensure that social inclusion is incorporated as a unifying theme of mental health service provision. Social inclusion in mental healthcare can be seen as part of a cultural shift towards patient/user choice, empowerment and partnerships between patients and carers, as opposed to the traditionally didactic and disempowered status of mental health users, particularly in relation to their consultant psychiatrists.

There has been a radical overhaul of postgraduate medical training, resulting in the development of specialty-specific training posts, a new curriculum and the development of competence-based assessments. The main psychiatric specialties, represented by the Faculties of the Royal College of Psychiatrists, have been involved in developing their own competence-based curricula and workplace-based assessments for trainees. Social inclusion competences need to be incorporated into these frameworks.

Undergraduate medical training

Medical students are trained to think of themselves as future team leaders with overall responsibility and ultimate say over treatment and care decisions, and some may find it hard to relinquish that role and sense of control over treatment decision-making. Trainees entering psychiatry may find the more egalitarian and multidisciplinary approach to patient care takes some adapting to, and some trainees may be better at this than others.

There are variations between medical schools in the amount of time allocated to, and integration between, core teaching in psychiatry and what is taught on related topics such as psychology, psychopharmacology and communication skills. Some schools have considerable vertical integration of aspects of psychiatry throughout the curriculum but in others psychiatry is taught as an isolated block.

What is required is an undergraduate curriculum that specifies the key aspects of knowledge, skills and attitudes related to psychiatry that medical students require for basic competence. There is also a need to meet the standards of *Tomorrow's Doctors* (General Medical Council, 2009), which forms the basis for subsequent training through the Foundation Programme and into Specialty Training. *Tomorrow's Doctors* was originally published in 1993 and has been reviewed and revised to adapt to modern medical practice. It reiterates the duties of a doctor registered with the General Medical Council, which stress the importance of working in partnership with patients (Box 16.1).

Specific to teaching in clinical psychiatry, the principal aims of the undergraduate medical course are:

- to provide students with knowledge of the main psychiatric disorders, the principles underlying modern psychiatric theory, commonly used treatments and a basis on which to continue to develop this knowledge
- to assist students to develop the necessary skills to apply this knowledge in clinical situations
- to encourage students to develop the appropriate attitudes necessary to respond empathically to psychological distress in all medical settings.

Box 16.1   The duties of a doctor registered with the General Medical Council

Patients must be able to trust doctors with their lives and health. To justify that trust you must show respect for human life and you must:

- make the care of your patient your first concern
- protect and promote the health of patients and the public
- provide a good standard of practice and care
  - keep your professional knowledge and skills up to date
  - recognise and work within the limits of your competence
  - work with colleagues in the ways that best serve patients' interests
- treat patients as individuals and respect their dignity
  - treat patients politely and considerately
  - respect patients' right to confidentiality
- work in partnership with patients
  - listen to patients and respond to their concerns and preferences
  - give patients the information they want or need in a way they can understand
  - respect patients' right to reach decisions with you about their treatment and care
  - support patients in caring for themselves to improve and maintain their health
- be honest and open and act with integrity
  - act without delay if you have good reason to believe that you or a colleague may be putting patients at risk
  - never discriminate unfairly against patients or colleagues
  - never abuse your patients' trust in you or the public's trust in the profession.

You are personally accountable for your professional practice and must always be prepared to justify your decisions and actions.

Source: General Medical Council (2009)

The medical school curriculum has the opportunity to influence the development of all future doctors in their knowledge and attitudes to mental illness. Future doctors need to be aware of the ignorance, prejudice and discrimination faced by people with mental ill health and to understand the importance of developing partnerships between health services and service users and carers. Training provides an opportunity for students to reflect on their preconceptions, assumptions and prejudices about people with mental health problems, particularly individuals who self-harm or abuse substances, who are often perceived as particularly unworthy of empathy. In addition, the nature of the association between social conditions and circumstances and ill health needs to be understood.

Undergraduate medical school teaching in psychiatry should emphasise the 'equal but different' roles of professionals within mental health multidisciplinary teams and the importance of moving away from the traditional hierarchical structure of doctor and patient. Undergraduates need to understand the rationale for social inclusion and the related policy drivers, as well as the adverse health consequences of social exclusion.

All undergraduate curricula contain a significant component of communication skills training. This should emphasise the importance of the narrative approach, which should sit alongside the diagnostic component of medical practice and culturally sensitive skills and the challenges of using interpreters and/or language line (telephone interpreting service). The need to understand the individual as part of a wider social network and to include carers, where appropriate, in illness education and treatment decisions, must also be emphasised in training.

Postgraduate medical training

Contemporary training for new roles requires the definition of new competences, which should include those underpinning socially inclusive practice. Social inclusion should be explicitly incorporated into these frameworks and competences, rather than being seen as a secondary or incidental output. Consultant psychiatrists have a responsibility to ensure they have the competences to deliver the practice and services related to social inclusion, alongside their non-medical colleagues, and to develop these competences through appropriate training. Inclusion is everyone's job rather than being left to inclusion 'specialists'. The curriculum should contain elements that overlap with the issues that have been under consideration in this book, examples of which are shown in Box 16.2.

The development of competences to promote self-management, self-care and self-help should be added to the curriculum (see also Chapter 14). Self-management programmes emerged concurrently with expert patient initiatives (Department of Health, 2001; see Chapter 4), which encourage people with specific conditions to teach others with the same condition to manage their illness. Understanding trigger and warning signs can be used to develop self-management strategies, in partnership with psychiatrists and other mental health professionals. Self-medication, advanced directives and the development of crisis plans are part of the same approach. All contribute to the need for change in the traditional therapeutic relationship; such change requires a shift in the nature of the therapeutic relationship, from powerful prescriber to partner, coach and mentor.

Competences that psychiatrists need

The competences relevant to socially inclusive practice should be covered in the postgraduate curriculum, including those relating to self-management. Many of these are general competences, applicable to all psychiatrists, but those particularly relevant to each subspecialty should also be included. It can be useful to consider these competences under several headings including knowledge, attitudes, skills and behaviour, and examples of these

---

Box 16.2   Elements of social inclusion to be incorporated into the postgraduate curriculum

- All therapeutic interventions are set within a framework that acknowledges and respects diversity, social background, race and culture. Particular attention should be given to the nature and consequences of stigma, discrimination and exclusion. We should recognise that social inequality and exclusion have a potentially devastating effect on the recovery process.
- Psychiatrists should apply knowledge of specific techniques and methods that facilitate effective and empathic communication between the psychiatrist, patient, carers, colleagues and the wider healthcare system.
- Psychiatrists should demonstrate respect for the patient, taking their cultural, ethical and economic background and its impact into account by: practising in a manner that demonstrates respect for the diverse cultures, beliefs and values of patients, and promoting patients' rights to choice, confidentiality and protection while also recognising the complexities of competing rights, responsibilities and demands.
- Psychiatrists should seek to promote recovery by creating, developing or maintaining valued social roles for patients in the communities they come from. We should work in partnership to provide care and treatment that enables patients and carers to tackle mental health problems with hope and optimism and work towards a valued lifestyle within and beyond the limits of any mental health problem.
- Psychiatrists should work in partnership with primary care and other support services, be open to new ideas and developments that will improve patient care, wherever and whenever possible, work with patients and carers to develop collaborative management plans, and engage and sustain relationships with service users in a manner that maximises their participating and optimises cooperation and consent.

---

are set out in Boxes 16.3–16.7). Central to these competences are the ten essential shared capabilities set out in Chapter 14.

Knowledge

Box 16.3 shows some of the areas of knowledge that psychiatrists need to be aware of to support their daily practice, but they also need a broader array of knowledge to aid them in developing a clear understanding of the concepts relating to social exclusion/inclusion and recovery. This may be provided through an understanding of public health and epidemiology and the developing literature on well-being, health inequalities and the social causes of ill health, the prevention of ill health, and the underlying principles of recovery. To this list may be added knowledge of the development of government policies and how they bear upon mental health services. This base of knowledge provides the broader picture of our day-to-day practice and places it in context to society and the individual. To this should be added a firm knowledge of research that will aid in the critical appraisal of evidence.

> **Box 16.3   Competences relevant to socially inclusive practice: knowledge**
>
> In order to promote socially inclusive practice, psychiatrists should:
>
> - know locality resources and how to access them
> - have knowledge of legal rights and obligations (including housing law, child care, welfare rights, the Mental Health Act and access to citizenship)
> - know key policy drivers – the Expert Patient, New Ways of Working, Ten Essential Shared Capabilities
> - be familiar with the evidence base linking social exclusion with poor mental health
> - know what helps and impedes recovery and be aware of the diversity of significant factors to specific individuals
> - understand the background and historical context of concern for social inclusion and the significance of the service user and recovery movements
> - know how to negotiate ceasing treatments and stepping down supports once they are no longer needed, with an understanding of how overprovision of treatment or support can promote an unproductive dependency and be an impediment to self-care
> - develop knowledge of the range of self-care and self-management tools, their strengths and limitations
> - know supports for self-directed care and how to access resources and integrate them with complex care plans, for example direct payments, individual budgets and the care programme approach
> - be fully aware of the risk of misunderstanding concerning diagnosis and treatment and be skilled in sharing professional knowledge with patients and their families in ways they will retain and understand
> - understand the pivotal significance of hope in supporting recovery and be able to cultivate and sustain hope for individuals, teams and services
> - remain up to date with emerging evidence concerning evaluation of self-care methods and the assessment of recovery outcomes and recovery-based practice for individuals and services
> - have a wide knowledge of patient or service user-led support structures, peer groups and self-help resources in the local community
> - have a broad understanding of mediating factors of social inclusion and exclusion in society
> - understand the significance of discovery or rediscovery of a personal framework for identity that is not centred on illness or participation in psychiatric services
> - recognise the role that medical practitioners can play, as members of society, in promoting social inclusion through their services, their practice and themselves, and create bridges and opportunities for their patients.

Attitudes

Values are central to the adoption of socially inclusive practice and it is important to consciously address these in a dynamic way (Fulford & Woodbridge, 2007). Values-based practice may be seen as 'a way of working in health and social care that starts from respect for individual differences and provides a clear process for coming to balanced decisions where values are in conflict' (Fulford & Woodbridge, 2007: p. 146). The ten principles of values-based practice are shown in Box 16.4. Some of the values for mental health were set out in the NIMHE emerging national framework (NIMHE, 2005), itself drawing on three principles of values-based practice: recognition (role of values alongside evidence in all areas of mental health policy and practice), awareness (of the values involved in different contexts, their role and their effect on practice) and respect (of the diversity of values). An overriding principle here is that of the service user as a central and unifying focus for practice, with the values of each individual user of services and their communities being a key determinant for all actions by professionals. This idea of respect for diversity of values covers many of the concepts outlined in Chapters 3 and 5, including equality, citizenship and opposition to discrimination. The NIMHE values framework also holds this respect for diversity to be user-centred, recovery-oriented, multidisciplinary, dynamic, reflective, balanced and relational (NIMHE, 2005; Fulford & Woodbridge, 2007). These values are reflected in the competences outlined in Box 16.5.

These attitudes and the knowledge base can be linked to a range of skills and practices (behaviours), some of which are set out in Boxes 16.6 and 16.7. These are predominantly reflected in communication and direct therapeutic skills, but are also concerned with skills concerning interaction and negotiation with other professional groups and people

---

Box 16.4   Ten principles of values-based practice

1   Awareness: to be aware (and raise awareness) of the values in a given situation
2   Reasoning: thinking about values when making decisions
3   Knowledge: knowing about values and facts that are relevant to a situation
4   Communication: using communication to resolve conflicts/complexity and to share values
5   Service user-centred: considering the service user's values as the first priority
6   Multiperspective (or multidisciplinary): using a balance of perspectives to resolve conflicts
7   Facts and values (the 'two feet' principle): all decisions are based on facts and values; evidence-based practice and values-based practice therefore work together
8   The 'squeaky wheel' principle: values are often noticed only when there is a conflict – values should not just be noticed if there is a problem
9   Science and values: increasing scientific knowledge creates choices in healthcare, which can lead to wider differences in values; this is leading to an increasing role for values in decision-making
10 Partnership: in values-based practice decisions are taken by service users working in partnership with providers of care

Adapted from Fulford & Woodbridge (2007)

Box 16.5 Competences relevant to socially inclusive practice: attitudes

- Respect for diversity of values and a willingness to work with these in daily practice
- Willingness to see patient as a partner and collaborator in treatment decisions and an expert in their own disorder
- A recognition that building on the personal strengths and resiliences of service users as well as on their cultural and ethnic characteristics can facilitate recovery
- Respecting the diversity of routes to personal recovery, even if service user choice is not congruent with that of the clinician
- Recognising the negative effects of social inequality and exclusion on the recovery process
- An attitude of hope and confidence that people can recover from the impact of severe mental illness in many ways, even in the presence of continuing incapacities
- Recognition that respect is reciprocal – at a personal level (between service users, family members, friends, communities and providers), across professional groups (nursing, psychology, psychiatry, social work, occupational therapy) and between different organisations (health, social care, local authority housing, voluntary organisations, community groups, faith communities and other social support services)
- Placing an emphasis on positive working relationships supported by good communication skills at the heart of professional practice
- An openness and willingness to be responsive to change
- A willingness to be reflective, combining self-monitoring and self-management with positive self-regard

---

in the working environment and with organisations beyond traditional mental health services. These skills and practices are directed towards the development of a therapeutic relationship with services users which is concerned with empowerment and choice. They must, however, be supported by a multidisciplinary team that is working in a similar way and where responsibility is distributed across team members, according to their skills and expertise. Beyond individual practice the skills are aimed at identifying and challenging discriminatory attitudes and practices towards people with mental health problems, including equality of access to physical healthcare, and identifying and addressing facilitators and barriers to social inclusion.

Training to develop these competences will need to be supported by changes to the organisations providing mental health services and this may be done along the lines outlined in Chapter 15, especially noting the ten organisational challenges outlined there (Box 15.1: p. 315). These broader system changes may be, for example, structures that support user involvement in decision-making and user-directed care, providing services that are personalised to the individual service user, development of evidence-based vocational services, employment of peer professionals, monitoring of discrimination, stigma and diversity leading to meaningful review and change, being outwardly focused, and building links with community partners and networks. Overall, it is important to develop a professional and service culture which supports personal recovery and social inclusion for people with mental health problems.

Box 16.6   Competences relevant to socially inclusive practice: skills

- Advanced consultation skills that elicit a person's strengths as well as their symptoms and disabilities together with their own understanding of their condition and their capacity and willingness to manage it themselves
- Ability to go beyond the traditional medical role, to act as coach or mentor to the person seeking to develop their own self-care framework in conjunction with treatment provided by others
- Capacity to learn from the patient concerning their own experience of their condition, what works for them and what are the mediating factors in their life that support or inhibit self-care
- Ability to broaden the discussion to discuss a broad range of social issues and life experiences with patients, outside a narrow focus on symptoms and medical treatment
- Ability to facilitate access to information which supports patients' rights
- Ability to promote active and informed engagement of the service user in their own care and management, and supporting them in taking responsibility for their recovery
- Ability to explore the treatment choices available to an individual and work with them to weigh up the evidence in support of different therapeutic options.
- Ability to negotiate respecting the experience of the person seeking help such that the consultation becomes a discussion between those who are expert by training and those who are experts by their own experience
- Ability to understand the beliefs and attitudes of the individual and their family towards treatment and self-care and be able to reframe the medical role as offering expert support to people gaining skill and confidence in their own self-management
- Ability to promote an active, valued and participating role in society whatever the persisting symptoms and disabilities the individual has
- Ability to support people to develop advanced agreements and crisis plans as a form of self-directed care, but with an understanding of the limits and constraints on such plans
- Developing skills and experience in supporting people in self-care, self-management and self-directed care as a means of improving quality of life and supporting a process of personal recovery
- Ability to support restoration and promotion of self-care and self-management at the earliest opportunity in circumstances of compulsory treatment, while recognising and accounting for impaired capacity
- Skilled in one's own self-care, such as sustaining a healthy relationship between one's own home and work life, managing the experience of occupational stress. This may include participating in peer groups and in using and providing mentorship

---

Box 16.7   Competences relevant to socially inclusive practice: behaviour

- Providing holistic care and treatment for service users and their families/carers across a range of settings
- Promoting the social inclusion and recovery principles through teaching, advocacy and research.
- Utilising socially inclusive and recovery-oriented practice (Ten Top Tips) at every clinical encounter (including care programme approach reviews)
- Encouraging people in self-care, self-management and self-directed care to support their experience of personal recovery and their capacity to escape the constraints of illness-defined roles and behaviours
- Supporting people in seeking a secure place of belonging in ordinary society on the basis of equality and being skilled in effectively supporting an individual's engagement with ordinary social resources
- Liaising across service boundaries and agencies
- Actively challenging barriers to social inclusion such as stigma and discrimination
- Ensuring that diversity issues are mainstream and not marginalised
- Directing people to sources of appropriate information
- Coaching and supporting people in learning about their own condition and its management
- Providing information, not only 'illness-specific' materials, but also narratives of self-help and recovery that offer a basis for identification, modelling and hope
- Reviewing the full range of skills within the team skills required for socially inclusive practice and planning to attain them
- Using principles of least restrictive form of treatment
- Working with lay and legal advocates and the engagement of peer mentors as a support for people being heard, valued and included

Service user and carer involvement in training

The involvement of service users and carers in the training of mental health professionals and other mental health service staff is an essential ingredient in the development of socially inclusive and recovery-oriented practice. Traditionally, patients have been involved in the teaching of medical students, but usually in a passive role, through the traditional 'bedside' approach to training, with the goal of the acquisition of knowledge and skills (Wykurtz & Kelly, 2002), and also in postgraduate medical training and general practice (Stacy & Spencer, 1999; Spencer *et al*, 2000; Coleman & Murray, 2002). But the role of service users and carers in training for socially inclusive practice requires that they play a more active part in the development of attitudes, skills and knowledge of mental health professionals.

There are many examples of initiatives to involve service users and carers in the education of health professions and a substantial part of the literature has focused on service users in mental health settings (Repper & Breeze, 2007). Involvement may be in the planning of curricula and courses (Greenfield *et al*, 2001), in the development of teaching aids such as videos and DVDs (Ah-Mane, 1999), in assessing students, through telling their own stories and in direct teaching (Cole, 1994; Chapman, 1996; Masters *et al*, 2002). The evidence for the use of service users in teaching is generally positive. They are genuinely enthusiastic, often motivated by a desire to improve services (Barnes *et al*, 2000; Forest *et al*, 2000; Masters *et al*, 2002). They describe their experiences as being cathartic, increasing not only their knowledge but also their confidence, self-esteem and sense of control (Repper & Breeze, 2007). Service users give emphasis to the humanistic and interpersonal components of care, rather than the professional and technical ones. The budding professionals' response is also on the whole positive (Curran, 1997; Turner *et al*, 2000; Costello & Horne, 2001). Participants in service user teaching benefit by improving their understanding of the service user's point of view, by developing a greater empathy and awareness of the importance of communication skills (Klein, 1999; Wood & Wilson-Barnett, 1999). Despite the fact that there may be a dearth of systematic studies in this area, particularly studies examining the effects of service user and carer involvement in influencing practice, this type of participation is increasingly accepted as good practice and service users and carers are more routinely involved in undergraduate and postgraduate teaching up and down the country. One important reason for orienting training in this way is that the priorities of service users can be covered in the curriculum, thus giving the potential to develop a new shift in the relationship between mental health professionals and service users and carers. The teaching itself can reflect this, offering reciprocal exchange of benefits between professionals and service users that mirrors the type of relationships that are required for socially inclusive practice.

To be effective in delivering change the involvement of service users in the education of professionals will need to be an integral part of the undergraduate and postgraduate training schemes of mental health professionals, be a part of day-to-day practice and become more systematically delivered. The delivery of service user-led education and training programmes will need to achieve a consistent change in staff attitudes and behaviour and to do this we will need to introduce comprehensive, service user-led education and training programmes for all staff, across all professions and at all levels. This requires a supply of trained service users to act as the 'champions of change' (Sainsbury Centre for Mental Health, 2009). One possible way to drive this forward would be to establish a recovery education centre in every NHS mental health trust in the country (Chapter 15).

Continuing professional development

Continuing professional development is a central requirement for all psychiatrists. It could be an important tool to promote the necessary cultural change in attitudes and practice required to implement the social inclusion agenda across the profession. The Royal College of Psychiatrists plays a leading role in prioritising themes for the training and education of psychiatrists and should focus on the development of socially inclusive practice as a professional priority. This priority would then cascade through general professional activities including developing the themes for College conference programmes, specific training events, audit, research and teaching. All such activities can be progressed from the socially inclusive and recovery-oriented perspective.

Consultant psychiatrists will be members of local peer review groups, who are responsible for monitoring the annual personal development plans of their group members. These groups could operate to a structured agenda, to ensure that all members consider their personal needs in relation to socially inclusive practice. Individual plans could then reflect development needs in this area and be subject to monitoring and peer review.

Professional training and educational activities should serve as a model for socially inclusive practice. Service users and carers may provide valuable input to the design and implementation of education, training schemes and some research and audit projects, an approach successfully pioneered by the Royal College of Psychiatrists (Livingston & Cooper, 2004; Royal College of Psychiatrists, 2008). All such socially inclusive initiatives may become part of the individual's personal development plan and therefore be subject to monitoring and analysis. As such they would be a powerful vehicle for socially inclusive practice development.

Moving to inclusive training

The psychiatric curriculum and postgraduate psychiatric training must be used to promote modern values-based practice, including the agenda for social inclusion and recovery. Little change will be achieved merely through prescription. A more fundamental winning over of hearts and minds and effective multidisciplinary team working is needed to ensure that inclusive practice is achieved.

Training and teaching can be done through example as well as didactically. It should be inter-professional and multidisciplinary in order to improve opportunities for the whole team to learn and develop the necessary skills and knowledge base for socially inclusive practice. Service users and carers are central to this process and we should move to embedding this in the daily running of mental health services. Each of the psychiatric subspecialties will need to ensure that relevant socially inclusive competences are included within their curriculum. Most will apply to all mental health practitioners, however, each specialty may also have particular issues that are particularly relevant to users of their service and these will need to be identified separately. Trainees should expect to develop and demonstrate their awareness and growing competences in socially inclusive practice though workplace-based assessments. Opportunities to develop socially inclusive practice can be linked to continuing professional development and should be audited as an aspect of clinical governance, serving as a driver for service improvement and practice.

Summary

In addition to providing the key aspects of knowledge, skills and attitudes relating to psychiatry, the undergraduate curriculum needs to make future doctors aware of the ignorance, prejudice and discrimination faced by people with mental ill health, the importance of developing partnerships and of helping students to review their preconceptions, assumptions and prejudices about people with mental health problems. Students need to understand the nature of the association between social conditions and ill health.

The competences relevant to socially inclusive practice should be included in the postgraduate curriculum for psychiatry, including those relating to self-management. Competences relevant to each subspecialty should be developed.

Service users and carers are central to the training of professionals and there is a need to develop a system to provide a cadre of service user trainers, possibly as part of a recovery education centre in each NHS service provider organisation.

Continuing professional development is a central requirement for all psychiatrists and is an important tool to promote the necessary cultural change in attitudes and practice, required to implement the social inclusion agenda across the profession.

References

Ah-Mane, S. (1999) Clinical view – learning from psychosis. *Nursing Times*, **95**, 43–47.

Barnes, D., Carpenter, J. & Bailey, D. (2000) Partnerships with service users in interprofessional education for community mental health: a case study. *Journal of Interprofessional Care*, **14**, 189–200.

Chapman, V. (1996) Consumers as faculty: experts in their own lives. *Journal of Psychosocial Nursing and Mental Health Services*, **34**, 47–49.

Cole, A. (1994) It was an education: service users assess student social workers. *Community Living*, January, 16–17.

Coleman, K. & Murray, E. (2002) Patients' views and feelings on the community-based teaching of undergraduate medical students: a qualitative study. *Family Practice*, **19**, 183–188.

Costello, J. & Horne, M. (2001) Patients as teachers? An evaluative study of patients' involvement in classroom teaching. *Nurse Education in Practice*, **1**, 94–102.

Curran, T. (1997) Power, participation and post modernism: user and practitioner participation in mental health social work education. *Social Work Education*, **16**, 21–36.

Department of Health (2001) *The Expert Patient: A New Approach to Chronic Disease Management for the 21st century*. Department of Health.

Forrest, S., Risk, I., Masters, H., *et al* (2000) Mental health service user involvement in nurse education: exploring the issues. *Journal of Psychiatric and Mental Health Nursing*, **7**, 51–57.

Fulford, B. & Woodbridge, K. (2007) Values-based practice in teaching and learning. In *Teaching Mental Health* (eds T. Stickley & T. Basset). John Wiley & Son.

General Medical Council (2009) *Tomorrow's Doctors*. General Medical Council.

Greenfield, S. M., Anderson, P., Gill, P. S., *et al* (2001) Community voices: views on the training of future doctors in Birmingham, UK. *Patient Education and Counseling*, **45**, 43–50.

Klein, S. (1999) The effects of the participation of patients with cancer in teaching communication skills to medical undergraduates: a randomised study with follow-up after 2 years. *European Journal of Cancer*, **35**, 1448–1456.

Livingston, G. & Cooper, C. (2004) User and carer involvement in mental health training. *Advances in Psychiatric Treatment*, **10**, 85–92.

Masters, H., Forrest, S., Harley, A., *et al* (2002) Involving mental health service users and carers in curriculum development: moving beyond 'classroom' involvement. *Journal of Psychiatric and Mental Health Nursing*, **9**, 309–316.

National Institute for Mental Health in England (2005) *NIMHE Guiding Statement on Recovery*. NIMHE.

Repper, J. & Breeze, J. (2007) User and carer involvement in the training and education of health professionals: a review of the literature. *International Journal of Nursing Studies*, **44**, 511–519.

Royal College of Psychiatrists (2008) *Fair Deal for Mental Health: Our Manifesto for a 3-year Campaign Dedicated to Tackling Inequality in Mental Healthcare*. Royal College of Psychiatrists.

Royal College of Psychiatrists (2009) *A Competency Based Curriculum for Specialist Training in Psychiatry: Core and General Module*. Royal College of Psychiatrists (http://www.rcpsych.ac.uk/PDF/Curriculum%20-%20core%20and%20general%20module.pdf).

Sainsbury Centre for Mental Health (2009) *Implementing Recovery: A New Framework for Organisational Change*. Position Paper. Sainsbury Centre for Mental Health.

Sayce, L. & Boardman, J. (2003) The Disability Discrimination Act 1995: implications for psychiatrists. *Advances in Psychiatric Treatment*, **9**, 397–404.

Sayce, L. & Boardman, J. (2008) Disability rights and mental health in the UK: recent developments of the Disability Discrimination Act. *Advances in Psychiatric Treatment*, **14**, 265–275.

Spencer, J., Blackmore, D., Heard, S., *et al* (2000) Patient-orientated learning: a review of the role of the patient in the education of medical students. *Medical Education*, **34**, 851–857.

Stacy, R. & Spencer, J. (1999) Patients as teachers: a qualitative study of patients' views on their role in a community-based undergraduate project. *Medical Education*, **33**, 688–694.

Turner, P., Sheldon, F., Coles, C., *et al* (2000) Listening to and learning from the family carer's story: an innovative approach in interprofessional education. *Journal of Interprofessional Care*, **14**, 387–395.

Wood, J. & Wilson-Barnett, J. (1999) The influence of user involvement on the learning of mental health nursing students. *NT Research*, **4**, 257–270.

Wykurtz, G. & Kelly, D. (2002) Developing the role of patients as teachers: literature review. *BMJ*, **325**, 818–821.

CHAPTER 17

Community mental health and the inclusion–exclusion seesaw

Tom K. J. Craig

According to one definition of social exclusion, 'An individual is socially excluded if he or she does not participate in key activities of the society in which he or she lives' (Burchardt *et al*, 2002, p. 30). These key activities include education, employment, access to leisure facilities and civic participation. As this book documents, people who have mental illness are often excluded from some if not all of these activities. Those with the more severe forms of disorder are unlikely to be employed, more likely to reside in shared and subsidised accommodation, live in material poverty, rely on welfare benefits, and have restricted social networks and limited access to opportunities and leisure facilities in the community. Explaining this exclusion is tricky because it clearly arises in part from the nature of mental illness. Some of the more severe disorders begin in childhood and impair educational attainment that in turn limits occupational opportunity in adult life; people with depression withdraw from social contact and those with chronic schizophrenia neglect their environment. But clearly, as the term exclusion implies, much of the problem lies not with the mentally ill person but with the rest of us – how we structure society, the rules and regulations that facilitate access to education and employment, and how we go about organising assistance for the disadvantaged. Some mentally ill people, coming from a migrant group perceived as competing for jobs and resources or who are marginalised because they do not speak English or have a black skin, can have a double or triple whammy, as evidenced by the striking over-representation of some of these groups in coercive treatment settings (Bermingham *et al*, 1996; Coid *et al*, 2000; Audini & Lelliott, 2002).

How we organise care is itself confounded by our prejudices and beliefs about the capabilities of the mentally ill person and how much we generalise from observing a specific impairment to an assumption of global incompetence. On the one hand is the view that the affected individual is essentially powerless to change their state and the caring response is therefore one of doing 'for' the individual. On the other hand is the belief that however profound is the appearance of the disability, people have the capacity to make positive adaptations, so that providing care is a matter of teaching and giving advice to help the individual solve or work round their problems. The recent emergence of the recovery approach and its wide adoption by mental health organisations is one very powerful manifestation of this view. Hope and optimism are at the heart of the approach that emphasises the possibility of success rather than failure, of looking forward not back, and of encouraging the taking of those risks where success would boost confidence and self-esteem (Anthony, 1993; Andresen *et al*, 2003; Roberts & Wolfson, 2004).

The extent to which these views dominate a mental health system has quite profound consequences. The first view leads inevitably to greater exclusion. If disorders are essentially incurable and all efforts in vain, then there is little point going beyond the provision of the very basic necessities of life and certainly no point in making life difficult for society by efforts to integrate. But before we get too carried away with our enthusiasm for the other view, recovery, consider that the inevitable consequence of empowering individuals to make and take decisions in life will be that some of these decisions will go horribly wrong. There is an abiding naive presumption that once discharged from the clutches of a repressive institutional 'system' individuals will flourish, needing just the gentlest of nudges to find useful things to do, to make use of a wide range of ordinary community facilities and to lead a fulfilling life. The reality, documented by several follow-up studies of patients discharged to the community, is often one of quite appalling levels of isolation, impoverishment and neglect (Melzer *et al*, 1991).

The story then, of the evolution of care of the mentally ill, is one of a tussle between a very powerful tendency in society to eject and exclude those who do not fit in and the counter force enshrined in moral teachings from time immemorial of human rights, compassion, acceptance and fair play. Each of us struggles with this tension to some degree. The relative dominance of exclusion or inclusion has much to do with the state of the economy including opportunities for employment, the availability of affordable housing and the extent to which mental illness is regarded as innate and incurable.

Residential exclusion

For the best part of the past 200 years, the approach to the mentally ill, as for many of those who society viewed as deviant, was one of active exclusion. Some of the early asylums, like the Retreat in York, demonstrated a relatively enlightened approach and produced remarkable results through a regime of occupation, amusements and kind but firm discipline. But the majority were little more than convenient warehouses for controlling those whose condition made them unsuitable for productive labour. By the end of the 19th century there were 100 000 people in these asylums and the numbers were steadily rising. Although there were critics from early on advocating more liberal approaches, these voices were overlooked, not least because many of the living conditions that so exercised the reformers were hardly different from those enjoyed by the sane working class. Also, the peak of the asylum era coincided with the emergence of a particularly bleak and hopeless view of mental illness as the product of irreversible degenerative or inherited brain disease and saw criminals and psychiatric patients as evolutionary failures for whom nothing much could be done (Warner, 1994; Porter, 2002).

The first stirrings of fundamental disillusion with the asylum mirrored wider societal change in attitudes to the poor between the two world wars. Disillusion was fed by scandalous reports of inhumane treatment and casual cruelty meted out to inmates. In 1949, the wards in Dingleton Hospital were thrown open, with Mapperley Hospital following in 1953 and Warlingham Park a year later. Also around this time, developments in psychotherapy and the discovery of new drug treatments gave new hope and confidence to the professionals and gave added impetus to these 'open door' experiments and milieu treatments. Finally, the development of out-patient care brought mental health professionals into closer contact with individuals with milder disorders who could be effectively managed without incarceration, prompting the development of clinics in general hospitals and other less stigmatising settings. So by the early 1960s the idea that mental healthcare could be better provided without the asylum was well under way. Enoch Powell, the then minister for health, announced a bold policy of 'the elimination of by far the greater part of this country's mental hospitals as they exist today'. He went on to envisage radical changes to the way mental illness would be managed in the future, with the medical profession accepting responsibility for more and more care of patients in the community and with the local authorities achieving 'an almost unlimited range of gradation between the complete independence of full mental and physical health and the almost complete dependence of the old or subnormal whose need for care and attention is little short of that which only a hospital can provide' (Powell, 1961).

Closing the asylum involved two challenges. First, what to do with the large numbers of institutionalised residents, and second, what could be done to manage or better prevent the future accumulation of people with severe disability. For the first challenge, things progressed reasonably well and a range of accommodation from highly staffed residential homes to independent flats with visiting support was provided in ordinary housing in the community. There were some concerns expressed of increased mortality among the elderly in the period immediately following transfer (Holloway, 1991) and of a reduction in meaningful day-to-day activity (Jeffreys et al, 1997), but the conclusions of the major English research study carried out to evaluate the closure of an asylum were reassuring, finding few adverse events, some clinical improvements and significant gains in social interaction and activity (Leff & Trieman, 2000). Furthermore, it turned out that although there had been considerable resistance from local communities who feared for the value of their property and the safety of their children (Wolff *et al*, 1996*a*), where some effort was put in by mental health professionals to involving local residents in the planning of the move and for neighbours to meet the patients, many of these concerns were dealt with and the public often turned out to be far more supportive of inclusion than the ex-institutional staff who accompanied residents into the community (Wolff *et al*, 1996*b*).

Despite the continuing advances in the treatment of severe mental illness and the fact that the majority of the old resettled asylum population are now dead, the need for long-term residential care seems to be just as great now as it has ever been. A survey in two areas of England found that a quarter of the asylum hospitals open at the time of Enoch Powell's speech were still operational 42 years later in 2003 (Chaplin & Peters, 2003). Furthermore, many patients with forensic histories and challenging behaviours still experience prolonged periods of incarceration, often housed miles away from their family and friends and offered very little by way of rehabilitation programmes aimed at returning them to their original neighbourhoods (Poole *et al*, 2002; Ryan *et al*, 2004). Even where local accommodation can be found, it is often in the form of shared living and hardly ideal as a model of social inclusion. Group living encourages services to provide block rather than individualised attention and some critics argue that the hospital asylum has been replaced by a patchwork of residential and nursing-home care that at best replaces the hospital ward with a more homely environments but at worst substitutes one level of neglect with another (Geller 2000; Priebe *et al*, 2005).

Despite these criticisms, many people who would formerly have been hospitalised for life now have tenancy agreements with the rights held by any other citizen to a place of their own where they can 'live peacefully and quietly' without harassment (Housing Corporation, 1998). The majority of people who have mental disorders live in their own homes, and where tenancy or daily living support is needed it is most commonly provided through mobile teams. It remains a fairly contentious issue as to the balance in these teams between unqualified general support workers and more skilled staff with some knowledge of the challenges of severe mental illness. In addition, such support is likely to be sufficient to meet basic living requirements but falls short of the level needed to achieve a meaningful social life. Even in a fairly high supported scheme, a resident might get a visit every few days for an hour or two focused on practical household chores interspersed with acres of idleness. Studies suggest that social isolation and the lack of recreational opportunity are the most frequently cited problems in these supported schemes (Friedrich *et al*, 1999). But despite these concerns, one of the significant achievements of deinstitutionalisation has been to increase the number of people who are able to live in settings that they value and to enjoy a substantially improved quality of life over that formerly available in the institution (Newman, 2001).

Organising care in the community

While beds continued to close through the 1970s and 1980s, alternative community provision increased by only a fraction of the need. For example, new residential care places fell short of the White Paper *Better Services for the Mentally Ill* (Department of Health and Social Security, 1975) target by 48 000, and as admissions to long-stay beds were halted in the first phases of asylum closure, patients who would have been shipped off to a long-stay now accumulated in acute beds or shuttled in and out of hospital. This 'revolving door' population had many of the disabilities of the old hospital population and soon came to be labelled the 'new long-stay' (Mann & Cree 1976; Clifford *et al*, 1991). Around the same time as the asylums were closing, there was a parallel run-down of many of the old reception centres and hostels for homeless people that had housed sizeable numbers of mentally ill people who had been discharged or fallen out of psychiatric care. The planned re-provision of these hostel places was slow in materialising and by the mid-1980s, while homelessness among those resettled from the asylums was extremely rare, significant numbers of the mentally ill ex-residents of these shelters began appearing on the streets of many British cities. Their numbers were swollen by younger people from the new long-stay that were also jamming up the acute wards (Craig & Timms, 1992). To add to the misfortunes of community care, a number of homicides involved cases where it was clear that there had been inadequate supervision and care. Although community mental health centres and teams had become the standard of non-hospital care, they were mostly dealing with common mental disorder and had little capacity to provide the intensive supervision or support that some patients needed. It was not long before vigorous voices in the profession were condemning community care as an abject failure and equally not long before these siren calls were picked up by the popular press and fed into the wider public and political prejudice and anxiety.

Although the more extreme clamour of the tabloid journalist could be dismissed as over-reaction, there is little doubt that it contributed to a corrosive message about the essential hopelessness and incompetence of the mentally ill, who, for better or worse, needed others to make decisions for them and required supervision for life. In response, new systems of care were introduced to focus attention on the severely mentally ill. Staff working predominantly with common mental disorder in primary care were pulled back to the specialist service and directed to concentrate their efforts on people diagnosed with psychosis. One manifestation of this redirection of effort was the care programme approach (CPA) and its implementation through case management, assertive outreach and (the now defunct) supervision register. The principles of the CPA also dovetailed with emerging models of clinical case management in the USA, where landmark research studies showed that intensive supervision of patients involving close attention to ensuring adherence to treatment could have a striking success in reducing reliance on hospitalisation (Stein & Test

1980). Impressed by these results, adaptations of the model were trialled in England (Marks *et al*, 1994) and subsequently fairly widely adopted, finally being re-branded as assertive outreach and introduced as a core service as one component of the National Service Framework reconfiguration of services alongside crisis home treatment and early intervention teams (Department of Health, 1999).

The assertive outreach team exemplifies the challenge facing mental health services of balancing practices that lie on the pathway to exclusion (segregation, paternalism and the use of enforced treatment) with those of inclusion (collaborative care planning, personal choice and empowerment). It also brings into sharp focus a particularly thorny issue of risk. The CPA was introduced in 1990 as a direct response to the perceived failure of the system to provide ongoing control over risky patients who went on to commit serious crimes. The problem with risk is that once identified, it is extremely difficult to ignore, even when years have passed without recurrence. The consequence has been for some teams a steadily growing population of patients with very little movement out of the mental health system, contained by mutual fears of relapse and risk. Although, logically, this should really apply only to those who have the worst risk histories, it nevertheless tends to colour how all people with severe mental illness are perceived and generates an understandable 'safe rather than sorry' response. As the numbers of patients trapped in this system grow, so the capacity to provide the more time-consuming family and psychological therapies that could make a difference to the chance of recovery diminishes and the mental health team becomes increasingly consumed with firefighting relapses and readmissions. This can have quite profoundly damaging effects on staff morale and patient outcome. Reversing this situation is possible, but it requires very strong leadership from senior staff who are prepared to take the decision to act and the responsibility to own the risk in the face of siren calls from the sidelines.

One of the themes of the early days of deinstitutionalisation was the importance of the district general hospital in the wider mental healthcare system. In part this was a nod in the direction of the social inclusion of the mental health practitioners themselves who were given a place alongside their counterparts in physical medicine. This was clearly good for the esteem of the professionals, but it also had benefits for the patients who could be treated and hospitalised where necessary in a less segregated settings. Odd, then, the current impetus to re-provide the ageing facilities on these sites in new mental health-specific buildings remote from the district general hospital. The shift may be justified in terms of expense of remaining on the acute site or perhaps the opportunity to create a more 'homely' environment in a new building or even on the grounds of distancing the wider provision of mental healthcare from a 'medical model', but whatever the justification, one is left with the uneasy feeling that it looks like a recreation of the segregated asylum and adds rather than detracts from exclusion.

Facilitating inclusion: the example of employment

Poverty is strongly associated with mental health problems. Most mentally ill people have much lower disposable income than others in society and even those on welfare benefits often do not receive the full amount they are entitled to (Becker *et al*, 1997). Most CPA care plans will contain some assessment of financial need, at least in very broad terms, and helping to improve a patient's income is often seen as something that a care coordinator can do that is helpful and a sure way to improve engagement (Frost-Gaskin *et al*, 2003). But paradoxically this can also be disempowering. Emphasising welfare benefits can reinforce the message of incapacity and should not be the only approach to increasing disposable income. A return to full- or part-time paid employment is one obvious alternative.

The importance of meaningful occupation to recovery has been at the heart of mental healthcare from the very beginnings of modern psychiatry. Paid employment not only brings material benefits to the individual and to society, but also makes a significant contribution to personal well-being and self-esteem. Work defines who we are, provides us with a structure to the day, provides social contacts and support and is a major source of the sense of personal achievement (Warr, 1987). So it seems blindingly obvious that the greater the extent to which a mentally ill person can successfully manage a job with an employer who is part of mainstream society in which they are treated just like any other worker, the greater the likely benefit. If this was recognised, it certainly was not a central theme of earlier employment programmes. Initially patients were engaged in tasks that were important to the institution, typically involving simple assembly-line activity such as preparing the folders for case notes or assembling treatment packs. The work was, by and large, boring, repetitive and unrewarding, but as several early studies showed, some activity was definitely better than none (Wing & Brown, 1970; Miles, 1971). By 1967, most hospitals had industrial therapy workshops and between these, the hospital laundry and the postal service, the majority of patients were employed in some capacity during the day. A small step towards social inclusion with the wider community was introduced in the form of contracts with companies based outside of the asylum system to deliver a very diverse range of products – from garden gnomes to electrical transformers. As the asylums closed, the more profitable elements of this assembly line moved to community locations and began setting up small not-for-profit businesses and charitable enterprises. All of these sheltered workshops continued to need a substantial contribution from hospital-based staff and thus considerable financial subsidy from government and charitable donation. The majority of the workers were at best marginally productive and the businesses themselves were, for the most part, not expected to compete in the open market against more efficient mainstream competitors. For the patient-employee, movement on to the open market was extremely rare.

351

The sheltered workshop gradually fell from favour for a variety of reasons. Even the most productive workshops were never able to survive very long without some state subsidy and even then, survival meant increasing productivity. This, in turn, could only really be achieved by cherry-picking the more able employee, which annoyed referrers in the mental health teams who wanted these services to take on their most disabled clients. So the sheltered workshop came to be identified as the rump of the old asylum, maintaining the social exclusion of its workforce from mainstream society, paying subsistence wages and providing little or no opportunity for advancement. In response, several of the organisations subsequently morphed into social firms – small companies in which about half the employees are disabled but who are regarded as equal partners and receive the going rate for the work they do. They operate as business ventures in the competitive marketplace without subsidy (Grove & Drurie, 1999).

Supported employment

Until the late 1990s, virtually all mental health occupational rehabilitation in Britain followed a model derived ultimately from the rehabilitation of physically disabled people, in which participants underwent a detailed evaluation of their abilities, followed by a period of training and finally a placement in a job that matched their skills. Most recently, and again hailing from the USA, there has been considerable interest in the supported employment approach that dispenses with the protracted assessment and pre-vocational training and instead goes for rapid job search and placement with in-job training. Although this has now by far the strongest research evidence base (Bond et al, 2008) and has been shown to be an effective intervention in several countries including in England (Burns et al, 2008), there remains a substantial gulf between its implementation in research and everyday practice. Many mental health professionals and employment advisors are very sceptical about the approach despite the evidence. They point to the consensual nature of research such that only the most able and interested take part, to the differences between societies in the extent to which employment per se is valued, to the preparedness of employers to take on someone with a mental illness, and to the perceived risks to the individual of the stress of employment. All these arguments can and have been rebutted by both research evidence and practice but remain a significant obstacle to the roll-out of the approach. One of the consequences of the reluctance to embrace supported employment is the way its implementation in routine services drifts away from the proven model, for example contracting the employment service from an employment organisation rather than embedding the employment specialist in the community mental health team or rebadging an occupational therapist to the role. The research constraints of limited case-loads and long-term follow-up are also frequently watered down in practice, so that it is not unusual to find employment specialists with 50 or more patients on their books and little capacity for continuing involvement with the worker for more than a few months post-placement.

Another criticism of the supported employment approach that has some merit is that significant numbers of mentally ill people have not got the inclination or confidence to try open employment directly, preferring a rather more gradual return to activity. Overlapping with the demise of the sheltered workshop, the 'clubhouse' model arrived in England from the USA in the early 1990s. The appeal of the model was partly that it offered a less obviously institutional approach to day care as well as a promise of greater access to ordinary jobs on a part-time or shared basis. People who go to clubhouse join as members not patients, and as members have a shared responsibility for the running of the organisation, helping to maintain the building, preparing meals, working in the office and greeting visitors. As members they also have responsibilities to look out for each other and to participate in social activities together. In addition, clubhouses arrange employment with mainstream employers, but it is the clubhouse that holds the contract, with the actual jobs being shared between members. At first sight this has all the appearances of a fairly institutional model with relative segregation of members from the local community, but recent research has shown comparable outcomes in terms of achieving off-benefit open employment to that achieved by supported employment (Macias *et al*, 2006; Schonebaum *et al*, 2006).

From patient to mental health worker

Given the large numbers of employees in the average mental health trust, it is perhaps surprising that more jobs are not made available in these settings. In the USA there has been some considerable experimentation with employing ex-patients as community case managers (Solomon & Draine 1995; Mowbray *et al*, 1998) or in peer support mentoring roles (Davidson *et al*, 1999). In the UK, experience is more limited, although some replications have been reported (Craig *et al*, 2004; Doherty *et al*, 2004). Perhaps the most well-known of these is the work of Rachel Perkins and colleagues (1997). They describe models of employment contracts where the personal experience of mental health problems is seen as an essential or at least desirable aspect for the post. The person works with exactly the same conditions as other healthy employees. Support for those who need it is built into the employment contract. The experience is not only good for the employee in these roles but can serve as a great morale booster for other patients in the system. Service users are also increasingly involved in the formal management arrangements of clinical teams and trusts as well as playing an important role in both conducting and advising on research (Rose *et al*, 2008).

One of the obstacles to a return to work for people who have been ill for many years is the potential loss of welfare benefit that may result. Changes to the benefit and employment rules have helped to ease what was an impossible 'benefit trap', but problems still remain, particularly for the young and for those who have been ill for many years and are in receipt of multiple assistance such as housing and council tax benefits that have a very low limit of earnings before being cut. For those for whom a return to paid employment seems some way off, having meaningful occupation is still among the most helpful interventions we can encourage and for many people, contributing in a voluntary capacity to an activity that is helpful to others is a great way of boosting esteem and promoting personal recovery. The default option of attendance at a social club as the sole activity outside the home is better than nothing but rightly comes quite far down the list of things to do.

Self-directed care: letting the person decide

In general, people with mental health problems are socially isolated and have a low level of participation in leisure activities outside the home. It is partly a consequence of illness, but also reflects structural barriers such as the lack of opportunities and discrimination. The response of services has tended to be to provide special facilities such as drop-in centres or organised programmes of outings and activities. The trouble with this, of course, is that these tie up considerable public financial resources in forms of care that perpetuate segregation. Recognising this, there is an important effort to shift financial resources out of the state and into the hands of individuals who have been assessed as eligible for receiving social care services so that they are empowered to purchase the care how and where they want (Department of Health, 2006a). For example, a statutory service may only be able to provide a visit from a support worker at a particular time of day, whereas given the resources, the individual may be able to find a friend or relative to provide the support and also reimburse them for their time. Similarly, payments might be used to pay for membership of a club or for access to some regular social activity. It is, of course, not entirely without strings, so there are qualifying criteria to be met and the care that is to be purchased has to be agreed with the care coordinator. On top of that, recipients may be required to keep records of how the money has been spent, care coordinators may not give advice on employment, and the implementation of the scheme including criteria for eligibility vary considerably around the country. But these caveats aside, it gives the individual considerable control over the way care is provided.

The personalisation agenda is also extending to healthcare (Department of Health, 2006b) but here the emphasis is on greater choice over access to the various components of healthcare and to earlier intervention closer to home than to personalised budgets. Welcome though this is, it does not address a more serious challenge to the physical healthcare of the mentally ill. People who experience mental illness have far higher rates of obesity, smoking, heart disease and diabetes, and greatly elevated mortality rates (Harris & Barraclough, 1998). Yet despite these higher rates of physical illnesses, there is good evidence that they are less likely to receive health screening and that they frequently fall between the cracks of primary and secondary care. Although physical healthcare is largely the responsibility of general practice, the specialist mental health service has to shoulder some of the responsibility for acting on the needs of their patients. Physical health needs are part of the CPA checklist but very few community mental health staff are competent or settings equipped to carry out even the most rudimentary health monitoring. It need not be this way as there are enough well-reported studies of successful shared-care agreements between primary care and secondary care and of physical health programmes run entirely within the mental health service that significantly reduce the level of cardiovascular risk factors (Ohlsen *et al*, 2005; Pendlebury *et al*, 2007; Smith *et al*, 2007). The challenge is now to up-scale these research-based interventions to a form that can be reliably delivered in routine care.

Conclusion

Considered over a 50-year period, one of the more striking changes in society has been the widespread shift away from an authoritarian 'doctor knows best' approach towards shared decision-making and the freedom of the individual to accept or reject advice. These changes are also apparent in mental healthcare, with an increasing emphasis on providing people with the information, the skills and the tools to manage their condition as well as the opportunities and resources they need to lead their lives. The inclusion–exclusion seesaw is, therefore, currently very definitely tipped towards greater inclusion, although it is a fragile balance and as this book shows, much remains to be done if people with mental health problems are ever to be accorded the same value and rights of access as other members of society.

Summary

The evolution of care of people with mental health problems has witnessed opposing social tendencies of rejection and of justice and compassion. This can be seen in the development of the asylums during the 19th century, their demise in the UK during the second half of the 20th century, the development of care based in community settings and the present debates about the importance of employment in facilitating inclusion.

References

Andresen, R., Oades, L. & Caputi, P. (2003) The experience of recovery from schizophrenia: towards an empirically validated stage model. *Australian and New Zealand Journal of Psychiatry*, **37**, 586–594.

Anthony, W. A. (1993) Recovery from mental illness: the guiding vision of the mental health service system in the 1990s. *Psychosocial Rehabilitation Journal*, **16**, 11–23.

Audini, B. & Lelliott, P. (2002) Age, gender and ethnicity of those detained under Part II of the Mental Health Act 1983. *British Journal of Psychiatry*, **180**, 222–226.

Becker, T., Thornicroft, G., Leese, M., *et al* (1997) Social networks and service use among representative cases of psychosis in south London. *British Journal of Psychiatry*, **171**, 15–19.

Bermingham, L., Mason, D. & Grubin, D. (1996) Prevalence of mental disorder in remand prisoners: consecutive case study. *BMJ*, **313**, 1521–1524.

Bond, G. R., Drake, R. E. & Becker, D. R. (2008) An update on randomized controlled trials of evidence-based supported employment. *Psychiatric Rehabilitation Journal*, **31**, 280–290.

Burchardt, T., Le Grand, J. & Piachaud, D. (2002) Degrees of exclusion: developing a dynamic multidimensional measure. In *Understanding Social Exclusion* (eds T. Hills, J. Le Grand & D. Piachaud), pp. 30–43. Oxford University Press.

Burns, T., White, S. J., Catty, J., *et al* (2008) Individual placement and support in Europe: the EQOLISE trial. *International Review of Psychiatry*, **20**, 498–502.

Chaplin, R. & Peters, S. (2003) Executives have taken over the asylum: the fate of 71 psychiatric hospitals. *Psychiatric Bulletin*, **27**, 227–229.

Clifford, P., Charman, A., Webb, Y., *et al* (1991) Planning for community care. Long stay populations of hospitals scheduled for rundown or closure. *British Journal of Psychiatry*, **158**, 190–196.

Coid, J. W., Kahtan, N., Gault, S., *et al* (2000) Ethnic differences in admissions to secure forensic psychiatry services. *British Journal of Psychiatry*, **177**, 241–247.

Craig, T., Doherty, I., Jamieson-Craig, R., *et al* (2004) The consumer-employee as a member of a mental health assertive outreach team. 1: Clinical and social outcomes. *Journal of Mental Health*, **13**, 59–69.

Craig, T. K. J. & Timms, P. W. (1992) Out of the wards and onto the streets? Deinstitutionalisation and homelessness in Britain. *Journal of Mental Health*, **1**, 265–275.

Davidson, L., Chinman, M., Kloos, B., *et al* (1999) Peer support among individuals with severe mental illness: a review of the evidence. *Clinical Psychology: Science and Practice*, **6**, 165–187.

Department of Health (1999) *National Service Framework for Mental Health: Modern Standards and Service Models*. Department of Health.

Department of Health (2006a) *Direct Payments for People with Mental Health Problems: A Guide to Action*. Department of Health.

Department of Health (2006b) *Our Health, Our Care, Our Say: A New Direction for Community Services*. Department of Health.

Department of Health and Social Security (1975) *Better Services for the Mentally Ill* (Cm 6233). HMSO.

Doherty, I., Craig, T., Attafua, G., *et al* (2004) The consumer-employee as a member of a mental health assertive outreach team. 2: Impressions of consumer-employees and other team members. *Journal of Mental Health*, **13**, 71–81.

Friedrich, R. M., Hollingsworth, B., Hradek, E., *et al* (1999) Family and client perspectives on alternative residential settings for persons with severe mental illness. *Psychiatric Services*, **50**, 509–514.

Frost-Gaskin, M., O'Kelly, R., Henderson, C., *et al* (2003) A welfare benefits outreach project to users of community mental health services. *International Journal of Social Psychiatry*, **49**, 251–263.

Geller, J. L. (2000) The last half century of psychiatric services as reflected in 'Psychiatric Services'. *Psychiatric Services*, **51**, 41–67.

Grove, B. & Drurie, S. (1999) *Social Firms: An Instrument for Economic Empowerment and Inclusion*. Social Firms UK.

Harris, E. C. & Barraclough, B. (1998) Excess mortality of mental disorder. *British Journal of Psychiatry*, **173**, 11–53.

Holloway, F. (1991) 'Elderly graduates' and a hospital closure programme: the experience of the Camberwell Resettlement Team. *Psychiatric Bulletin*, **15**, 321–323.

Housing Corporation (1998) *The Shorthold Tenant's Charter*. Housing Corporation.

Jeffreys, S. E., Harvey, C. A., McNaught, A. S., *et al* (1997) The Hampstead Schizophrenia Survey 1991. 1: Prevalence and service use comparisons in an inner London health authority, 1986–1991. *British Journal of Psychiatry*, **170**, 301–306.

Leff, J. & Trieman, N. (2000) Long-stay patients discharged from psychiatric hospitals: social and clinical outcomes after five years in the community. The TAPS Project 46. *British Journal of Psychiatry*, **176**, 217–223.

Macias, C., Rodican, C. F., Hargreaves, W. A., *et al* (2006) Supported employment outcomes of a randomized controlled trial of ACT and Clubhouse models. *Psychiatric Services*, **57**, 1406–1415.

Mann, S. A. & Cree, W. (1976) 'New long stay' psychiatric patients: a national sample survey of fifteen mental hsoptials in England and Wales. *Psychological Medicine*, **6**, 603–616.

Marks, I. M., Connolly, J., Muijen, M., *et al* (1994) Home-based versus hospital-based care for people with serious mental illness. *British Journal of Psychiatry*, **165**, 179–194.

Melzer, D., Hale, A. S., Malik, S. J., *et al* (1991) Community care for patients with schizophrenia one year after hospital discharge. *BMJ*, **303**, 1023–1026.

Miles, A. (1971) Long-stay schizophrenic patients in hospital workshops: a comparative study of an industrial unit and an occupational therapy department. *British Journal of Psychiatry*, **119**, 611–620.

Mowbray, C. T., Moxley, D. P. & Collins, M. E. (1998) Consumers as mental health providers: first-person accounts of benefits and limitations. *Journal of Behavioural Health Services and Research*, **25**, 397–411.

Newman, S. J. (2001) Housing attributes and serious mental illness: implications for research and practice. *Psychiatric Services*, **52**, 1309–1317.

Ohlsen, R. I., Peacock, G. & Smith, S. (2005) Developing a service to monitor and improve physical health in people with serious mental illness. *Journal of Psychiatric and Mental Health Nursing*, **12**, 614–619.

Pendlebury, J., Bushe, C., Wildgust, H., *et al* (2007) Long term maintenance of weight loss in patients with severe mental illness through a behavioural programme in the UK. *Acta Psychiatrica Scandinavica*, **115**, 286–294.

Perkins, R., Buckfield, R. & Choy, D. (1997) Access to employment. *Journal of Mental Health*, **6**, 307–318.

Poole, R., Ryan, T. & Pearsall, A. (2002) The NHS, the private sector and the virtual asylum. *BMJ*, **325**, 349–350.

Porter, R. (2002) *Madness: A Brief History*. Oxford University Press.

Powell, E. (1961) *Address to the National Association of Mental Health Annual Conference, 9 March 1961*. National Health Service History (www.nhshistory.net/watertower.html).

Priebe, S., Badesconyi, A., Fioritti, A., *et al* (2005) Reinstitutionalisation in mental health care: comparison of data on service provision from six European countries. *BMJ*, **330**, 123–126.

Roberts, G. & Wolfson, P. (2004) The rediscovery of recovery: open to all. *Advances in Psychiatric Treatment*, **10**, 37–48.

Rose, D., Fleischman, P. & Wykes, T. (2008) What are mental health service users' priorities for research in the UK. *Journal of Mental Health*, **17**, 520–530.

Ryan, T., Pearsall, A., Hatfield, B., *et al* (2004) Long term care for serious mental illness outside the NHS: a study of out of area placements. *Journal of Mental Health*, **13**, 425–429.

Schonebaum, A. D., Boyd, J. K. & Dudek, K. J. (2006) A comparison of competitive employment outcomes for the clubhouse and PACT models. *Psychiatric Services*, **57**, 1416–1420.

Smith, L., Yeomans, D., Bushe, C., *et al* (2007) A well-being programme in severe mental illness. Reducing risk for physical ill health: a post programme service evaluation at 2 years. *European Psychiatry*, **22**, 413–418.

Solomon, P. & Draine, J. (1995) The efficacy of a Consumer Case Management Team: 2-year outcomes of a randomised trial. *Journal of Mental Health Administration*, **22**, 135–146.

Stein, L. I. & Test, M. A. (1980) Alternative to mental hospital treatment. I: Conceptual model, treatment program and clinical evaluation. *Archives of General Psychiatry*, **37**, 392–397.

Warner, R. (1994) *Recovery from Schizophrenia: Psychiatry and Political Economy*. Routledge & Kegan Paul.

Warr, P. (1987) *Work, Unemploymnet and Mental Health*. Oxford University Press.

Wing, J. K. & Brown, G. W. (1970) *Institutionalism and Schizophrenia: A Comparative Study of Three Mental Hospitals, 1960–1968*. Cambridge University Press.

Wolff, G., Pathare, S., Craig, T., *et al* (1996a) Who's in the lion's den? The community's perception of community care for the mentally ill. *Psychiatric Bulletin*, **20**, 68–71.

Wolff, G., Pathare, S., Craig, T., *et al* (1996b) Public education for community care: a new approach. *British Journal of Psychiatry*, **168**, 441–447.

CHAPTER 18

Socially inclusive practice and psychiatry in the 21st century

Jed Boardman, Alan Currie, Helen Killaspy and Gillian Mezey

In this book we set out to define social exclusion in the context of people with mental health problems, look at how such people are excluded, why this matters to psychiatry and what can be done to improve their inclusion. Central to social exclusion and inclusion is the idea of participation in the key activities of society and this has brought us to the importance of: agency and the social barriers to inclusion, especially stigma and discrimination; the multiple causes of exclusion and their dynamic impact over the life course; the role of equality, human rights and citizenship; and the importance of social capital, support and networks. Many of these concepts are also embedded in the principles of recovery.

We have found that people with mental health problems and those with learning disabilities are excluded on a range of different indices and some, particularly those with long-term mental health problems, are more likely to be excluded than others. The implications of the exclusion of many people with mental health problems for psychiatry are manifold, but the experience of exclusion is profoundly negative, has consequences for health and well-being, and carries a high cost for society and individuals. However, this does not have to be the case and psychiatry and mental health services can have a positive impact on the problems of exclusion. This final chapter will give an overview of the arguments, examining where we stand now and how policy and practice will need to change in the future.

Social changes and exclusion

When Joseph Rowntree set up his eponymous trusts in 1904 he was concerned that they 'search out the underlying causes of weakness or evil in the community' (Watts, 2008: p. 6). He identified war, poverty, slavery, excessive drinking, gambling and the drugs trade as central to these 'social evils' (Mowlam & Creegan, 2008). He believed that it was possible to define and measure such evils (or perhaps what we would now call social problems) and subject them to systematic study (Harris, 2009). At that time, two surveys carried out in London and York (Booth, 1889; Rowntree, 1901) identified that 25–30% of people lived in absolute poverty, had an income insufficient to maintain good health, and that the worst poverty was seen among families with young children and older people who lived alone (Harris, 2009). Since these early attempts at the systematic study of poverty matters have changed: incomes have increased and absolute poverty is virtually unheard of; indeed, even by 1936 Rowntree found poverty in York to be half that of a previous generation and in his final post-war survey he noted that absolute poverty was almost gone (Rowntree, 1941; Rowntree & Lavers, 1951). Access to consumer goods and leisure has increased, the overall quality of life for the UK population has improved, and during the second half of the 20th century we have seen continued economic growth and prosperity (Ryder & Silver, 1970; Marwick, 1990; Rose, 2002; Layard, 2005; Wilkinson & Pickett, 2009). Despite these advances and the removal of absolute poverty, substantial numbers of people lack the material resources to maintain 'the living conditions and amenities which are customary, or at least widely encouraged or approved' in society (Townsend, 1979: p. 31). This relative poverty is as common today as absolute poverty was in Victorian Britain just over 100 years ago. The same groups, families with children and the elderly, are still among the most vulnerable, and many people live on incomes that are not adequate to maintain good health. To this list of high-risk groups we can now clearly add people with mental health problems.

British society has gained from the increases in affluence seen in the 20th century, but there seem to be limits to these gains and many believe that we have now reached a time when we no longer benefit from these levels of economic growth and prosperity (Layard, 2005; Harris, 2009; Wilkinson & Pickett, 2009). These limits are reflected in the high levels of self-interested consumerism, individualism and materialism, as well as increasing levels of inequality. A hundred years after Joseph Rowntree identified his social evils, the British population has recently examined contemporary social evils and identified a number of dominant themes (Mowlam & Creegan, 2008; Watts, 2008) (Box 18.1). High among these were individualism, consumerism and a decline of community, and a decline of values. Interestingly, the problems of drugs and alcohol and inequality and poverty remained as much a concern to contemporary Britons as they were to Rowntree in 1904.

Along with the changes in affluence we have seen a shift in social relations and social consensus (Harris, 2009). This may be seen in the changes to the structure of our working population; for example, in 1951 skilled and semi-skilled industrial workers made up 70% of the adult male population employed in Britain, but by the end of the 20th century this had fallen to 15% (Harris, 2009). These demographic and cultural changes may determine our collective responses to the prevailing current social problems as, unlike in Joseph Rowntree's day, our awareness of them may not be balanced by an optimism in our collective capacity to solve them. Indeed,

> some of the distinctly 'communitarian' features of earlier British historic culture – which had militated against many of the more dire social evils earlier experienced on the continent – may have declined or been irrevocably lost (Harris, 2009: p. 16).

> **Box 18.1 Contemporary social evils**
>
> In a survey by the Joseph Rowntree Foundation, the British public identified social evils associated with:
>
> - individualism, consumerism and a decline of community
> - drugs and alcohol
> - decline of values
> - families and young people
> - inequality and poverty
> - institutions, apathy and a democratic deficit
> - violence and crime
> - gender inequality
> - religion
> - social diversity, immigration and intolerance
> - health and care
> - environmental issues.
>
> Source: Watts (2008)

The response to these problems thus remains a challenge to contemporary Britain. At their heart are the levels of inequality now experienced in modern society and, as was argued in Chapter 5, this inequality not only undermines social justice but also the social solidarity that makes human lives worthwhile and contributes to the possibility of change through collective action. Nonetheless, before this begins to sound impossibly pessimistic we may wish to reflect that our current social and economic conditions are not fixed but rather,

> reflect the characteristics of the societies in which we find ourselves and vary even from one rich market democracy to another. At the most fundamental level, what reducing inequality is about is shifting the balance from a divisive, self-interested consumerism driven by status competition, towards a more socially integrated and affiliative society. Greater equality can help us develop the public ethos and commitment to working together which we need if we are going to solve the problems which threaten us all. As wartime leaders knew, if a society has to pull together, policies must be seen to be fair and income differences have to be reduced (Wilkinson & Pickett, 2009: pp. 227–228).

Policies for social change

Although it has not been our objective in this book to examine the social and economic policies required to achieve reductions in inequalities and begin to rebuild social cohesion, it is worth considering some general strategies at this stage, before moving to examine policies directed at increasing the social inclusion of people with mental health problems. What would such policies look like? For some commentators, policy and practice should aim at creating sustainable social justice. The New Economics Foundation

(2009) have proposed that three sources of wealth (the 'three economies') should be harnessed: the resources of people, the planet and markets. They argue that the purpose of a 21st-century welfare state is to 'harness and distribute the resources of these "three economies" in order to enable people to live their lives in ways that are satisfying and sustainable' (p. 11). There is an emphasis here on growing the 'core economy', one that is concerned with the resources of people and driven by social capital. Central to this is the concept of 'co-production', the production of public services through the contribution of service users and communities, making use of their resources and expertise, together with professional service providers (Ostrom, 1973; Cahn, 2004; New Economics Foundation, 2008). The New Economics Foundation set out five principles for sustainable social justice: building on the assets of people; protecting the planet's natural resources; fostering and regulating markets; creating inclusive, participatory and accountable systems of governance; and use of the best available knowledge (Box 18.2). These principles are based on the Department for Environment, Food and Rural Affairs (2005) policy on sustainable development. The New Economics Foundation also propose steps to begin developing public policies in this direction (Box 18.3).

These policy initiatives, although not spelled out in detail, contain many of the elements of change that have been proposed in this book, including the development of partnerships between service users and health services (co-production), the valuing of lived experience in addition to scientific evidence, the importance of social capital, the role of prevention and early intervention, and the need to improve people's well-being.

Policies for inclusion of people with mental health problems

By the very nature of the problem, the policies designed specifically to focus on the social inclusion of people with mental health problems should

---

Box 18.2   Five principles for sustainable social justice

1   People: strong, healthy and just society, fair distribution of power, resources and opportunities, equal life chances and well-being for all
2   Planet: safeguarding natural resources
3   Markets: promoting a sustainable economy, fostering and regulating markets to enhance the well-being of people and the planet
4   Governance: inclusive, participative and accountable; engaging the resources of people to define and realise the lives they wish to live
5   Knowledge: using the best available knowledge, drawing on robust evidence and the lived experience of people

Adapted from Coote & Franklin (2009)

Box 18.3   Six steps towards sustainable social justice

1 Aim for well-being for all: put equality at the heart of social policy, create conditions for people to flourish, tackle economic factors that impede life chances
2 Put prevention before cure: introduce cross-sectoral and departmental policies, promote resilience, act to lower poverty and to stop wealth escaping from poor neighbourhoods
3 Grow the core economy: employment policies, income support, childcare and family support – redesign these to support and nurture people
4 Make carbon work for social justice: public investment in 'green collar jobs', developing green technologies, redistribute carbon and income
5 Make public services sustainable: public services to give priority to cutting carbon, promote activities (e.g. travel) that are green
6 Value what matters: welfare system judged by longer-term social, economic and environmental returns, evaluate services by their impact on people, planet and markets, account for negative social, economic and environmental consequences of public investment

Adapted from Coote & Franklin (2009)

be cross-sectoral, covering not only health and social services but also education and training, employment, housing, transport, leisure, and civil and human rights. Some examples of these can be seen in the proposals put forward by Mental Health Europe (2008) and the UK Social Exclusion Unit (Office of the Deputy Prime Minister, 2004) (Boxes 18.4 and 18.5). In addition, there needs to be a set of comprehensive policy measures instituted to reduce stigma and discrimination. Some examples of possible strategies in this area have been put forward by Thornicroft (2006) (Box 18.6).

At present, there are no definite comprehensive mental health service policies aimed at social inclusion, but as we saw in Chapter 4 there are clear examples of Department of Health initiatives aimed at recovery, New Horizons being just one of them (Department of Health, 2009a). The Future Vision Coalition (2009) has proposed four main directions for mental health service policy: call for actions to be coordinated across government departments, a focus on promotion, prevention and early intervention, a greater emphasis on social outcomes, and a change in the nature of relationships between mental health services and service users.

Public mental health services are in their infancy and central to this is the development of well-being in the population (Department of Health, 2009a; see also Chapter 10). The government has proposed some steps that can be taken (Department of Health, 2009b) (Box 18.7). Key interventions here include: integrating physical and mental health and well-being, developing sustainable connected communities, and promoting meaning and purpose. These require community action and individual behavioural changes. Aked et al (2008) suggest five actions that may be used to communicate to

Box 18.4 Recommendations for promoting social inclusion of people with mental health problems

In health and social services:

- strengthen communication and interaction between the health and social sector and ensure more integrated actions
- ensure involvement and participation of people with mental health problems and their families in policy and decision-making
- complement the de-institutionalisation process with increased development of alternative solutions for health and social services in the community.

In education and training:

- promote early prevention of mental disorders in schools and develop specific education policies targeting pupils with mental health problems
- create information and support services in schools and universities supporting students with mental health problems to complete their education
- increase (financial) support for NGOs and other providers of vocational training and rehabilitation for people with mental health problems.

In employment:

- raise awareness among employers of the employment potentials of people with mental health problems
- create decent job opportunities in sheltered/adapted employment or social firms as well as in the open labour market
- ensure a decent minimum income for people with mental health problems as well as a fair regulation of the compatibility between work and social benefits.

In housing:

- promote legal regulations promoting housing rights of people with mental health problems and prohibiting discrimination
- prevent homelessness of people with mental health problems by supporting the development of affordable and adequate housing
- provide (financial) support to NGOs and other providers of alternative housing solutions such as sheltered living opportunities.

In transport:

- provide people with mental health problems, who rely on social assistance, with price reductions and support for access to public transport
- pay special attention to people living in rural areas with limited access to public transport.

In leisure activities:

- provide concessions and price reductions for social and leisure activities to people with mental health problems who rely on social assistance
- support the establishment and sustainability of self-help groups and social clubs for people with mental health problems as well as initiatives aimed at bringing people with mental health problems together with other people who live in the community.

In civil and human rights:

- ensure people with mental health problems are informed about their rights

Box 18.4 *(contd)*

- enforce the implementation of anti-discrimination legislation in all areas
- support the creation of contact points for legal advice for people with mental health problems.

In other important areas:

- ensure the involvement of people with mental health problems and their families in relevant policy and decision-making as well as in ongoing monitoring and evaluation of services
- seek partnership with NGOs and other grass-roots providers of services in mental health to ensure adequacy, flexibility and sustainability at the local level
- provide an adequate financial frame for the development of sustainable community-based mental health services
- guarantee equal treatment for people with mental health problems with regard to insurance coverages.

In vulnerable groups:

- pay special attention to the mental health and social needs of migrants and invest in culturally sensitive approaches to mental health and social services
- adopt a gender-based approach in mental health and social support services
- invest in mental health promotion and early prevention of mental disorders and drug abuse in children and young people
- create spaces for meeting others and living in the community for older people and fight social isolation.

In good practices:

- adopt the principles of person-centredness, independence, empowerment and community orientation
- invest in social activities in the community as well as in initiatives promoting labour market integration of people with mental health problems
- fight stigma and prejudice in society through realistic messages in the media
- support NGOs and other voluntary providers of mental health and social services.

In the National Action Plans on Social Inclusion:

- include people with mental health problems in the framework for the National Action Plans on Social Inclusion in all countries as a separate group from people with other disabilities
- involve NGOs and other civil society organisations, especially mental health associations, in the discussion, drafting, implementation and monitoring of the national reports on strategies for social protection and social inclusion
- enforce an integrated approach to tackling the needs of people with mental health problems in all areas of the national reports, social inclusion, health and long-term care, and pensions
- assume and promote ownership and responsibility for the national reports as well as for all other OMC-related instruments, such as mutual learning and peer reviews
- ensure an effective implementation of agreed strategies and actions as laid down in the national reports.

NGO, non-governmental organisation; OMC, open method of coordination
Source: Mental Health Europe (2008)

Box 18.5   Summary of the UK government's Social Exclusion Unit's 27-point action plan to reduce social exclusion of people with mental health problems

1   Stigma and discrimination – a sustained programme to challenge negative attitudes and promote awareness of people's rights:
   • programme backed by £1.1 million investment in 2004–05 to challenge discrimination against people with mental health problems, with closer co-ordination across government and the voluntary sector
   • practical teaching resources to challenge the stigma surrounding mental health from an early age through schools
   • planning for vigorous implementation of the proposed new public sector duty to promote equality of opportunity for disabled people.
2   Role of health and social care in tackling social exclusion – implementing evidence-based practice in vocational services and enabling reintegration into the community:
   • modernised vocational services which reflect evidence-based practice and provide a choice of services to meet diverse needs
   • access to an employment adviser and social support for everyone with severe mental health problems
   • redesigning mental health day services to promote social inclusion
   • improved access to vocational and social support in primary care
   • strengthened training on social inclusion for health and social care professionals
   • measures to tackle inequalities in access to health services, and
   • closer working with the criminal justice system, including strengthened police training on mental health issues.
3   Employment – giving people with mental health problems a real chance of sustained paid work reflecting their skills and experience:
   • improved training on mental health issues for Jobcentre Plus staff
   • £1.5 million from the Phoenix Fund to improve support for adults with mental health problems who are interested in enterprise and self-employment
   • clearer guidance on the use of Access to Work to fund adjustments for this client group, and on the continuing needs of disability living allowance claimants upon returning to work
   • consideration of further improvements to the linking rules and permitted work rules to support the transition from benefits to work
   • improved support for employers and job retention through the government's new vocational rehabilitation framework.
4   Supporting families and community participation – enabling people to lead fulfilling lives the way they choose:
   • improved support to access education and training opportunities
   • strengthened evidence base to enable wider roll-out of arts interventions
   • targeted family support to meet the needs of the many parents with mental health problems and their children
   • removal of unnecessary barriers to community roles such as jury service, and more consistent practice on paying people with experience of mental health problems to advise on service design.
5   Getting the basics right – access to decent homes, financial advice and transport:

Box 18.5 *(contd)*

- new guidance to housing authorities on lettings and stability for adults with mental health problems
- improved access to financial and legal advice, and affordable transport.

6 Making it happen – clear arrangements for leading this programme and maintaining momentum:
- cross-government team tasked with driving implementation, with progress overseen by ministers
- independent advisory group to advise the government on progress
- local implementation led jointly by primary care trusts and local authorities, supported by the National Institute for Mental Health in England
- better use of the expertise in the voluntary and community sector.

Source: Office of the Deputy Prime Minister (2004)

Box 18.6 Strategies to reduce discrimination

Action to support service user advocacy groups. Provide specific financial support to increase empowerment in people with mental health problems, for example:

- participating in formulating care plans and crisis plans
- using cognitive–behavioural therapy to reverse negative self-stigma
- running regular assessments of consumer satisfaction with services
- creating user-led and user-run services
- developing peer support worker roles in mainstream mental healthcare
- advocating for employers to give positive credit for experience of mental health illness
- taking part in treatment and service evaluation and research.

Action to support individuals and their families:

- develop new ways to offer diagnoses
- actively provide factual information against popular myths
- develop and rehearse accounts of mental illness experiences that do not alienate other people.

Action to support people with mental illness at work. Measures for 'reasonable adjustments' in the Disability Discrimination Act:

- improve environment for people with concentration problems (quieter workplace with fewer distractions, rest area)
- supervision to give feedback and guidance on job performance
- use of headphones to block out distracting noise
- flexibility in work hours to attend their healthcare appointments, or work when not impaired by medication
- external job coach for counselling and support, and to mediate between employee and employer
- buddy/mentor scheme to provide on-site orientation and assistance
- clear person specifications, job descriptions and task assignments
- contract modifications to allow whatever sickness leave they need
- gradual induction phase

Box 18.6 *(contd)*

- improved disability awareness in the workplace to reduce stigma and to underpin all other accommodations
- reallocation of marginal job functions that are disturbing to an individual
- allowing use of accrued paid and unpaid leave for periods of illness.

Action at the local level:

- commission and provide supported work schemes
- increase the availability of psychological treatments to improve cognition, self-esteem, confidence and social functioning
- health and social care employers give recognition to the expertise by experience through positive encouragement and support in recruitment and staff management practices
- ensure people with mental illness and employers are properly informed of their rights and obligations
- mental health agencies and advice organisations actively encourage and support service users in securing their rights under the Disability Discrimination Act
- more widespread implementation, evaluation and impact assessments of focused anti-discrimination interventions
- provide accurate data on mental illness recovery rates to mental health practitioners and to service users and carers
- encourage and support greater service user involvement in local speakers' bureaux and other anti-sigma and anti-discrimination initiatives.

Action at the national level:

- promote a social model of disability that incorporates human rights, social inclusion and citizenship
- provide accurate data on mental illness recovery rates to the media
- promote service user-defined outcomes
- ensure adequate funding is available and used for new supported employment schemes and greater availability of psychological treatments
- make available and disseminate widely information, guidance and advice on the Disability Discrimination Act
- audit compliance with codes of good practice in providing insurance
- review law on jury eligibility criteria
- any new mental health legislation should include a principle of non-discrimination (people with mental disorders should, wherever possible, retain the same rights and entitlements as those with other health needs).

Adapted from Thornicroft (2006)

the public the behavioural changes required at the individual level, all of which are based on evidence from the research literature (Box 18.8). The outcomes of public mental health policy would be based on measures of the population's subjective well-being and regular monitoring of these metrics could form a new way of measuring societal progress, an alternative to the usual economic indicators of gross domestic product (GDP) and growth (Layard, 2005; New Economics Foundation, 2009). These measures of well-being could form a cross-cutting and more informative approach to directing policy-making and produce an altered dynamic between the government and the public (New Economics Foundation, 2009).

Future mental health services and practice

In the final section of this book we have been concerned with what the future of mental health services should look like. Presently, the services are at a point of change, having moved from an institutional and asylum-based service to a community-based system (Chapter 17). Future changes

---

Box 18.7   Key interventions for promoting well-being

Ensure a positive start in life:

- promote good parental mental health – identify and treat poor parental mental health and relevant risk factors both antenatally and in later years with universal and targeted approaches
- promote good parenting skills – universally as well as targeting high-risk families with more intensive interventions
- develop social and emotional skills – for example, via mental health promotion in schools (universal) and targeted skills development in high-risk children
- intervene early with conduct and emotional disorders – with parenting programmes, school behaviour approaches, cognitive–behavioural therapy and wilderness programmes.

Build resilience and a safe, secure base:

- develop violence and abuse prevention skills – universal programmes in schools and colleges and target high-risk young people
- poverty reduction – interventions to assist people back into employment and address fuel level poverty, for example.

Integrate physical and mental health and well-being:

- target those with mental health problems – for health improvement programmes and physical health checks
- identify and treat mental health problems – in those presenting with chronic illness/coronary heart disease.

Develop sustainable, connected communities:

- use community participative approaches to develop safe, green community spaces – targeting areas of urban deprivation/discriminated groups, with inter-generational and cross-cultural components.

Promote meaning and purpose:

- create community and organisational values – to aid inclusion and bring people together with a common sense of purpose
- improve access to psychological therapies – to assist in developing meaning from adversity.

Source: Department of Health (2009*b*)

Box 18.8   Five ways to well-being

Five actions into our day-to-day lives are important for well-being:

1   Connect... With the people around you. With family, friends, colleagues and neighbours. At home, work, school or in your local community. Think of these as the cornerstones of your life and invest time in developing them. Building these connections will support and enrich you every day.
2   Be active... Go for a walk or run. Step outside. Cycle. Play a game. Garden. Dance. Exercising makes you feel good. Most importantly, discover a physical activity you enjoy and that suits your level of mobility and fitness.
3   Take notice... Be curious. Catch sight of the beautiful. Remark on the unusual. Notice the changing seasons. Savour the moment, whether you are walking to work, eating lunch or talking to friends. Be aware of the world around you and what you are feeling. Reflecting on your experiences will help you appreciate what matters to you.
4   Keep learning... Try something new. Rediscover an old interest. Sign up for that course. Take on a different responsibility at work. Fix a bike. Learn to play an instrument or how to cook your favourite food. Set a challenge you will enjoy achieving. Learning new things will make you more confident as well as being fun.
5   Give... Do something nice for a friend, or a stranger. Thank someone. Smile. Volunteer your time. Join a community group. Look out, as well as in. Seeing yourself, and your happiness, linked to the wider community can be incredibly rewarding and creates connections with the people around you.

Source: Aked *et al* (2008). Reprinted with permission, New Economics Foundation (www.neweconomics.org)

may require that mental health services move to being socially inclusive, with recovery orientation playing a central role. Across the world there are many examples of specific services that embrace these approaches (Slade, 2009) but, as yet, there are no examples of a nationally comprehensive service that is recovery-oriented. This is the challenge for the future. To make this happen there need to be changes at the practice, service delivery and service culture level as well as changes to the training of mental health professionals and others working in mental health services (Sainsbury Centre for Mental Health, 2009; Shepherd *et al*, 2010). One key change required is a transformation of the existing workforce, giving greater emphasis to the role of peer professionals (Ashcraft & Anthony, 2005; Shepherd *et al*, 2008; Sainsbury Centre for Mental Health, 2009).

In developing such services we should consider the principles and values that may lie behind the creation of socially inclusive mental health services (some of these are laid out in Box 18.9). These are based on the discussions in previous chapters, the New Economics Foundation (2009) principles for sustainable social justice, and the recovery principles of hope, agency and opportunity (Chapter 3). Slade (2009) also makes five suggestions for how mental health services and professionals can improve social inclusion for mental health service users: spending resources differently, for example by shifting money into employment services; organising community-based events to help alter the perceptions of 'them' and 'us'; educating employers about workplace accommodations; getting mental health service staff to run groups in mainstream community settings; and finally, promoting the voice of mental health service users in society.

Mental health professionals will inevitably be uneasy about some of these proposed changes, anxious that their expertise and authority will be undermined. In previous chapters we have set out the reasons why social inclusion and personal recovery are desirable outcomes for people with mental health problems and have outlined the deleterious effects of exclusion. Many mental health professionals will recognise that the values of recovery often reflect the reasons why they committed themselves to working in mental health services and that these principles support our professional values of respect, collaboration and social justice (Chapter 1). For professionals the challenge is to utilise the value that they already give to their relationship with the service user and to shift this to one of partnership where the key ingredients are openness, reciprocity, collaboration as equals, a willingness to go the extra mile, and a focus on the individual's inner resources (Borg & Kristiansen, 2004; Shepherd *et al*, 2008). In this shift in the way professionals approach their work, they will remain important, but they will have to recognise that their contribution needs to be made in a different way, one that acknowledges the service user's self-defined priorities. There have been many purported obstacles to recovery-oriented practice, all of which may be challenged (Box 14.3: p. 306). Yet moving to a recovery-oriented approach can have advantages for both service users and professionals, a situation where 'everyone has won and all must have prizes'.

Box 18.9 Principles for socially inclusive mental health services

- Place people at the forefront of services – aiming to build meaningful and satisfying lives
- Adopt the organisational aim of supporting personal recovery
- Embed recovery principles (hope, agency, opportunity) at all levels of the organisation and services
- Use best available knowledge in service and treatment developments to improve clinical and social outcomes
- Give primacy to outcomes valued by service users
- Emphasise prevention, promotion and early intervention
- Place an emphasis on co-production, developing partnerships with service users and partnerships between all provider and commissioning agencies
- Focus on inclusion in the community, not just integration
- Fight discrimination and champion respect, rights and equality for people with mental health problems
- Challenge and dismantle barriers to recovery and inclusion

In Chapter 14 we set out the ten top tips for recovery-oriented practice. Many psychiatrists may recognise that these are what they already sometimes do or aspire to do, but the challenge here is to adopt these behaviours as part of core practice. How many of us ask service users about their hopes, fears and aspirations or go beyond the deficits in people's lives that brought them into contact with services? To adopt the behaviours of the ten top tips would mean shifting from a deficit-based approach to one that focuses on people's strengths. It means we must question the validity of our diagnostic systems, strengthen their scientific basis and examine their utility in communicating with service users and society (Bentall, 2003; van Os, 2009). A move to a recovery-oriented approach would also mean acknowledging the limits of our current treatments. Although both pharmacological approaches and psychological therapies may be considered to be generally effective, they are limited, as revealed by their low overall effect sizes, their side-effect profiles and their problems with individual level applicability (Rush *et al*, 2006; Scott, 2006; Lewis & Lieberman, 2008; Bentall, 2009). Moving services and practice to be more inclusive could go some way to make up for these limitations in conventional practice.

Financial challenges for mental health services

Since 1999, we have seen significant rises in NHS funding generally and in mental health services too (Boardman & Parsonage, 2007; Sainsbury Centre for Mental Health, 2008; Appleby *et al*, 2009). However, this is unlikely to continue as the UK government faces significant challenges as a result of the current economic recession and a growing national debt, predicted to rise from 59% of GDP in 2009 to 79% of GDP in 2013/14 (Chancellor of the Exchequer, 2009). This puts the funding of public services under threat and marks a period of increasing uncertainty, despite the prior rises in NHS funding. The NHS Confederation (2009) predicts a £8–10 billion real-terms cut in NHS funding between 2011 and 2015 and the King's Fund (Appleby *et al*, 2009) a reduction across government spending departments of 2.3% per year in the same period. Mental health services will be subject to these resource pressures, perhaps amplified by their historical low funding base and also by the likely cuts to social service provision which may be felt more sharply by community services. They will also face demand pressures as a result of changes in morbidity and demography (McCrone *et al*, 2008) and the possibility that the effects of the recession will increase demands for services (Catalano, 1991; Murphy & Athanasou, 1999).

These pressures force us to think about the future funding of mental health services and whether the argument can be made for investing in them in order to safeguard the future. As the effects of exclusion on people with mental health problems are profound, can we afford to have another generation of young people left to face long-term unemployment, another generation of people with mental health problems on long-term incapacity benefits, ending in the criminal justice services or failing to reach their potential? The possibility is that socially inclusive and recovery-oriented services can significantly add to improved outcomes for people with mental health problems and can do this without profound increases in funding or by providing initial increases in spending in an attempt to create longer-term savings. This would require improving the quality of mental health services and increasing productivity, improving commissioning and examining the current workforce (NHS Confederation, 2009; Royal College of Psychiatrists *et al*, 2009).

Conclusion

Trying to predict the future may be thwarted with difficulties, but one thing we know is that mental health services must and will change. Future changes are necessary to accommodate the advances seen in the 20th century, from asylum to community-based system. But these changes must also recognise the voice and needs of mental health service users and carers; they must pay heed to the continuing exclusion of many people with mental health problems in contemporary society, to the limitations of our current treatments and to the evolving evidence base for approaches that can improve both clinical and desirable social outcomes. The creation of more socially inclusive and recovery-oriented approaches in mental health services is core to these changes. However, these approaches are not yet fully developed or tested and more work needs to be done to create a more comprehensive picture of what these may look like. This should not be a barrier for delaying their development as there is sufficient evidence and experience to begin their implementation and to evaluate and learn from this and our future experience. But if these approaches are to be given any chance of success, they must be backed by broader health service policies and by economic and social policies that value and support a more equal and inclusive society. It is the role of governments to create policies that benefit society.

Summary

The social and economic changes of the 20th century have brought increasing affluence to British society, but not without some cost, particularly that of increasing inequality. Policies for social change and those to improve the inclusion of people with mental health problems must be coordinated across all sectors and government departments and must be aimed at sustainable social justice. The future development of socially inclusive and recovery-oriented mental health and social services can have mutual benefits for professionals and for service users and their carers. Such services can be developed in spite of the threats to public service funding and must be supported by broader economic and social policies that support a more equal and inclusive society.

References

Aked, J., Marks, N., Cordon, C., *et al* (2008) *Five Ways to Wellbeing*. New Economics Foundation (http://www.neweconomics.org/publications/five-ways-well-being-evidence).

Appleby, J., Crawford, R. & Emmerson, C. (2009) *How Cold will It Be? Prospects for NHS Funding 2011–2017*. King's Fund.

Ashcraft, L. & Anthony, W. A. (2005) A story of transformation: an agency fully embraces recovery. *Behavioural Healthcare Tomorrow*, **14**, 2–22.

Bentall, R. P. (2003) *Madness Explained: Psychosis and Human Nature*. Penguin.

Bentall, R. (2009) *Doctoring the Mind: Why Psychiatric Treatments Fail*. Allen Lane.

Boardman, J. & Parsonage, M. (2007) *Delivering the Government's Mental Health Policies: Services, Staffing and Costs*. Sainsbury Centre for Mental Health.

Booth, C. (1889) *Labour and Life of the People (Vol. 1: Of Life and Labour of the People in London)*. Williams and Norgate.

Borg, M. & Kristiansen, K. (2004) Recovery-oriented professionals: helping relationships in mental health services. *Journal of Mental Health*, **13**, 493–505.

Cahn, E. (2004) *No More Throwaway People: The Co-Production Imperative*. Essential Books.

Catalano, R. (1991) The Health Effects of Economic Insecurity. *American Journal of Public Health*, **81**, 1148–1152.

Chancellor of the Exchequer (2009) *Chancellor of the Exchequer's Budget Statement: Check against Delivery*. HM Treasury, 22 April (http://www.hm-treasury.gov.uk/bud_bud09_speech.htm).

Coote, A. & Franklin, J. (2009) *Green Well Fair: Three Economies for Social Justice*. New Economics Foundation.

Department for Environment, Food and Rural Affairs (2005) *Securing the Future: Delivering UK Sustainable Development Strategy* (Cm 6467). HM Government (http://www.defra.gov.uk/sustainable/government/publications/uk-strategy/index.htm).

Department of Health (2009a) *New Horizons: Towards a Shared Vision for Mental Health*. Consultation. Department of Health.

Department of Health (2009b) *Flourishing People, Connected Communities: A Framework for Developing Well-Being*. Department of Health.

Future Vision Coalition (2009) *A Future Vision for Mental Health*. NHS Confederation.

Harris, J. (2009) 'Social evils' and 'social problems' in Britain, 1904–2008. Joseph Rowntree Foundation.

Layard, R. (2005) *Happiness: Lessons from a New Science*. Allen Lane.

Lewis, S. & Lieberman, J. (2008) CATIE and CUtLASS: can we handle the truth? *British Journal of Psychiatry*, **192**, 161–163.

Marwick, A. (1990) *British Society Since 1945* (2nd edn). Penguin.

McCrone, P., Dhanasiri, S., Patel, A., *et al* (2008) *Paying the Price: The Cost of Mental Health Care in England to 2026*. King's Fund.

Mental Health Europe (2008) *From Exclusion to Inclusion – The Way Forward to Promoting Social Inclusion of People with Mental Health Problems in Europe*. Mental Health Europe.

Mowlam, A. & Creegan, C. (2008) *Modern-Day Social Evils: The Voices of Unheard Groups*. Joseph Rowntree Foundation.

Murphy, G. C. & Athanasou, J. A. (1999) The effect of unemployment on mental health. *Journal of Occupational and Organizational Psychology*, **72**, 83–99.

New Economics Foundation (2008) *Co-Production: A Manifesto for Growing the Core Economy*. New Economics Foundation.

New Economics Foundation (2009) *National Accounts of Well-Being: Bringing Real Wealth onto the Balance Sheet*. New Economics Foundation.

NHS Confederation (2009) *Dealing with the Downturn*. NHS Confederation.

Office of the Deputy Prime Minister (2004) *Mental Health and Social Exclusion: Social Exclusion Unit Report*. Office of the Deputy Prime Minister.

Ostrom, E. (1973) *Community Organization and the Provision of Police Services*. Sage Publications.

Rose, J. (2002) *The Intellectual Life of the British Working Class*. Yale.

Rowntree, B. S. (1901) *Poverty: A Study of Town Life*. Macmillan.

Rowntree, B. S. (1941) *Poverty and Progress: A Second Social Survey of York*. Longman's.

Rowntree, B. S. & Lavers, G. R. (1951) *Poverty and the Welfare State: A Third Social Survey of York Dealing only with Economic Questions*. Longman's.

Royal College of Psychiatrists, NHS Confederation & London School of Economics and Political Science (2009) *Mental Health and the Economic Downturn: National Priorities and Economic Solutions*. Royal College of Psychiatrists.

Rush, A. J., Trivedi, M. H., Wisniewski, S. R., *et al* (2006) Acute and longer-term outcomes in depressed outpatients requiring one or several treatment steps: A STAR*D report. *American Journal of Psychiatry*, **163**, 1905–1917.

Ryder, J. & Silver, H. (1970) *Modern English Society*. Methuen.

Sainsbury Centre for Mental Health (2008) *Spending on Adult Mental Health Services in England*. Sainsbury Centre for Mental Health.

Sainsbury Centre for Mental Health (2009) *Implementing Recovery: A New Framework for Organisational Change*. Position Paper. Sainsbury Centre for Mental Health.

Scott, J. (2006) Depression should be managed like a chronic disease. *BMJ*, **332**, 985–986.

Shepherd, G., Boardman, J. & Slade, M. (2008) *Making Recovery a Reality*. Sainsbury Centre for Mental Health.

Shepherd, G., Boardman, J. & Burns, M. (2010) *Implementing Recovery: A Methodology for Organisational Change*. Sainsbury Centre for Mental Health.

Slade, M. (2009) *Personal Recovery and Mental Illness: A Guide for Mental Health Professionals*. Cambridge University Press.

Thornicroft, G. (2006) *Actions Speak Louder… Tackling Discrimination Against People with Mental Illness*. Mental Health Foundation.

Townsend, P. (1979) *Poverty in the United Kingdom*. Penguin.

Van Os, J. (2009) 'Salience syndrome' replaces 'schizophrenia' in DSM–V and ICD–11: psychiatry's evidence-based entry into the 21st century. *Acta Psychiatrica Scandinavica*, **120**, 363–372.

Watts, B. (2008) *What are Today's Social Evils? The Results of a Web Consultation*. Joseph Rowntree Foundation.

Wilkinson, R. & Pickett, K. (2009) *The Spirit Level: Why More Equal Societies Almost Always Do Better*. Penguin.

Index

Compiled by Linda English